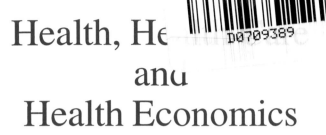

Health, Health Care and Health Economics

Perspectives on Distribution

Edited by

Morris L. Barer
Centre for Health Services and Policy Research,
University of British Columbia, Vancouver, British Columbia, Canada

Thomas E. Getzen
Department of Risk, Insurance, Health Management and Actuarial Science,
Temple University, Philadelphia, Pennsylvania, USA

and

Greg L. Stoddart
Centre for Health Economics and Policy Analysis,
McMaster University, Hamilton, Ontario, Canada

JOHN WILEY & SONS

Chichester · New York · Weinheim · Brisbane · Singapore · Toronto

Copyright © 1998 by John Wiley & Sons Ltd,
Baffins Lane, Chichester,
West Sussex PO19 1UD, England

National   01243 779777
International (+44) 1243 779777
e-mail (for orders and customer service enquiries): cs-books@wiley.co.uk
Visit our Home Page on http://www.wiley.co.uk or http://www.wiley.com

Reprinted October 1999

Other Wiley Editorial Offices

John Wiley & Sons, Inc., 605 Third Avenue,
New York, NY 10158-0012, USA

WILEY-VCH Verlag GmbH, Pappelallee 3,
D-69469 Weinheim, Germany

Jacaranda Wiley Ltd, 33 Park Road, Milton,
Queensland 4064, Australia

John Wiley & Son (Asia) Pte Ltd, 2 Clementi Loop #02-01,
Jin Xing Distripark, Singapore 129809

John Wiley & Sons (Canada) Ltd, 22 Worcester Road,
Rexdale, Ontario M9W 1L1, Canada

Library of Congress Cataloging-in-Publication Data

Health, health care and health economics : perspectives on
    distribution / edited by Morris L. Barer, Thomas E. Getzen, and Greg
    L. Stoddart.
        p. cm.
    Includes bibliographical references (p.   )
    ISBN 0–471–97879–5 (cased)
    1. Medical economics—Cross cultural studies. 2. Health services
accessibility—Cross-cultural studies. I. Barer, M.L. II. Getzen,
Thomas E. III. Stoddart, G. L.
    RA410.H424 1998
    338.4´33621—dc21   98–19860
                                                                CIP

British Library Cataloguing in Publication Data

A catalogue record for this book is available from the British Library

ISBN 0–471–97879–5

Produced from camera-ready copy supplied by the editors
Printed and bound in Great Britain by Biddles Ltd, Guildford and King's Lynn
This book is printed on acid-free paper responsibly manufactured from sustainable forestry, in which at least two trees are planted for each one used for paper production.

Contents

About the Editors

Morris L. Barer is the Director of the Centre for Health Services and Policy Research, and a Professor in the Department of Health Care and Epidemiology, at the University of British Columbia. He is also an Associate of the Population Health Program of the Canadian Institute for Advanced Research. He served for five years as the senior editor for Health Economics with *Social Science and Medicine*, where he remains an Advisory Editor. He is also on the editorial board of the *Journal of Health Politics, Policy and Law*. He is co-editor of the recently published *Why Are Some People Healthy and Others Not: The Determinants of Health of Populations* (Aldine de Gruyter, 1994). He has published extensively on issues ranging from the determinants of health to health human resource policy, health services utilization analysis, international comparative health care policies, economic evaluation, and health care financing, and has consulted widely on policy issues related to these areas. He has played a key role in the development of a population-based linked health database for the province of British Columbia, and the development of protocols for facilitating access to that database for the health research community.

Thomas E. Getzen is Professor of Health Care Finance in the Department of Risk, Insurance, Health Management, and Actuarial Science at Temple University, and the founding Director of the International Health Economics Association (iHEA). He is the author of a recently published textbook, *Health Economics: Fundamentals and Flow of Funds* (Wiley, 1997). He is on the editorial board of *Health Economics*, and has published extensively on transactions costs in health manpower and contracting, price indexes, forecasting, aging and long-term care financing, and the analysis of national health expenditures. He has served as chair of the health economics committee of the American Public Health Association, and of the Finance Forum of the Association of University Programs in Health Administration. He has consulted widely, both within the United States and internationally, and has been a visiting professor at the Centre for Health Economics, University of York, and at the Wharton School, University of Pennsylvania.

Greg L. Stoddart is a member, and was the founding coordinator, of the Centre for Health Economics and Policy Analysis at McMaster University, where he is also a Professor in the Department of Clinical Epidemiology and Biostatistics, and an Associate Member of the Department of Economics. He is a Fellow in the Population Health Program of the Canadian Institute for Advanced Research, and serves on the editorial board of the *Journal of Health Economics*. His publications include works on health-care financing, utilization analysis, human resource planning, alternative delivery modalities, and methods and applications of economic evaluation of health services. Among those publications is the international best selling textbook, *Methods for the Economic Evaluation of Health Care Programmes* (Oxford, 1987, 1997), on which he is one of the co-authors. He has served as a consultant to the World Bank, the World Health Organization and to several Canadian Ministries of Health and task forces.

Contributors

David Bishai
School of Hygiene and Public
Health
The Johns Hopkins University
Baltimore, Maryland, USA

Han Bleichrodt
iMTA
Erasmus University
Rotterdam, The Netherlands

Dov Chernichovsky
Health Policy Program for
Economies Under Stress
Health Policy and Management
Unit
Ben-Gurion University of the
Negev
Be'er Sheva, Israel

Anthony J. Culyer
Department of Economics and
Related Studies
University of York,
Heslington, York, UK

Shelley Derksen
Manitoba Centre for Health Policy
and Evaluation
University of Manitoba
Winnipeg, Manitoba, Canada

Jane Doherty
Centre for Health Policy
Department of Community Health
University of the Witwatersrand
Johannesburg, South Africa

Robert G. Evans
Centre for Health Services and
Policy Research; and
Department of Economics
The University of British
Columbia
Vancouver, B.C., Canada

Wei Fu
National Health Economics
Institute
Ministry of Health
Beijing, P.R. China

Ulf-G Gerdtham
Centre for Health Economics
Stockholm School of Economics
Stockholm, Sweden

Unto Häkkinen
STAKES
National Research and
Development Centre for Welfare
and Health
Helsinki, Finland

John Horne
Department of Community Health
Sciences
University of Manitoba
Winnipeg, Manitoba, Canada

William C. Hsiao
Department of Health Policy and
Management
School of Public Health
Harvard University
Cambridge, Massachusetts, USA

Shanlian Hu
Training Center for Health
Administrators
Shanghai Medical University
Shanghai, P.R. China

Jeremiah Hurley
Centre for Health Economics and
Policy Analysis
McMaster University
Hamilton, Ontario, Canada

Tatiana Kirsanova
New Economic School
Moscow, Russia

Jan Klavus
STAKES
National Research and
Development Centre for Welfare
and Health
Helsinki, Finland

Yuanli Liu
Department of Health Policy and
Management
School of Public Health
Harvard University
Cambridge, Massachusetts, USA

David Mayston
Department of Economics and
Related Studies
University of York
Heslington, York, UK

Gavin Mooney
Department of Public Health and
Community Medicine
University of Sydney
Sydney, NSW, Australia

Cameron A. Mustard
Manitoba Centre for Health Policy
and Evaluation; and Department
of Community Health Sciences
University of Manitoba
Winnipeg, Manitoba, Canada

Joseph P. Newhouse
Harvard University
Cambridge, Massachusetts, USA

Elena Potapchik
New Economic School
Moscow, Russia

Uwe E. Reinhardt
Woodrow Wilson School of Public
and International Affairs
Princeton University
Princeton, NJ, USA

Thomas Rice
Department of Health Services
School of Public Health
University of California
Los Angeles, California, USA

Jack Rodgers
Price Waterhouse LLP
Health Policy Economics Group
Washington, D.C., USA

Claude Schneider-Bunner
LATEC
Université de Bourgogne
Dijon, France

Marian Shanahan
Manitoba Centre for Health Policy
and Evaluation; and Department
of Community Health Sciences
University of Manitoba
Winnipeg, Manitoba, Canada

Karen Smith
Price Waterhouse LLP
Health Policy Economics Group
Washington, D.C., USA

Elena Sosenskaya
New Economic School
Moscow, Russia

Gun Sundberg
Department of Economics
Uppsala University
Uppsala, Sweden

Alex van den Heever
Centre for Health Policy
Department of Community Health
University of the Witwatersrand
Johannesburg, South Africa

Eddy van Doorslaer
Department of Health Policy and
Management
Erasmus University
Rotterdam, The Netherlands

Adam Wagstaff
School of Social Sciences
University of Sussex
Brighton, UK

Alan Williams
Centre for Health Economics
University of York
Heslington, York, UK

Foreword

This book recognizes a milestone in the evolution of health economics as a discipline, the founding conference of the International Health Economics Association. Both the Association and the conference built on past efforts. More or less formal health economics groups had existed for several years in a variety of countries, and there had been prior international conferences as well, most notably at Tokyo in 1973, Leiden in 1980, and Zurich in 1990. However, there had been no prior health economics organization at the international level. This book contains selected papers from the conference held at Vancouver in May of 1996. The theme of the conference and the subject of the book's papers -- equity in health, health care services and health care financing -- is certainly of interest in all countries (more on that in the editors' forward). The International Health Economics Association can claim only some of the credit for the organization of the conference -- it was originally conceived during a telephone conversation between Tom Getzen, the Association's founding President, and Morris Barer, at a time when the Association was little more than a good idea. The lion's share of the organizational effort was undertaken by Morris Barer, Karen Cardiff and their planning team at the University of British Columbia; the immense task of creating a scientific program was ably handled by the editors of this volume, with the generous assistance of an illustrious international scientific program committee. The Conference itself was, in some ways, the official launch of the Association; indeed, the Association held its first board meeting at the conference. Economists are trained in the concept of horizontal equity - equal treatment of equals - and vertical equity - equitable treatment of unequals, usually meaning different income groups. Health economics poses an additional dimension of vertical equity, however, namely equitable treatment of those in different health states. Because of scarce resources, not all potentially useful health care will be delivered. Hence, resources must be allocated across individuals, but this is typically not done by standard market mechanisms. For example an individual may have a private or public insurance contract that is incompletely specified. A typical American insurance contract might agree to cover all necessary care, but leave that definition in the hands of the insurer and the medical profession, subject to possible appeal to the courts. Or a public health service and its physicians may face the issue of how to allocate across individuals without an explicit contract. The technical capabilities for health care to remedy or palliate illness have clearly increased over time and so correspondingly have the costs of care. As larger fractions of GDP are devoted to health care, questions of who gets what, who pays, and how improved health is distributed as a result, are likely to become more insistent. It is to those intriguing questions that the papers in this volume are devoted.

Joseph P. Newhouse

Preface

Health economics is becoming an increasingly prominent "discipline" in the evolution of health care systems around the world. The centrality of schemes developed by health economists in reform initiatives in a number of countries, and the growing importance of methodologic advances that will assist in the critical process of evaluating alternative social interventions intended to promote health, suggest that health economics is a discipline "on the rise." This emergence of interest in the work and results of health economics research has given rise to a need for new and better ways to communicate, both within the health economics community, and from that community to the health policy community.

It has also given rise to a need for a refocusing or rebalancing of the research interests of the health economics community. Issues of distribution, of health, health care, and health care costs, have long been of central importance to policy-makers, but have tended to get short shrift (assumed away or, worse, simply ignored in the pursuit of the keys to "efficiency") by whole segments of the health economics research "agenda." This collection of papers, selected from a much larger group of presentations at the inaugural conference of the International Health Economics Association (iHEA), and indeed the themes of the conference itself, were and are intended as small contributions toward achieving that rebalancing. The seeds for this inaugural conference were sown back in 1990, during the so-called Second World Congress on Health Economics (University of Zurich). During a corridor conversation, one of us (MLB) suggested to one of the Zurich Conference organizers (Peter Zweifel), that it should not be another ten years before the next such meeting (the first Congress was held in Leiden in 1980), and went on to suggest that in order to ensure that another decade did not pass, he would commit himself to organizing a 1995 Vancouver meeting. Feeling that such promises should be widely shared, Peter proceeded to close the Zurich conference by making public this offer.

In the interim, iHEA was founded in 1993 by Alan Maynard, Joe Newhouse, Mark Pauly, Jim Burgess and Tom Getzen. Cam Donaldson and the HESG network were a source of inspiration and provided an important boost in the initial efforts to ascertain the level of interest in an international organization. Cooperation from the publishers of two leading journals in the field, Wiley *(Health Economics)* and Elsevier *(Journal of Health Economics)* made it possible to offer a bundle of services that was cost-effective and widely appreciated. In less than two years, iHEA grew to more than 500 members in 34 countries. A seminal event in the formation of iHEA was the presentation of the first Kenneth J. Arrow Award for best paper in health economics. The presentation, to Richard Hirth, occurred at the 1993 meeting of the American Public Health Association.

Meanwhile, that idle 1990 promise was still out there, and its perpetrator received periodic reminders in various newsletters of health economics or related organizations from around the world, and a small but irritating trickle of requests for further information on dates, venue, and the like. But it was not until one of us (TEG) made a fateful phone call to another (MLB), who was hiding in California on sabbatical in the winter of 1994, that the necessary fertilizer was applied to those initial seeds. The offer from TEG, to organize the inaugural conference of the Association, and in so doing to discharge MLB's 1990 commitment, was too enticing to refuse. A 1995 conference was, by that time, impossible, but 1996 seemed conceivable (and by the time 1996 rolled around, thankfully no one except MLB seemed to recall the precise date attached to the original promise).

From this humble beginning began the immense task of creating an international event that would serve multiple purposes: formally launching the International Health Economics Association; initiating a regular series of international conferences that would bring together practitioners of, and those interested in the results of, health economics research; creating opportunities for truly international exchange of information; creating a forum for the presentation of new research in areas representing the broad range of interests of the health economics research community.

But the organizers (now including GLS, recruited by MLB to make good on the Canadian offer to host the conference) wanted something more for this event, so that it would not be, or be remembered as, just one more in a series of meetings of health economists (see below). The international health economics community, that is, those involved in what might be thought of broadly as research in health and health care economics, tends to be a bit xenophobic. While some interesting comparative research gets done, and there is a fair bit of cross-boundary consulting activity, a glance at any of the professional journals in which health economists publish makes clear that the bulk of their work is very narrowly focused, if not within their own state/province, then at least within national borders. There is plenty of methodologic exchange, but much less exchange of the critical institutional, regulatory, financial and historical details that make policy extrapolation so risky and often unrewarding.

The creation of groups, and the structuring of conferences, have historically done little to break down these geographic barriers. We have formal organizations of health economists from the U.K., Scandinavia, Europe, Australia, Canada and Thailand, to cite a few examples. Each of these organizations sponsors periodic (often annual) conferences, dealing largely with issues of import to the "host" organization's members, which tend predominantly to be "home" issues.

Prior to the iHEA conference, there had been few, and then quite random, conference events structured to try to bring this international community together in fora that would facilitate cross-border learning, and encourage new international collaboration on problems of common interest in diverse health care systems. The first such gathering was in 1973 in Tokyo, sponsored by the International Economic Association. It was then another seven years until the World Congress on Health Economics, held in the Netherlands, in the fall of 1980. There was no organizational connection between these two events. And it was to be another ten years before the next such exchange -- the second world congress took place in the fall of 1990 in Zurich, largely due to the initiative of Peter Zweifel.

But the lack of regularity of such meetings would not have provided sufficient impetus for the huge investment necessary to creating an event of this scale. The inaugural iHEA conference was, from the outset, structured to be truly international, not only in the themes it addressed, but in the audiences which it tried to reach. One of the key intents of the conference organizers was to create opportunities for the health economics community in the "developed world" to get more involved in the health care system problems of developing and emerging economies around the world. The major themes of the conference (one of which is featured in the contents of this collection) were carefully chosen not because they are the sub-areas in which most health economists work, but because they are areas of critical importance to health policy evolution around the globe in which health economists have as yet not made the sorts of critical contributions which are both possible and necessary -- the themes represented areas of opportunity and challenge, rather than areas of familiarity, intended in part to stimulate new work in these areas. The themes were:

• Distributional Issues in Health and Health Care Financing
• The Boundaries of Health Care: What's In, What's Out, and Why Does it Matter?
• Toward a Better Understanding of Objectives and Motivations (of providers, payors, and users)
• Health Care Reform -- Why is Everyone Doing It? Who Gains, Who Loses? General Lessons
• Payoffs in Health and Wealth, or the Opportunity Cost of Health Care

As might be expected with such objectives, we were more successful in attracting work in some areas than in others. But as the conference program (see the Appendix) attests, the conference attracted a remarkable breadth of work, including some significant contributions in all the chosen thematic areas. The program owes a considerable debt to a committed and conscentious scientific program committee: William Hsiao, Naoki Ikegami, Bengt Jönsson, Pierre-Jean Lancry, Willard Manning, Alan Maynard, Anne Mills, Gavin Mooney, Michael Morrisey, Charles Normand, Jean-Pierre Poullier, Thomas Rice, Jeff Richardson, Joan Rovira, Frans Rutten, J.-Matthias Graf von der Schulenburg, George Torrance, and Peter Zweifel. We received about 325 abstract submissions, each of which underwent scientific review. About 250 of them were assembled into thematic clusters (usually of three papers), which were then mapped into a program that had to accommodate the vagaries of various travel schedules and constraints.

One of the other objectives of the conference organizers was to encourage participation by graduate students in health economics. With that in mind, we organized a student competition, inviting the submission of abstracts, then complete papers, from graduate students involved in health economics research (again encouraging papers on the above themes), and we were able to provide travel support and registration fee waivers to the authors of the papers judged to be the best of a very good group. We are grateful to Andrew Jones for agreeing to chair the committee charged with the difficult task of judging the submissions, and to David Feeny, Bengt Jönsson, Thomas Rice and Alan Shiell for working with Andrew. Three of the "prize" papers (Bleichrodt, Bishai, Schneider-Bunner) are included in this volume.

Of course creating a conference requires much more than simply assembling a scientific program. The challenge of planning the event, getting delegates accommodated, ensuring on-site logistics were seamless, in short creating a positive conference experience, was borne by the conference Planning Committee, ably chaired by Karen Cardiff from the Centre for Health Services and Policy Research at the University of British Columbia (CHSPR). She was assisted by the local conference organizer (MLB), Mary Brunold (CHSPR), Susan Isaacs (B.C. Ministry of Health), and Steve Kenny (B.C. Health Industry Development Office), and by the talented and enthusiastic staff of International Conference Services, particularly Sarah Lowis. And creating an edited collection requires much more than simply choosing which papers to include. Without the heroic efforts of Connie Koran, Lebby Balakshin, Juliet Ho and Kimberlyn McGrail, this book would never have seen the light of day.

The conference represented without a doubt a watershed for the organization and, in a very real sense, brought closure to the "fomative years." Over 600 delegates from close to 40 countries attended the inaugural meeting, and almost 300 papers and poster presentations were featured over a period of five days. The first day was taken up with pre-conference sessions, ably presented by Sam Sheps, Robin Hanvelt, Willard Manning, Mark McClellan, John Mullahy, Clyde Hertzman, Michael Wolfson, George Torrance, William Furlong, David Feeny, Lauren Cuddy, and Wynand van de Ven. These pre-conference sessions were a mix of traditional health economics preoccupations ("Advances in Health Econometrics," "Risk-Adjustment," "Health Utilities"), and issues and methods that represented opportunities for health economists to look beyond the techniques and questions of their own discipline ("Critical Appraisal," "Determinants of Health of Populations").

The plenary sessions were designed to feature some of the themes noted above. Uwe Reinhardt from Princeton led off with a stimulating (and entertaining) presentation entitled "The New Social Contract for Health Care: Should Economists Write It or Merely Describe It?" On the second day of the conference, Adam Wagstaff, Eddy van Doorslaer and Alan Williams presented papers in a plenary session devoted to issues of distribution and equity. The conference closed with Robert Evans' introspective look at the profession of health economics, "Toward a Healthier Economics."

In the midst of the post-conference euphoria (that it had gone so well, and that it was over!), there was one small matter left for the conference organizers -- how to create a conference proceedings. During the discussions that led, eventually, to the present volume, there were considerations of a book series (each book on a theme), and of special journal issues. It was clear that there were too many papers for a traditional "Proceedings." But that was about all that was clear. In the end, we felt that there was no satisfactory way, in one book, to capture the full breadth of papers presented at the conference. We also kept coming back to where we had begun in the process of deciding on featured themes, to the fact that we should use this book, as we had tried to use the conference, as a vehicle for communicating something about what health economics *could* offer (rather than what it has, and continues to, offer). As a result, we decided to create this, a volume containing selected papers on *one* of the chosen themes.

Several considerations had led to the choice of "equity" or distribution, of health, health care, health care costs, as one of the featured themes for the Conference:

1. The important association between income and income inequalities on the one hand, and health inequalities on the other;

2. The persistence of inequalities despite policy interventions designed specifically to remove or reduce economic barriers to access to care;

3. The potential for economists to improve on existing measures of an often contentious construct of central importance to health and public policy;

4. The under-emphasis on matters of distribution, relative to issues of efficiency, in much of the health economics research to date.

The book opens, as did the conference, with a "rap on the knuckles" to professional health economists, about the use (and particularly misuse) of the concept of efficiency. Reinhardt leaves no doubt that notions of equity are central (even if not explicit) to the "misconstruction of economic analysis by the laity," and economists' complicity in this phenomenon. The book closes, again as did the conference, with Evans' exploration of the "persistent, illogical and unsound analysis by competent professionals," on issues of distribution, and his constructive suggestions for beginning to remedy this.

Between the "book-ends," are a number of papers that do take up the task of examining the extent and effects of inequities or inequalities from a variety of perspectives and in different contexts. David Mayston's study of aboriginal populations in Australia demonstrates large health differentials, and then attempts to determine the mechanisms by which inequalities are generated, maintained, and magnified. David Bishai, drawing on the "health capital" model of Michael Grossman, provides a detailed empirical examination of intergenerational transfers, revealing one aspect of the production process, "quality" of parental time. Ulf Gerdtham and Gun Sundberg's study of Swedish health inequalities demonstrates the sensitivity of current econometric techniques by showing that even small differentials can be reliably measured even in a relatively homogenous population. The study by Jan Klavus and Unto Häkkinen extends the analysis into the temporal dimension, examining the dynamics of inequality in response to the severe Finnish recession of 1990-1993. Cam Mustard *et al.* delve into the micro-level interaction of income, medical care utilization and incidence of payment burden among a stratified random sample of Manitoba households. Eddy van Doorslaer and Adam Wagstaff present summary data from the Euro-ECuity project, the most comprehensive examination of equity in health, health care use and health care financing undertaken to date. These six papers demonstrate the range and technical sophistication which health economists and others are beginning to bring to the empirical analysis of equity.

These empirical papers lead to the next set of questions, regarding implementation and evaluation. Jack Rodgers and Karen Smith use simulations of MSAs for a Medicare population to demonstrate numerically the type of favorable/unfavorable selection which can cause insurance to have unintended side-effects. MSA premium simulations may seem far removed from the study of mortality among groups of aboriginals, but both address differential risks, and the effects of public and private interventions which amplify or moderate the pre-existing inequities. Liu *et al.* examine the collapse of the Cooperative Medical System in rural China, and use simulations to evaluate the feasibility of risk-pooling. Chernichovsky *et al.* use the sharp increase in regional funding inequalities after the break-up of the Soviet Union as a natural experiment. They find that although education and life-styles created differences in mortality, changes in the availability of health care financing and medical resources had no effect, at least in the short run. Jane Doherty and Alex van den Heever use a case study of post-reform South Africa to argue that sudden changes in regional financing to correct prior inequities led to a waste of resources and bureaucratic disruption. A centrally mandated attempt to rapidly reverse decades of inequality that was not sensitive to local conditions and organizational constraints may have reduced efficiency and political support for more durable, albeit slower, reform. The lesson from these studies in the managerial economics of health is that inequalities are important, and are difficult to change. That such lessons are predictable does not mean that they have been well appreciated by policy makers or the public.

It is these problems of how we frame and think about issues of inequality that are addressed in the philosophical contribution of Claude Schneider-Bunner, the analysis by Alan Williams on the notion and measurement of "a fair innings," or equity in opportunities for life-time health, and Han Bleichrodt's examination of the logical requirements for QALY aggregation.

The next four papers are the set from one of the most well-attended, and introspective, parallel sessions of the conference, "Reconsidering the Theoretical Foundations of Health Economics." As chair of this session, Anthony Culyer was invited to introduce the papers. He offers some personal reflections on the nature and potential of the extra-welfarist approach, which each of the papers in this group at least in part addresses. Hurley critically examines two evaluative frameworks used by health economists – welfare economic and extra-welfarist – and argues that both frameworks exhibit important incongruities with deeply-held values in many societies. Mooney points out that economists have neglected the "community commodity" health care, and the role of health care systems as social institutions *per se*. Rice examines the desirability of market-based health care reforms through a reconsideration of economic theory and its limitations, which are thrown into sharpest relief by scrutiny of the assumptions made in welfare economics theory.

Readers may notice some overlap among the papers of this last group, and with the opening and closing papers of the volume. For this we offer no apologies -- we think it both interesting, and significant, that six authors asked, independently, to reflect on how we do our work as health economists made strikingly similar observations, often citing the same references (and occasionally even the same passages from those references).

Equity is a consideration that has tended to be neglected in the work of health economists. This volume represents one small step toward redressing the imbalance. We hope it will stimulate further interest by health economists in issues with which policy-makers and the general public tend to be pre-occupied. The tools of economics offer some promise in this effort, from the econometric techniques and indexes for measurement, to the ability of economic analysis to reveal the operation of rational self interest in the swirl of forces hidden under the seemingly bland assumption of "initial endowments." This inaugural iHEA conference provides evidence that health economists have more answers, and yet more questions, than were previously known.

Morris L. Barer
Tom E. Getzen
Greg L. Stoddart

1

Abstracting from Distributional Effects, this Policy is Efficient

UWE E. REINHARDT

Woodrow Wilson School of Public and International Affairs
Princeton University
Princeton, NJ, USA

When health economists started to meet formally sometime during the 1960s, they were a ragtag appendage to more general meetings of economists. Usually they held a session or two in a small room, often during lunch. In those days, economic growth in the industrialized world was strong, and the main problem in health policy was to develop the real resources capable of meeting the growing demand for health care that society was more than willing to underwrite financially. Consequently, health economists concentrated on the search for methods to enhance the supply of health-care resources and to improve the productivity of these resources. In the United States, health economists also participated actively in the search for an optimal universal health insurance system that was then thought to be just around the corner in the United States, but that, in the end, never came. By that

Health, Health Care and Health Economics: Perspectives on Distribution
Edited by Morris L. Barer, Thomas E. Getzen, and Greg L. Stoddart
Copyright 1998 John Wiley & Sons, Ltd.

time, of course, the European nations already had implemented universal health-insurance coverage decades before, and Canada was in the process of doing so. Remarkably, Canada accomplished that monumental task with a simple design that was fully fleshed out in the span of a few years, without the help of large numbers of health-economists and management consultants.

Today, the supply of real resources willing to meet the demand for health care tends to exceed society's willingness to pay for these resources almost everywhere in the world. Put another way, a voracious demand for health-care incomes everywhere taxes society's willingness to meet that demand. Because health care is still widely regarded in most nations as a so-called "merit" or "social" good that ought to be made available to all members of society, regardless of ability to pay, politicians naturally find themselves in the middle of this sandwich. Beset by the thankless task of limiting access to plentiful resources with appeal to limited budgets, these hard-pressed politicians increasingly turn to economists for advice. They do so presumably in the sincere belief that economists know how to allocate scarce resources smartly to competing ends. They may also do so, however, because they have come to appreciate the economist's ability to couch tough policies in felicitous language.

Whatever the motivation among policy makers may be, the exponential growth in the size of annual meetings of health economists attests to this growing demand for their services. These days, health economists no longer meet as afterthoughts to someone else's meeting. Now they organize their own meetings. Instead of booking merely a room or two for a small luncheon, they book entire hotels!

ECONOMISTS AND HEALTH POLICY

Economists do, indeed, have much to offer public and private decision makers who jointly determine the allocation of resources to and within an economic sector that now represents anywhere from 7 to 14% of the gross domestic product (GDP) in the industrialized nations and is pressing hard on the economies in the newly industrialized countries and the developing economies as well. To list but a few of the profession's strengths:

o   Economists know how to define and measure the cost of alternative courses of action with greater sophistication than any other profession. Even a first-year undergraduate course in economics can take the typical health-care executive far beyond the realm of the customary thinking in corporate board rooms--for example, by driving home the crucial distinction between fixed and variable costs, the irrelevance of sunk costs and the power of marginal analysis. It is astounding how many executives in the health-care industry are totally innocent of these basic concepts.[1] It is equally astounding how many management consulting firms now sell as "cutting edge technology" ideas that have been standard fare in economics for almost a century.[2]

o   Economists probably are better than any other profession--actuaries included--at structuring information properly for decision-making under uncertainty. In particular, economists have been instrumental in developing the markets in which risks are traded far beyond what might have been imagined only a few decades ago.

o   With their powerful analytic framework, economists can help force public discourse on health policy into the confines of logic. In the process, economic analysis helps debunk many of the illusions that drive public health policy. For example, economists can lay bare the hidden and often contradictory valuations implicit in the decisions of private and public decision makers in the economy, thereby debunking the myth that "human life" is priceless.

o   Through detached empirical research on the behavior of the various agents in the health economy, economists can vastly improve the prevailing folklore on which decisions in the private and public sector necessarily are based -- for example, the erstwhile folklore that the demand for health care is perfectly price-inelastic or the flattering notion that health professionals are impervious to economic incentives.

---

[1] For an illustration, see Reinhardt, 1996
[2] For an illustration, see Pallarito, 1997.

o   Economists can make very useful contributions to the field of "evidence-based" medicine -- including the relatively new field of pharmaco-economics -- as long as economists do not impose their own subjective valuations on alternative clinical outcomes and, equally important, as long as they make crystal clear to the users of their analyses precisely whose valuations they do use.

o   Most importantly, through detached analysis economists can be instrumental in identifying the trade-off frontiers at which moral choice comes into play -- trade-offs that must properly be left to someone else.

It will be noted that these and many other contributions one could enter in such a list have in common that they all represent *positive* economic analysis. That form of analysis merely seeks to explain, through deductive logic, how rational individuals will respond to changes in the constraints that impinge upon their actions; through empirical research, how decision makers in the economy actually do react to such stimuli, how particular markets work; and through computer simulations based on empirically estimated response coefficient, how the health care system is likely to respond to the exogenous changes wrought by public policy. Economists are at their best in the realm of positive analysis.

Even positive economic analysis, of course, is not immune to the analyst's predilections, which may enter in subtle and not so subtle ways. The empirical estimates by which economists seek to describe the behavior of agents in the health care sector almost inevitably become amalgams of preconceptions and observed data. Rare is the case in which an hypothesis is stated in testable form and then confronted *only once* with a body of empirical information. More common is the practice of restating the underlying equation, transforming the data some more and sometimes even truncating them, in an iterative search for "plausible" coefficients. As one scientist producing ostensibly positive analysis is reported to have put it candidly: "I wouldn't have seen it if I hadn't believed it" (Cohn, 1989).

The potential for bias in ostensibly positive health-economics can be amplified by the funding of that research. Increasingly, health-economic research is commissioned not by disinterested parties, but by partisan causes seeking scientific support for a particular point of view. During the debate over the health-reform proposed by President Clinton in 1993-94, for example, the opponents of a government mandate on employers to provide their employees with health insurance had no trouble finding respected economists who imputed to that mandate large losses in employment. In their simulations, these economists assumed, as most economists do, that, over time, the cost of the mandate would be passed to employees through lower take-home pay, and that the supply of labor is highly sensitive to changes in take-home pay. On the other hand, policy makers who favored the employer mandate had no trouble finding equally respectable economists who assumed the supply of labor to be rather insensitive to take-home pay, in which case the mandate would lead to only a modest reduction in employment, albeit more steeply reduced take-home pay. The econometric literature offers a sufficiently broad palette of estimates of the wage-elasticity of labor supply to support quite a range of simulated predictions (Krueger and Reinhardt, 1994).

Economists may bristle at the innuendo that they would bend their positive analysis to a client's whims. That would be an odd posture for a profession that thinks nothing of modeling the behavior of physicians by the simple utility function

[1]
$$U = f(Y, L) \, ,$$

(where Y is income and L is time available for leisure),

and that would deny that an increase in the physician-population ratio in a given market area might lead to a supplier-induced upward shift in the demand for physician services, presumably on the theory that the Y/L-maximizing physicians already in the area would already have pushed out the demand for their services to the highest position tolerated by patients and their insurers. If economists assume that physicians would behave thus, why would they not assume also that economists would behave likewise in structuring information for use by others?[3] It may be

---

[3] The associations of most other professions have formal codes of professional ethics and committees to watch over these codes. Furthermore, the sessions at their meetings and their literature in general exhibit a deep concern with their profession's ethics. Remarkably, the American Economics Association (AEA) does not have a formal committee on professional ethics, and rarely, if ever, does the AEA feature sessions devoted to, say, the "Professional Ethics of Economic Analysis." A case can be made for developing more explicit codes of professional ethics -- certainly in as sensitive a field as health economics -- and for establishing formal committees to stand guard over those codes. Perhaps the International Health Economics Association (IHEA) can take a lead in this quest.

countered that standard peer review and professional reputation are sufficient to assure ethical conduct in health-economic research. Policy makers, however, are no longer buying that thesis, at least not in the United States. Why else, for example, would the reigning majority party in the United States Congress insist that the head of its Congressional Budget Office -- a body created strictly for the purpose of ostensibly positive economic analysis -- be staffed at the top by economists of the majority party's own choosing?

To enhance their reputation as producers of positive policy analysis, and the general quality of that analysis, health economists the world over would do well to mimic more routinely than the profession now does the approach to auditing employed by the accounting profession.[4] This could be accomplished by opening all empirical research in health economics to full and complete external audit. In principle, that audit should go beyond the traditional boundary of peer review -- the evaluation merely of the theory and econometric method that underlies the analyses. It should extend *routinely* also to the raw data and to the transformed data that drove the findings and recommendations. Ideally, there ought to be a formal audit capacity enabling researcher A *easily* and quickly to get access to the very data tape used by researcher B to produce particular results subject, of course, that such data be used by others strictly for the purpose of audit, and not to grind out publishable work in competition with the researcher whose labor produced the empirical base. If such audits were routinely feasible, their mere threat probably would enhance the accuracy of the ever-growing flood of analysis that now informs health policy as much as it merely buffets that policy.

The potential for unwitting or purchased bias in *positive* health economics is one potential pitfall in the burgeoning field of health economics. Health economists enter even more treacherous ground when they seek to offer decision makers *normative* prescriptions, unless in so doing they take as given to them the clearly stated goal or goals the decision maker seeks to pursue, and the economist merely helps the decision maker identify the least-cost method of reaching the stated goals. Economists are not licensed, so to speak, to posit these goals for decision makers, or to set the relative weights that ought to be attached to each of multiple goals -- for example, to each of the twin-goals of "equity" and "efficiency," as these terms

---

[4] That proposal is developed in the author's "Making economic evaluations respectable," *Social Science and Medicine*, Vol. 45, No. 4, pp. 555-562.

may be understood.

Unfortunately, it is child's play to infuse normative economic analysis with the analyst's own preferences. It can be done by the way economists structure their information for decision makers. It can also be done simply with the idioms economists select to communicate their analyses to decision makers. As Kenneth Arrow (1963) has observed on this point in his classic "Uncertainty and the Welfare Economics of Medical Care," in connection with the economist's use of the word "optimal":

> A definition is just a definition, but when the *definiendum* is a word already in common use with highly favorable connotations, it is clear that we are really trying to be persuasive; we are implicitly recommending the achievements of optimal states (p.942).

In the vernacular, the word "optimal" is generally taken to mean unquestionably "the best." To economists the word connotes no such thing. Inspired by the writings of the nineteenth century Italian economist Vilfredo Pareto (1897), modern economists have fallen into the habit of treating the term "Pareto optimality" as a synonym for "Pareto efficiency,"[5] a concept to be revisited further on in this essay. As Francis Bator had beautifully demonstrated in his earlier classic on the "Simple Economics of Welfare Economics," however, a given resource base can be allocated in infinitely many different Pareto efficient ways, and economists have no objective method of determining which among these alternatives truly is the best (Baumol, 1977, pp. 530-531). Worse still, if one were given a choice only between two allocations, one Pareto efficient (alias Pareto optimal) and the other not, the first would not necessarily be "better" than the second. Any properly trained economist knows this. Most lay persons probably would be surprised to hear it.

The remainder of this essay will focus, in the main, on the role language plays in coloring the advice economists give policy makers. The language economists use intra-professionally has precise meaning that often is at variance with the connotation lay people put upon the same words. That circumstance alone can lead quite innocently to serious distortions in communicating ideas to the public. But the problem goes beyond mere differences in the meaning put upon particular sequences of letters. As Arrow points out, many times economists deliberately use carefully chosen language to sell others on a particular point of view.

---

[5] See, for example, Baumol, 1977; Landsburg, 1995; and Browning and Browning, 1986.

When health economists adopted the habit of referring to, say, cancer stricken human beings as "consumers" rather than as "patients," they were not just innocently adapting a real-world context to their standard analytic framework. They were actively seeking to replace the image of a frightened individual who more or less passively accepts whatever treatment the attending physician recommends, with the image of a rational buyer who does (or should) shop around for cost-effective health care. Wittingly or unwittingly, they were conjuring up a distinct normative framework for the allocation of health-care resources. When economists describe the rationing of scarce resources by price and ability to pay as a "free-market allocation" and the allocation through non-market mechanism as "rationing," they are not acting as neutral observers. They implicitly express their preference for rationing by price and ability to pay. It can even be argued that economists are treading on dangerous ground when they emphasize "economic efficiency" in their prescriptions, with the caveat "abstracting from distributional effects." In so doing, economists may make the studied pretense that the decision makers using the analysis will automatically take care of any untoward "distributional effects." If economists know with reasonable certainty that this will not be done, however, then such a posture is tantamount to the mantra among American vendors of assault rifles that "guns don't kill people; people do."

In his presidential address to the 1996 annual meeting of the American Economics Association, Victor Fuchs (1996) argued that American health economists far too frequently let their own ideology temper their policy recommendations during the debate on the Clinton health-reform bill, on both sides of the political divide. I shall join Fuchs in pleading that, if we do feel called upon to offer *normative* recommendations on public policy as professional economists -- rather than as mere citizens -- we scrupulously reveal, to the extent it is humanly possible, the prior normative propositions that drive our recommendations, so that their users stand properly apprized of the ideology these recommendations embody. It is one thing to advocate or to enlist market forces in health care, after honestly confronting and revealing the likely distributive implications of that approach. It is quite another to do so in blissful ignorance of these implications or, worse still, by carefully camouflaging these implications with the often misleading technical yet soothing jargon of our profession. By the same token, it is misleading to advocate non-market algorithms for the distribution of health care without alerting users of one's analysis to certain hidden economic costs implicit in such algorithms, costs that may fall heavily on particular individuals as well.

The remainder of the essay proceeds as follows. The section immediately following presents a homework exercise taken from a first year course in economics. That exercise is designed to highlight both the precision and the limits of certain words used in economic analysis and widely misunderstood among lay persons. The exercise also illustrates dramatically the role of normative economics -- particularly the use of the word "efficiency" -- in a concrete policy setting. Teachers of undergraduates may find the exercise useful in their own class rooms, and so may students who might perchance read this essay. The essay is written with students very much in mind. Walking through that warm-up exercise may be particularly illuminating to health-policy analysts from the formerly socialist nations. The essay is written with these readers very much in mind as well. It is not uncommon in these nations that policy makers and their economic advisers see in the magic of "the market" a virtual panacea for most of the problems faced by their health care systems. They are encouraged in that regard by the roving bands of "experts" from the established market economies -- notably from the United States -- who spread the gospel of "the market" for health care with almost missionary zeal. To be sure, it is important that hard-pressed policy makers in these nations allocate scarce health-care resources "efficiently." But it is equally important to understand fully what the concept of "efficiency" that the foreign "experts" try to sell actually means, and does not mean, in the context of health care. Many novices to market economics may be surprised to learn that "more efficient" does not necessarily mean "better" and might even mean "worse."

Following this warm-up exercise is a brief comment on the current transformation of the American health care system and its implications for the role of health economists. That section draws on a lengthier treatment of that subject published elsewhere (Reinhardt, 1996). For better or for worse, the American health care system seems to be regarded by the rest of the world with much fascination and, one suspects, as an inspiration for health care reform at home. Because national health policy and health care systems ought to reflect the social ethic nations wish to impose upon the distribution of health care, it is important for health economists elsewhere to understand the social ethic that now drives American health care policy. It would be dangerous to import from the United States ideas not suitable for transplantation into the soil of a different social ethic.

This commentary on transformation of the American health care system is followed by an exploration of certain pitfalls of welfare economics, drawing mainly on the classic but now somewhat neglected literature -- notably the definitive writings of Bator (1958), Baumol (1969), and Arrow (1963) -- that had settled decades ago many of the arguments on welfare economics that still occupy us today.

That more philosophical literature does not appear to be given quite the prominence that it once had in the typical graduate program in economics, perhaps because room had to be made for the growing and highly demanding field of data analysis.

Finally, I offer some observations on the pitfalls of cross-national comparisons of entire health care systems.

A WARM-UP EXERCISE IN WELFARE ECONOMICS

In my first-year undergraduate course in micro-economics at Princeton University, I sometimes introduce students to the welfare-economic implications of free markets with the aid of the following stylized illustration:

> Consider a two-family society composed of the Chens and the Smiths. Both families have identical incomes and wealth. Members of the Smith family all are wild about jelly beans. Members of the Chen family will eat jelly beans, but none of them is wild about them. Not surprisingly, at any quantity of jelly beans demanded per period, Q, the Smith family's marginal-value curve for jelly beans (more familiar to you as the household's "demand curve" for jelly beans) sits higher in a graph of P (price per pound of jelly beans) on Q than does the Chen family's marginal-value curve. Put another way, at any volume of jelly beans they already consume in a given period, the Smiths are willing to pay more for an additional package of jelly beans than are the Chens, because the Smiths "value" jelly beans more in the sense that they genuinely appreciate them more.

Equipped with a graph of the two demand curves, we begin our analysis with the initial situation in which an ostensibly benevolent government distributes an identical quantity of jelly beans per period to each of the two families, free of charge at the time of delivery. To pay the foreign suppliers of jelly beans, the government levies an identical tax on both families. Because the benevolent government deems jelly beans to be good for people and therefore wants each family to consume its allotment, the two families are not allowed to trade their jelly-bean ration for money or vice versa.

We calculate the total consumers' surplus enjoyed by the two families under this restricted, initial condition.[6] Next, we relax the government's strictures and allow the families freely to trade jelly beans for money, assuming zero transactions costs.

---

[6] To make this calculation clear and easy, we assume that jelly beans are traded in discrete, standard packages.

We calculate the total consumer surplus that will obtain after all trading has stopped. We discover, naturally, that it exceeds the total attained under the initial "no-trade" condition. Furthermore, we discover that the equilibrium reached under the relaxed rules will be the same as that which would have obtained, had government not implemented its tax- and "free"-jelly-beans program in the first place.

Thus do we celebrate the beneficence of the legendary Invisible Hand doing its good work in a free market, without even having debited to the government's ill conceived scheme certain other costs it imposes on society, including the deadweight loss from taxation that we explore earlier in the course.

Programmed with these fundamental insights, my students are then sent home to exercise these insights on the following problem (to which suggested answers are supplied in the appendix of this paper).

Econ 102

EXERCISE IN "WELFARE ECONOMICS"

In an editorial entitled "Gammon's Law Points to Health-Care Solution" that was published by the prestigious *The Wall Street Journal* (November 12, 1991), Nobel Laureate economist Milton Friedman, formerly of the University of Chicago and now at the Hoover Institute of Stanford University, sharply attacked the government-run Medicare program for the elderly and the Medicaid program for the disabled and the poor. He concluded thus:

> The *inefficiency*, high cost and inequitable character of our medical system can be fundamentally remedied in only one way: by moving in the other direction, toward re-privatizing medical care. ... The reform has two major steps: (1) End both Medicare and Medicaid and replace them with a requirement that every U.S. family unit have a major medical insurance policy with a high deductible, say $20,000 a year or 30% of the unit's income during the prior two years, whichever is lower. (2) End the tax exemption of employer provided medical care. ... Each individual or family would, of course, be free to buy supplementary insurance, if it so desired (Emphasis added).

The "deductible" in a health insurance policy is the annual amount the family must finance with its own resources before any insurance coverage begins. To put Friedman's policy recommendation into perspective, review tables 18.1 and 18.2 of your textbook (Stockman, 1996). The tables indicate that in 1990, at about the time Friedman formulated his recommendation, median pretax income in the United States was $29,943 for all households and $35,353 for "families," that is, for households with two or more members. If we assume that Friedman meant to base the recommended deductible not on the <u>sum</u> of the family's income during the past two years but only the *average* annual family income over the prior two years, then that deductible in 1990 would have been $10,500 per year for a family with median pretax income of $35,353. The outlays on health care of a relatively health family probably would not have reached that deductible. A family stricken with serious illness almost surely would have had to pay that much out of pocket before insurance coverage would set in. In addition, each family would have to pay the premium for the catastrophic insurance policy.

Professor Friedman injected his editorial into the presidential election campaign of 1991-92, during which health policy had moved to center stage. He acknowledged the contribution to his editorial by fellow Nobel Laureate economist Gary S. Becker of the University of Chicago and by economist Thomas Moore, Ph.D., formerly of President Reagan's Council of Economics Advisors and now at the Hoover Institute of Stanford University. In short, we may regard the editorial as a significant statement made by prominent American economists who sought to influence with their normative analysis both the election and the path of public health policy.

To appreciate better the use of the word "efficiency" in this context, consider now two families, the Chens and the Smiths. The Chens are wealthy and the Smiths are poor. Into each family there has just been born a baby. As it happens, Baby Chen is perfectly healthy. Baby Smith, alas, is somewhat sickly. Both families live in Professor Friedman's ideal world, that is, neither family has health insurance covering visits to the physician's office, although they may have the kind of catastrophic coverage he would allow above the deductible of 30 percent of income. The diagram below depicts these two families' marginal-value curves for visits by the infant with a physician per year (hereafter referred to simply as "visits"). Recall that we refer to these curves as "demand curves." Yet another name for them would be "willingness-to-pay curves." Assume that, if their incomes and the health status of their babies had been identical, the two families' marginal-value curves for visits would have been identical[7] as well.

With these preliminaries, answer the following set of questions, drawing in the process on the jelly-bean case we had discussed in class and on Chapter 11, "Economic Efficiency and the Gains from Trade," of your textbook (Stockman, 1996), especially pp. 304-309.

---

[7] I do not explicitly mention the possibility of positive externalities in consumption at this stage, but do invite students to discover these on their own in parts (g) and (j) of this exercise.

FIGURE 1

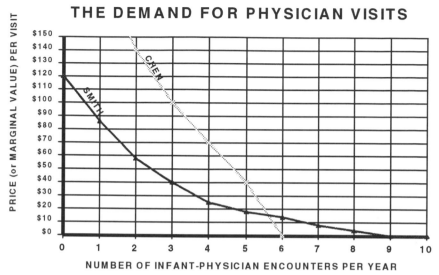

THE DEMAND FOR PHYSICIAN VISITS

NUMBER OF INFANT-PHYSICIAN ENCOUNTERS PER YEAR

QUESTIONS

a. Why, do you suppose, do the two families' demand curves for physician visits not coincide? Why do the Smiths seem to value visits less than do the Chens at visit rates up to about 5.5 annual visits and why do they value visits more than do the Chens at visit rates above that level? (Not a silly question. Many seasoned adults in the so-called "real world" seem to have trouble with that question. Even some economists, who should know better, appear to confuse in their analyses "tastes" with other factors that may enter a consumer's demand function).

b. If these two families could procure physician visits in a freely competitive market, at a price of, say, $40 per visit, then the allocation of physician visits to the two babies in the free market envisaged by Professor Friedman and his colleagues would be

_____ **visits/year to healthy Baby Chen**

_____ **visits/year to sickly Baby Smith**

c. Accept for the moment the normative proposition adopted by many practicing economists and by the politicians they inspire that the marginal-value curves of individual consumers or households signal the marginal *social* value of commodities. [Note that not every economist and politician subscribes to that proposition, although Professor Friedman and his colleagues most probably do.] Also assume that the free-market price of $40 per visit reflects the social marginal cost of producing visits, including the opportunity cost of the physician's time. Then, would the free-market allocation of visits you have identified in Part (b) be "economically efficient" as the author of your text (and virtually all other introductory textbooks in economics) defines that term? Explain.

d. Continue with the proposition and assumptions made in Part (c). Then the marginal social value of, say, the 3rd visit per year by a baby to the physician is

$$\$\underline{\hspace{2cm}} \text{ if it is made by healthy Baby Chen}$$

$$\$\underline{\hspace{2cm}} \text{ if it is made by sickly Baby Smith}$$

e. Suppose now that, for some reason, physician visits in this society were not allocated through a free-market algorithm, but instead were allocated to the two families by the government, under some administrative algorithm, and in a way that had allocated to the sickly Baby Smith 4 visits to the physician per year and to the healthy Baby Chen only 2 visits per year. Would such an allocation be **Pareto efficient** as your text defines that term?

f. Would it be a **Pareto improvement** if, in the situation described in part (e), one visit were taken away from sickly Baby Smith and given instead to healthy Baby Chen? Explain, in a sentence or two.

g. Would it be a **potential Pareto improvement** if, in the situation described in part (e), one visit were taken away from sickly Baby Smith and given instead to healthy Baby Chen? Explain, in a sentence or two.

h. Would the reallocation of one physician visit from sickly Baby Smith to healthy Baby Chen described in parts (e) represent an **increase in economic efficiency** as the author of your text defines that term? Explain, in a sentence or two. Be sure to define all of the terms you use in your answer, including "economic efficiency."

i. Would the reallocation of one visit from sickly Baby Smith to healthy Baby Chen described in part (e) be a **better** allocation of resources? Would the author of your text say so? Explain, in a sentence or two.

j. Could the government-administered allocation of physician visits described in part (e) above be properly described as "rationing"?

k. Could the rationing of physician visits in this case be avoided if the government refrained from intervening in the market for physician visits and instead let free market forces determine their allocation? (Not a silly question; many seasoned adults seem to have trouble with it.)

l. Start with the free-market solution under Part (b) as the initial position. Suppose now the government used general tax revenues to grant the low-income Smith family a subsidy of $30 per visit and that the market price of $40 per visit reflects the marginal social cost per visit. Economists would impute a "welfare loss" (alias "deadweight loss) to such a policy. In a properly executed graph, show the size of this "welfare loss." In your own view, is this really a "welfare loss"? Defend your conclusion as best you can.

m. Finally, in the light of the preceding exercise, comment briefly on the following statement: "Freely competitive markets allocate scarce resources to those who value them the most."

==

Evidently, this exercise is designed to drive home forcefully the highly circumscribed role that value-laden terms such as "value," "efficiency," "rationing" and "welfare gain or loss" play in economic analysis. I consider it important that my students -- future users of economic analysis or future practitioners of the craft -- be aware of the distortion that our technical jargon tends to pick up as it goes beyond the confines of our discipline.

In this respect, the current transformation of the American health care system is instructive. The language and imagery of economics reign triumphant in that transformation; but often they have served merely to put a civilized spin on policies that might not be viewed as such by the American public, if those policies were described to the public forthrightly. For example, one must wonder how ordinary Americans would react to the forthright proposition that health care in the United States should be more widely rationed by price and ability to pay. Similarly, one wonders how ordinary Americans would react if they were told bluntly that more of the nation's health spending should be shifted from the shoulders of healthy Americans onto the shoulders of chronically ill Americans. As Victor Fuchs reminds us (1997), however, that shift is precisely the result of the current trend in the United States to give "the *coup de grace* to community rating" in private health insurance, in favor of "actuarially fair" health-insurance premiums.

ECONOMISTS AND THE TRANSFORMATION
OF AMERICAN HEALTH CARE

To the American media, the general American public and possibly to the rest of the world, the torturous debate over American health reform during the past several years may have come across as a mere disagreement over the best administrative mechanism of implementing a shared distributive ethic for health care. "We all want the same thing in health care," American politicians are wont to intone. "We merely quibble over how best to get there, without wrecking the economy."

Nothing could be further from the truth. The debate was only tangentially over alternative means to reach a common goal. Seemingly technical arguments over methods merely served to camouflage far more troublesome disagreements over the distributive ethic that ought to govern American health care. The decade-old struggle over the proper ethical foundation for American health care can be distilled into the following pointed question:

> To the extent that a nation's health care system can make it possible, should the child of, say, a low-income waitress or gas station attendant have the same chance of avoiding illness and, if afflicted by illness, of surviving and fully recuperating from it as does the child of a better-off middle- or upper-middle class American?

Most Canadians and Europeans -- probably even most Canadian and European economists -- would answer that question resolutely in the affirmative. The health care systems of these nations stand as a concrete testimony to that professed ideology. Although in these countries a small minority of very well-to-do families do have private health insurance[8] and fancy themselves to be getting superior health care with that coverage, families in the bottom 90% or so of these nations' income distribution have long tended to share one health-insurance and one health-care delivery system, on virtually identical terms.

Public opinion surveys have consistently shown that, at the superficial and facile level of such surveys, the overwhelming majority of the American public also

---

[8] Canada does not have a flourishing private health insurance system (although there are pressures in that direction, and it may yet come); but Canadians with the means to do so can avail themselves of the American health care system at any time they choose, and a few (although less than commonly claimed) Canadians are known to do so. In a sense, then, the United States can be viewed as Canada's upper-tier health care system.

professes to favor the highly egalitarian Canadian and European social ethic on health care, as is illustrated in Table 1 (Taylor and Reinhardt, 1991). For the purpose of public consumption, the dominant players who actually determine health policy in the United States -- chiefly the elected representatives in government and the handful of financially powerful interest groups to whom the elected officials are beholden -- tend to profess that ethic as well. One would be hard put to find instances in which American politicians or, say, American corporate executives allowed themselves to be quoted as openly advocating a health care system that rations health care by income class.

Table 1 Attitudes Toward "Equity" in Health Care
Selected Countries, 1991

Question:
People who are unemployed and poor should be able to get the same amount and quality of medical services as people who have good jobs and are paying substantial taxes.

	United States	Great Britain	France	Canada	West Germany
Agree strongly	61%	79%	67%	79%	69%
Agree, but not strongly	23%	16%	24%	15%	19%
Disagree, but not strongly	8%	2%	4%	3%	5%
Disagree strongly	6%	1%	3%	2%	2%
Not sure	2%	2%	2%	1%	5%

Source: Humphrey Taylor and Uwe Reinhardt, 1991, Table B, p. 8

Tacitly, however, a working majority of these powerful players appear to subscribe to just such a health care system. After the dust stirred up by the last round of debate on the issue finally had settled in late 1994, it should have become evident to any perceptive observer that the United States now *officially* countenances an income-based health care system in which the rationing of health care will increasingly be based on the individual household's ability to pay for its own health care (Taylor and Reinhardt, 1991). Consequently, the American system will, indeed, offer the child of a well-insured or high-income family more, and better timed, health care than it will offer the child of an uninsured gas station attendant or waitress. Precisely what impact such a differential in health care will have on the probability of avoiding illness, or of surviving and fully recovering from a given illness, is not clear, but is eminently researchable.

This dominant social ethic in American health care is clearly apparent in the support many American policy makers give the concept of the Medical Savings Accounts (MSAs) -- an idea actively being marketed under the banner "Putting People First in Health Care" (Council for Affordable Health Insurance, 1993). Central to the MSA concept are catastrophic health-insurance policies with very high deductibles -- say, $5,000 per family per year. Families could meet the bulk of these deductibles from funds in their own medical savings accounts into which families could make tax-deductible deposits up to a certain limit -- say, $4,000 per family per year. As the American Academy of Actuaries (1995) and others (Moon *et al.*, 1996) have pointed out, however, that approach would shift more of the financial burden of ill health from relatively healthy Americans to relatively sicker Americans. Furthermore, the tax subsidies proposed for the MSAs would be highly regressive, because the tax-deductibility of the deposits into the MSAs would, in effect, lower the after-tax, out-of-pocket payments for health care much more for high-income families than it would for low-income families (Pauly, 1994). The many American policy makers who favor MSAs -- now the majority in the Congress -- seem not to be troubled at all by these regressive distributional effects.[9] It is hard to imagine that, at this time, Canadian or European policy makers would exhibit a similar enthusiasm for so regressive a health-insurance scheme.

It is reasonable to suppose that this politically triumphant social ethic is likely to remain a permanent foundation for American health care for the foreseeable future. Just what has forged and cemented that ethic among the decision-making elite is the stuff for political scientists and sociologists, as is the question whether the implied social ethic actually is shared by the plebs or merely has been crammed down their throats by the dominant elite. Be that as it may, however, it is almost surely the case that the *official* embrace of income-based rationing of health care in the United States has been driven in good part by the marked secular widening of the nation's distribution of income during the past several decades. Health economists the world over will do well to follow these trends closely, for the

---

[9] In fairness it should be mentioned that the current method of financing comprehensive, employer-provided health insurance, which excludes premiums paid by employers on behalf of employees from the latters' taxable compensation, is also highly regressive.

widening of income distributions is not confined solely to the United States. It has been and will continue to be paralleled elsewhere in the industrialized world. To the extent that it does, health-policy makers elsewhere in the industrialized world will find it ever more difficult to preserve for their health care systems what Europeans call the *Principle of Solidarity*. They will abandon that principle the more quickly, the more enthusiastically they look to the United States for guidance on health policy.

Now, it can be argued that economists probably could do little to alter these megatrends, even if they wanted to. Nor is that their proper role as social scientists and policy analysts. Economists must search their souls, however, on the role they ought to play in this transformation. Should they become its energetic cheerleaders, because that transformation yields higher "economic efficiency," as textbooks define that term? Should economists deplore that transformation, because it may be judged inequitable, as many people would define income-based rationing of health care? Or should economists merely chronicle that transformation as faithfully and as objectively as they can, pointing out to policy makers and to the general public, in unvarnished prose, the full economic and ethical implications of that transformation, both those that the public may deem desirable or those it may deem deplorable?

The growing acceptance of income-based rationing of health care in the United States undoubtedly has found inspiration in the writings, teachings and punditry of economists in their *normative* mode, of which Friedman's previously cited editorial is an example. As already noted, in that literature "patients" have become "consumers," health care is treated as just another "private consumer good" -- certainly no different from food, clothes and shelter -- and physicians and hospitals as mere purveyors of that good. Hand in hand with these terms has come the proposition that a free market can produce and distribute the private consumption good "health care" more "efficiently" than can any other imaginable arrangement, because a free market can tailor the delivery of health care more closely to the consumers' idiosyncratic "tastes" than can a government program. Hand in hand with that proposition, in turn, has come the tacitly held ethical tenet that the quantity and quality of health care received by individuals can properly vary with their ability to pay for that care.

The proposition that health care, like food and housing, ought to be rationed by ability to pay is purely a moral judgement. As such, it is neither right nor wrong, and it must be respected in a debate on health policy. But surely it would have been appropriate, in a democracy, to debate this important question more explicitly than it has been debated in the United States. There the idea to ration health care by income class was not sold to the public in appropriately forthright terms. Instead, politicians painted the preferred health care system as a "free market" in which individuals are endowed with "responsibility" for their own health status and their own health care, and in which individual "consumers" are "empowered" to exercise "free choice" among "health-insurance products" and among the "consumer goods" that constitute health care. It was then predicted that such a health care system would be more "efficient" (that is, "better") than any other alternative system, and that it would even obviate the need for "rationing" health care.

This language, borrowed from our profession's lexicon is, of course, one felicitous way to describe the emerging transformation of the American health care system. But to tell an uninsured, low-income family with possibly sickly children that it is "empowered" by government to exercise "free choice" in health care, with its meager budget, is not much of a liberation, unless that proclamation were accompanied by public subsidies truly to empower that mother (which, alas, the proclamation has not been and in all likelihood will not be in the foreseeable future). While the policy envisaged by that proclamation could be styled as efficient in a purely technical sense -- as Milton Friedman and his colleagues evidently would -- it represents rationing by income class, pure and simple, even if to this day few American politicians would have the temerity to advocate income-based rationing openly.

Economists may properly protest that the problem in this regard lies not with economists, but in the misconstruction of economic analysis by the laity, and in the politicians' refusal to endow low-income families with the fiscal means to exercise meaningful choice in health care. *Entre nous*, for example, we might agree that within the context of the homework assignment presented above, the redistribution of a physician visit from sickly Baby Smith to health Baby Chen can be properly described as an increase in "economic efficiency," as we tend to define that term in our textbooks. We can also agree that that redistribution enhances "social economic welfare," as we commonly define that term at the technical level. On the other hand, how many of us would go on to argue that, therefore, such a "welfare enhancing" change necessarily would be an *improvement* upon the *status quo* -- that "greater efficiency" and added "economic welfare" is, *ipso facto*, "better"? But would non-economists be sophisticated enough to grasp these subtle distinctions within our lingo? Would not most of them automatically view a "more efficient" allocation of health-care resources as *ipso facto* a "better" one and, likewise, a state of "enhanced economic welfare" as ipso facto a "better" state of affairs? Would it be reasonable to expect lay persons to think otherwise? And if it is so, does that not impose upon the economics profession the moral burden to be ever so circumspect in the use of professional jargon when it is communicated across the divide between economists and non-economists?

In careless discourse, economists sometimes assert that markets allocate resources to those who *value* them the most. According to *Webster's*, the verb "to value" is a synonym of "to appreciate" (Webster's *New World Dictionary of the American Language*, 1966). But surely no economist would seriously propose that markets allocate scarce resources to persons who "appreciate" these resources the most? When economists use the verb "to value" in this context, they expect that verb to act like the analogue of a subroutine in a computer language that should read into one's mind the following larger text:

> Markets allocate resources to those individuals or other entities who are willing and able to bid the highest prices for these resources, regardless of the process by which the ability to pay the highest prices was amassed -- that is, regardless of the question whether the underlying distribution of income to which the market plays was an ethically acceptable starting point -- and regardless of the process that may have shaped the willingness to pay for these resources -- that is, regardless of what process shaped the bidders' "taste" for particular resources.

In the context of health care, the point regarding the formulation of "tastes" is particularly important, because a patient's "taste" for a particular medical procedure at a particular moment can be so powerfully shaped by the physician treating the patient.

It can be doubted that any lay persons not schooled in the technical jargon of our profession -- particularly politicians -- would ever read the same elaborate text into their brains when economists utter the verb "to value" before them. For example, few lay persons probably would think that, if scarce transplantable organs were simply auctioned off to patients willing and able to bid the highest money prices for them, a beneficent market had allocated these organs to patients who truly appreciated them the most **or who could benefit most from them** in a clinical sense. That being so, is it ever excusable for economists to use the verb "to value" as they are wont to do in the debate on health care policy, especially when they communicate with lay persons in the political arena?

Consider next the following statement, offered by an economist at the end of the 1980s, in the foreword to a compendium of papers seeking to assess the impact of a presumed shift of the American health care system towards a more market-oriented approach during the 1980s:

It appears that competition has increased substantially among providers and among insurers and health plans since 1977, perhaps more than anyone predicted or thought possible. Economic theory would suggest that this increase in competition should have resulted in a more *efficient* allocation of health services. ... But competition may have succeeded only in *improving* the allocation of health resources. In the next ten years, I believe, we will have to combine a better allocation of resources with a more equitable distribution of these resources (Emphasis added) (Greenberg, 1988).

That assessment can be questioned on both factual and interpretative grounds.

First, as those words were penned, private health-insurance premiums in the United States were rising at annual rates in the high double digits (between 15% to 20% per annum!), driving to utter despair the business sector that was paying these premiums on behalf of employees. During the period covered by the compendium, total national health spending rose from about 9% of the GDP in 1980 to close to 13% by 1990 while, at the same time, the number of Americans without any health insurance whatsoever had risen substantially as well.

Second, during the 1980s the excess capacity of the American health care system had grown apace. That excess capacity did not lead, as economic theory would have predicted, to a decline in the prices of health care services. On the contrary, the excess capacity served to drive up prices enough to prevent the elimination of the excess capacity. At that time, for example, the United States was found to have about four times as many mammography machines as would have been required to meet the prevailing use rates. That circumstance drove up the average cost per mammogram. The market for health care then was such that it also drove the prices charged per image to a level more than twice the price level that would have been needed to amortize a fully used machine over its useful life, along with a handsome built in profit per image (Brown *et al.*, 1990). Through the high prices triggered by that excess capacity, the American health care system in effect denied uninsured women who could not afford these high prices access to mammography *because there were too many mammograph machines!* Many economists may sincerely believe that it would be efficient to deny mammograms to uninsured, low-income women unwilling to cover with their own resources the *marginal* cost of those mammograms. Judging by his previously cited editorial, Milton Friedman evidently would. But no economist would define as efficient a market in which price-rationing occurs routinely at prices in excess of marginal costs.

The deviation of prices from marginal costs aside, however, one might agree that, in the purely technical sense of the term "efficiency" that many economists seem to favor, the American health care system probably did become somewhat more "economically efficient" during the 1980s, because in that decade the system probably did redistribute access to health care away from families who "valued" health care less (mainly the millions of uninsured Americans who were not able to pay for health care at its ever rising price) to those who "valued" health care more (well-insured or well-to-do Americans who were able to pay for health care even at its higher price). One might style such a redistribution a "potential Pareto improvement" (Stockman, 1996) and, therefore, an "increase in economic efficiency (Stockman, 1996) and, therefore, a net "social gain" (Landsburg, 1995) or "enhancement of economic welfare," as those terms tend to be defined in the textbooks that now inform undergraduates in economics. (In this connection, see the Appendix to this paper).

Suppose one grants all that. Even then one is left to wonder on what authority the author of that passage felt entitled to declare an arguably more "efficient" allocation of health care resources, *ipso facto* a "*better* allocation," especially in view of the possibility that this allocation became less equitable during the 1980s? Indeed, that greater inequity may not have been coincidental. In a classic trade-off between equity and efficiency (as economists define it), a less equal distribution of access to healthcare may well have been the price that had to be paid for the greater "efficiency" the author claims to have detected in American health care.

Now it may be countered that the implied trade-off between equity and efficiency (as economists define it) is actually specious, because a basic theorem in welfare economics suggests that considerations of equity in policy analysis can be separated from considerations of economic efficiency (Arrow, 1963). This is true, under certain conditions, in theory. The question is whether this basic theorem of welfare economics can survive in the practical world of policy analysis.

THE NARROW LIMITS OF
WELFARE ECONOMICS

Welfare economics is the branch of economics concerned with the "social desirability" of an "economic change." A well-defined "economic change" of this sort, for example, occurred in the Canadian Province of Quebec in 1970, when that province complemented a previously introduced hospital-insurance program with a program of universal health insurance coverage for all services provided by physicians in the home, office or hospital. Physician fees under this program were constrained by a fee schedule uniformly applied across the entire province. In many areas, certainly in the higher-income areas of the city of Montreal, that fee schedule is apt to have acted as a binding price ceiling.

Fortunately for the research community, a group of health-services researchers in Montreal had the foresight to survey large random samples of residents in Montreal about one year prior and one year after the implementation of the program in 1970 (Enterline *et al.*, 1973). It was found that the average number of physician visits per capita remained roughly constant, but that there was a marked redistribution of visits from higher-income to lower-income families, and that the average number of days wait for a routine appointment with a physician rose for all income groups, with the largest percentage increase in the higher-income groups.

What normative economic assessment might economists be able to offer about this dramatic "economic change"? By the definition of "efficiency" customarily offered in textbooks of economics, the change might be judged "inefficient," if for no other reason than that physician visits were diverted from higher-income families who had "valued" them more to lower-income families who evidently had "valued" them less in the previously unconstrained market for physician services. By that same line of reasoning, one would have judged the abolition of universal coverage and a return to the previous market environment an "increase in efficiency," as one might judge a partial return to the regime through the reintroduction of substantial cost sharing at point of service in Canada. Ideally, however, economists would like to be able to offer more. They would like to be able to rank these alternative regimes not only in terms of their relative "economic efficiency," as textbooks define that term, but also in terms of their "social desirability," as lay persons might understand that term. Is standard welfare economics as we know it and teach it up to that task?

Although every professional economist will at some point have been exposed to the subtle assumptions and tenets underlying conventional welfare economics, and although it may be deemed condescending to review them here, the casual use of the terms "efficiency" and "welfare gain" in the modern literature of economics suggests that something might be gained from a quick review of these pillars of welfare economics.

Pareto Efficiency

As already noted in the introduction to this essay, the most rigorous definition of "economic efficiency" is named after Vilfredo Pareto who first formally proposed it. According to that concept, an allocation of resources is said to be

Pareto efficient if it is impossible to make one person in society better off by reallocating these resources without making someone else worse off.

It is hard to disagree with that definition, as it borders on a tautology. As such, it tends to be generally useless in the world of practical affairs, as is illustrated in Figure 2. The solid curve in the graph depicts the maximum happiness that a two-person society, with its available resources, can bestow upon person A at a given

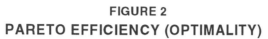

FIGURE 2
PARETO EFFICIENCY (OPTIMALITY)

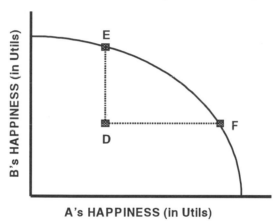

A's HAPPINESS (in Utils)

level of person B's happiness. It is society's happiness-trade-off-possibility frontier (not ever to be confused with the so-called "production possibility frontier"). Any point on the frontier is Pareto-efficient, which is also usually called "Pareto-optimal." Any point in the interior of the set bounded by the frontier evidently is Pareto inefficient.

All economists and, indeed, all lay persons ought to agree that any policy that would move the economy from the interior point D to the frontier between (and including) points E and F is a Pareto improvement, an increase in Pareto efficiency. We can say unambiguously that such an "economic change" is "socially desirable."

Alas, we cannot be so unequivocal about a policy that might move the economy from the Pareto-inefficient, interior, point D to Pareto-efficient points on the frontier, if those points lie outside the line segment EF. The Pareto criterion itself does not offer us any way to assess the "social desirability" of such a policy or, for that matter, of any move along the Pareto-efficient frontier, although public policy typically involves precisely just such moves. That is why Pareto's concept of "efficiency" or "optimality" is typically useless in the world of practical affairs. As William Baumol has observed on the Paretian construct:

> Pareto optimality analysis sidesteps the issue of income distribution....[Optimality rules resting on a Paretian foundation] remain either silent or prejudiced in favor of the *status quo* on the issue of income distribution and are, therefore, necessarily incomplete or unsatisfactory even on matters for which distribution is not the primary issue. Ultimately, the Paretian criterion can be considered the welfare economists' instrument *par excellence* for the circumvention of this issue. (Baumol, 1969)

It is illuminating to depict Pareto efficiency graphically, if only to expose the crucial difference between "Pareto optimality" and what is called "productive Pareto efficiency." The first concept deals with levels of human happiness; the second deals with rates of output of commodities. That crucial distinction sometimes gets lost in the heat of normative policy analysis.

Thus, in Figure 3 the coordinates represent not degrees of human happiness, as they do in Figure 2, but merely rates of output of two goods or services, X and Y. The solid frontier depicts the maximum output rate of Y the economy can grind out at any given output rate of X with the physical resources available to the economy. It is the production-possibility frontier to which every first-year student in economics is introduced in Chapter 1 of the text. Now, one may define as efficiently produced any combination of outputs X and Y situated on the production-possibility frontier, and any interior point as production-inefficient. But production-efficiency has only a tenuous relationship to the concept of overall Pareto efficiency (alias Pareto optimality), because a mere combination of two goods or services implies nothing precise about the distribution of human happiness it generates, nor can we know what happens to the degree of happiness enjoyed by individual members of society as the economy is moved from an inefficient point (such as output combination D in Figure 3) to an efficient output combination on the production possibility frontier. This is so even if the economy moves from, say, the interior point D to point E or to point F or to any point on the frontier between points E and F. That problem has vexed economists for over a hundred years. It has not been resolved, at least not to everyone's satisfaction.

To be sure, if the happiness of every member of society were a function solely of that individual's own rates of consumption of X and Y, or if there were only *positive* externalities in consumption (in the sense that individual A might derive satisfaction from seeing individual B consume more of either X or Y), then one could argue that the added output yielded by a move from point D to, say, point E in Figure 3 could always be distributed in a way that represents a genuine Pareto improvement. The simplest such algorithm would be to give the extra output of Y to just one person, without giving anyone else any less of either commodity X or Y. Indeed, there would be infinitely many different ways of distributing the added

FIGURE 3
EFFICIENCY IN PRODUCTION

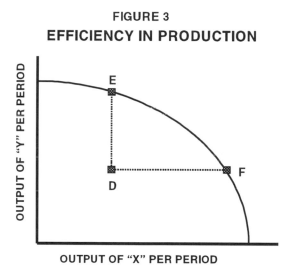

OUTPUT OF "X" PER PERIOD

output of Y among members of society without leaving anyone with any less of either commodity Y or X.

Things become much murkier, but also much more realistic, when we allow *negative* externalities in consumption -- when the happiness of one individual is affected not only by the rate of his or her own consumption of commodity X and Y, but also by the level of those rates *relative* to the rates of consumption enjoyed by other consumers in the peer group. The vernacular for that sort of sentiment is "social envy." Curiously, the role of envy in welfare economics is not much discussed in textbooks of economics. It is remarkable that economists, most of whom have had experience with raising children, tend to be so impervious to this basic human trait in their professional work. To illustrate, if one brings two well-behaved siblings each a chocolate bar on Day 1, both will be happy. If one brings each of them two chocolate bars on Day 2, both are likely to be even happier. But if, on Day 3, one brings one of them three chocolate bars and the other one four, two otherwise adorable siblings are bound to ruin the day.

Envy is common among human beings. Normally, the trait has its onset in early childhood and lingers until about, say, age 100, even among economists. It is the reason, for example, why people pay enormous prices for numbered lithographs, or for designer fashion, or for automobiles with limited editions, or why people in general work themselves to exhaustion merely to keep up with the Joneses. Envy probably is among the most basic of all human traits. It is the very engine of economic growth. Normative economic analysis that abstracts from this common human trait, because it is deemed unsavory, might be useful on other planets. It misses the core of the human experience on planet Earth.

Certainly in the context of health care, economists cannot abstract from either *positive* or *negative* externalities in consumption, because both forms of externality typify common attitudes towards health care. Most ordinary citizens in any country profess to derive positive utility from knowing that suffering fellow human beings receive appropriate health care, even if that care must be collectively financed. At the same time, social envy drives peoples' attitudes toward their health care system as well. Citizens in many countries tend to take umbrage at the thought that well-to-do citizens can obtain life-saving or health-restoring care not available to the average citizen, even if the well-to-do were made to purchase that care with their own money. Thus, the relative use of health care by the typical individual is likely to enter that person's happiness (utility) function in quite complex ways. Let R be the ratio of the use of health care by other, similarly sick or similarly healthy persons to the individual's own use of health care. If R is very low, increases in that ratio probably tend to increase the better-off individual's happiness, at least up to a point beyond which further increases in the ratio are likely to decrease the individual's happiness once again. There is no reason to suppose, of course, that the turning point occurs when the ratio is 1 -- when perfect equality is attained. Quite possibly, it occurs when R is below unity.

Given the presumably widespread existence of both *positive* and *negative* externalities in the use of health care, it would be reckless to interpret a move from the interior point D in Figure 3 to, say, point E as *ipso facto* an increase in general economic well being, even though we may call it an enhancement in productive efficiency. Suppose, for example, that such a move represented a rearrangement of the economy such that it would make available to severely ill patients a highly effective but also very expensive, high-tech procedure (perhaps a new drug, or new imaging machine, or the artificial heart), but that was accessible only to well-to-do families who can pay for it with their own resources. Economists can label this rearrangement as an increase in "production efficiency." Given current attitudes towards health care in most modern nations, however, could an economist in good conscience label that change also as a genuine "Pareto improvement," that is, as a genuine increase in social economic well being? Might it not be that, as a result of this increase in productive efficiency, and the associated distribution of that productivity gain solely to high-income families, middle- and lower-income Americans might feel disillusioned with their health care system and feel significantly worse off with the (presumably unchanged) health care resources they have hitherto enjoyed? How would one know, then, whether an increase in production efficiency also represented an increase in "social welfare?" As Pauly (1995) has remarked on this point:

> If higher than average health benefits for those willing to pay for them with their own money are regarded as unfair -- unless all are able and willing to pay for similar benefits -- then the welfare economics-based measure [of benefit-cost analysis] will not be acceptable. The United States generally seems to accept a minimum benefits view of equity, but other countries are alleged to take a view that spending one's own resources on more medical care for oneself or one's family is socially undesirable.

Pauly is correct in asserting that the current working majority of American *policy makers* accept the "minimum benefits view of equity," by which he appears to mean that citizens feel an entitlement to a basic minimum package of health benefits, but do not view as unfair a health care system that permits the well-to-do to procure for themselves, with their own money, superior health benefits. How well ingrained that attitude is among the American public is an open question. Close to two thirds of Americans disagreed with the statement "People,who pay more should get better care" in a 1991 national survey on attitudes towards health care (Taylor and Reinhardt, 1991), 44% of them strongly. On the other hand, about one third did agree with the statement, 20% of them strongly. By contrast, a much smaller percentage of respondents in Great Britain, France, Canada and (then) West Germany agreed with the statement. Fewer than 10% agreed with it strongly in those countries. In the meantime, attitudes may have shifted on this question in all countries.

In a more recent cross national survey of this sort, a higher percentage of American respondents felt that they were "treated unfairly" by their own health care system than did citizens in other countries, and a much larger proportion of Americans declared themselves dissatisfied with their health care system than did citizens in other countries with theirs (Blendon *et al.*, 1995), in spite of the relatively much higher per-capita spending on health care in the United States and the easy access to high-tech medicine (for those who can afford it). Although these are only opinion surveys and not preferences actually revealed in market transactions, these data nevertheless ought to give economists pause. They point to the role that negative externalities in consumption appear to play in health care. The general public even in the United States tends to view the health care system as something more than an industry that produces a variety of private consumer goods. They expect their health care system also to produce an intangible public good -- part of the cement that binds a group of people sharing a geography into a nation. Normative health economics ought not to abstract from that public good.

The Kaldorian Criterion (alias "Potential Pareto Improvements" [Stockman, 1996])

Frustrated by the narrow limitations inherent in the formal concept of Pareto efficiency, our profession has searched long and hard for alternative criteria by which one might judge the "social desirability" of policies that trigger economic change. Eager to get on in the world of practical affairs, the profession appears to have permanently settled on a rather dubious criterion originally proposed by Nicholas Kaldor (1939) and sold to policy makers ever since, *to wit*:

> The economic change wrought by a particular policy represents a "social gain" if those who gain from the reallocation value that gain sufficiently so that they could, in principle, bribe the losers into accepting that change, even if that bribe actually is not paid.

Translated into the realm of standard benefit-cost analysis, for which the Kaldorian criterion has become the gold standard of analytic platforms, the criterion might be expressed as follows:

> If those who stand to gain from a proposed change in the economy would maximally be willing to pay \$B to see that change made, *whoever these people may be, and given their tastes and their particular position in society's income distribution*, and if those who stand to lose from the change would maximally pay \$C to prevent that change, *whoever they may be, and given their tastes and particular position in the nation's income distribution*, then the proposed

change represents a "social gain" or "increase in social economic welfare" if the amount $B exceeds the amount $C.

On its face, this is quite a mouthful!

Some textbook writers refer to the Kaldorian criterion as a "potential Pareto improvement" and define the latter as *ipso facto* an "increase in economic efficiency" (Stockman, 1996). That appears to have become the common usage in our profession. For example, as Steven Landsburg instructs students in his introductory textbook *Price Theory and Applications* (Landsburg, 1995):

> According to the **efficiency criterion**, any change in policy that makes George $2 richer and Martha only $1 poorer *is a good thing*. Any change in policy that makes George $1 richer and Martha $2 poorer *is a bad thing*. More generally, the efficiency criterion pronounces that between two policies, we should always prefer the one that yields the higher *social gain*. The preferred policy is said to be more efficient than its rival (Emphasis added; bold print in the original).

It is useful to write out the Kaldorian criterion in full, if only to be reminded of the tenuity of its ethical foundation. One may call it, tongue-in-cheek, the "punch-in-the-nose" criterion, because it permits one literally to prove that, depending upon what compensation one might sincerely offer *ex ante* to someone whom one would like to punch in the nose (but who would not actually have to be compensated, *ex post*, for receiving that punch in the nose), throwing that punch might be judged "welfare enhancing" in a purely Kaldorian sense, as might be pumping a bullet into someone's leg in a similarly contrived experiment or, the more realistic environmental analogue, as might be shooting carcinogenic particles into someone's lungs. In the latter case, economists might convince themselves and those who might purchase their analyses that, if the recipients of the carcinogenic pollution collectively would be *willing to pay* only, say, $1 million to stop the pollution, but it would cost $1.1 million to achieve that goal, then that environmental protection would not be "socially desirable." That conviction, however, does not avoid the ethical implications of such a decision, and it would not make a do-nothing policy in this instance "socially desirable." The matter would remain a purely political problem. Economists might apprise politicians of the relevant cost data, but they cannot solve the problem for politicians with appeal to some "scientific" benefit-cost criterion.

In their professional writings, economists tend to apply the Kaldorian criterion with abandon and with nary a thought or apology for its shaky ethical foundation. How unwise that practice is depends, of course, on the particular context to which the criterion is applied. Within the context of health care, I would judge it reckless.

It has not always been so. Earlier economists were far more circumspect in the use of the criterion, and they agonized over its validity. In one of the more trenchant reviews of welfare economics in general, for example, William J. Baumol explored our profession's quest for an objective social-welfare criterion. His conclusion warrants extensive citation:

> In my view, the Kaldor test operates on the basis of an implicit and unacceptable value judgement. By using a criterion involving potential money compensation, [it] sets up a concealed interpersonal comparison of utility on a money basis. If [individual] Y's gain is worth $200 to him whereas [individual] X evaluates his loss at $70, we are not entitled to jump to the conclusion that there is a net [social] gain in [the associated change in the economy]. If X is a poor man or a miser, $70 may mean a great deal to him, whereas if Y is a rich man or profligate, $200 may represent a trifle hardly worth his notice. ... It is no answer to this criterion that these criteria are just designed to measure whether production, and hence potential welfare, are increased by the policy change -- that these criteria disentangle the evaluation of a production change from that of the distribution change by which it is accompanied (Baumol, 1977).

Years earlier, in the ominously titled chapter "'The Wreck of Welfare Economics" in his *Welfare Economics and the Theory of the State*, Baumol had concluded his long search for a value-neutral welfare criterion:

> The problem in sum is this: so long as we recognize the existence of particular types of interdependence in the results of activities of our economic units [such as positive or negative externalities in consumption], our analysis is likely to break down completely. We know, moreover, that the simplifying premise that these types of interdependence are negligible or non-existent is misleading. Such an assumption is not neutral; rather it leads inexorably to the acceptance of *laissez-faire* (Baumol, 1969).

To my knowledge, no one in the meantime has invalidated Baumol's assessment, although many economists have tried and others simply disregard it.

One defense of the Kaldorian welfare criterion is that, while its application in particular instances may redistribute economic privilege in undesired ways, its consistent and repeated application to public policy across the economy is bound to have a portfolio effect under which individual instances of injustice cancel one another out so that, in the end, all boats can be made to rise, so to speak, through policies driven by welfare-economic analysis. The most elegant version of this defense is the *expected-utility* or *constitutional* standard originally proposed by Buchanan and Tullock (1962). As Pauly has described the constitutional standard:

> This standard asks: given a wide variety of decisions to be made and a wide variety of individual circumstances for any member of a given group, what method would maximize the average or

expected well being of a person in that group? In effect, this standard assumes/argues that each person has the group-average probability of being in each of the circumstances that might occur. ... The constitutional perspective ... makes the [Kaldorian] potential compensation test more attractive. If society follows the benefit-cost rule [that test implies], on average every person can expect to be better off; the chance that the person will win will more than offset, in expectational terms, the chance that the person will lose (Pauly, 1995).

There clearly is something to that argument, although, as Pauly mentions, the same analytic construct was employed by Rawls (1971) to justify policies for a more egalitarian distribution of income. The construct has not carried conviction in that realm any more than it can in health policy. The standard raises two questions.

First, is it in fact the case that each member of society has the group-average probability of being in each circumstance that might occur, or does consistent application of the Kaldorian benefit-cost rule consistently favor one socioeconomic class over the other, or healthy people over chronically sick people? Second, even if the group-average probability of being in each circumstance were the same for all members of society, over what span of economic activity should policy makers and the affected individuals average (in their minds) the wins and losses from the "variety of decisions" that are to be adjudicated by the Kaldorian benefit-cost rule. Is it good enough when the disadvantages that the rule may visit on an individual in one economic sector (*e.g.*, health care) are offset, in "expectational terms," through advantages the rule bestows on the same individuals in another sector (*e.g.*, transportation or entertainment)? Or should the assumed portfolio effect take place within sectors (*e.g.*, within health care proper)? For example, if an application of the Kaldorian benefit-cost rule shifts more of the financial burden of ill health onto the shoulders of the chronically ill, is it good enough to tell the chronically ill that, on average, in expectational terms, a consistent application of a rule that hurts them in health care will bestow offsetting special benefits on them in other sectors? Would a consistent application of the Kaldorian benefit-cost rule in health policy not be likely to drive the entire health care system inexorably towards systematic income-based rationing and visit the economic cost of ill health more heavily on the sick than is the case even now in the United States? If that be the goal, or if it be judged an acceptable outcome, then economists using that line of defense had better articulate their acceptance of that outcome *in health care* very explicitly, at the outset, in any normative analysis they base on the Kaldorian criterion, so that users of the analysis can make their own moral judgement on the matter.

The Separation of "Equity" from "Efficiency" in Policy Analysis

Various arguments have been used to defend the proposition that considerations of "efficiency" in economic welfare analysis can be treated separately from considerations of "equity." For economic analysis in general, one might look to Francis Bator's previously cited article on "The Simple Economics of Welfare Maximization" (1958a), although one would be wise always to read also his important sequel entitled "The Anatomy of Market Failure" (Bator, 1958b). Within normative *health economics* proper, the separation of "efficiency" from "equity" appears to have its roots in Kenneth Arrow's classic "Uncertainty and the Welfare Economics of Medical Care," published in 1963 (Arrow, 1963). In that paper Arrow had written:

> I will hold that virtually all the special features of [the medical care] industry, in fact, stem from the prevalence of uncertainty. ... It is contended here that the special structural characteristics of the medical care market are largely attempts to overcome the lack of optimality due to nonmarketability of the bearing of suitable risks and the imperfect marketability of information (Arrow, 1963, pp.16-17).

Arrow did remark in passing upon externalities in the production of health caused by communicable diseases and upon a "more general interdependence, the concern of individuals for the health of others" which create "a theoretical case for collective action if each participant derives satisfaction from the contribution of all" (Arrow, 1963, p. 954). He did not specifically address the case of negative externality in consumption, namely, the role that social envy may play within a modern health care system, and the welfare loss envy may trigger when a health care system distributes health care resources manifestly unequally among individuals with the same illness. Perhaps he felt, along with countless disciples thereafter, that none of these problems seriously impaired the Second Theorem of Optimality, described by him as follows:

> If there are no increasing returns to production, and if certain other minor conditions are satisfied, then every [Pareto] optimal state is a competitive equilibrium corresponding to some initial distribution of purchasing power. Operationally, the significance of this proposition is that if the conditions of the two optimality theorems are satisfied, and if the allocation mechanism in the real world satisfies the conditions of a competitive model, then social policy can confine itself to steps taken to alter the distribution of purchasing power. For any given distribution of purchasing power, the market will, under the assumptions made, achieve a competitive equilibrium which is necessarily optimal; and any optimal state is a competitive equilibrium

corresponding to some distribution of purchasing power, so that any desired optimal state can be achieved.

The redistribution of purchasing power among individuals most simply takes the form of money: taxes and subsidies. The implications of such a transfer for individual satisfactions are, in general, not known in advance. But we can assume that society can ex post judge the distribution of satisfactions and, if deemed unsatisfactory, take steps to correct subsequent transfers. Thus, by successive approximations, a most preferred social state can be achieved, with resource allocation being handled by the market and public policy confined to the redistribution of money income (Arrow, 1963, p.943).

This important passage, written by one of the economic profession's most distinguished members, appears to have been taken by later generations of health economists as the much sought professional license to separate equity from efficiency in the formulation of health policy. If one accepts that dichotomy as legitimate, then one can in good conscience advocate reliance on "the market" as the best means to attain economic efficiency in the allocation of health-care resources, leaving it to the political process to recalibrate the distribution of income so as to render the market's verdicts ethically acceptable.

In fact, however, Arrow did not offer nearly so soothing an ointment for the problem of distributive justice in health-policy analysis. Even in the main text of his paper, he had observed that

If, on the contrary, the actual market differs significantly from the competitive model, or if the assumptions of the two optimality theorems are not fulfilled, the separation of allocative and distributional procedures becomes, in most cases, impossible (p. 943).

In my view, it would be stretching things to read into Arrow's article the conclusion that the health care market does not stray significantly from the competitive model. Even more destructive to the assumed separation of equity and efficiency, however, is the footnote Arrow felt compelled to append to this passage, *to wit*:

The separation between allocation and distribution even under the above assumptions [*i.e.*, even if the conditions of the two optimality theorems are met] has glossed over problems in the execution of any desired redistributive policy; in practice, it is virtually impossible to find a set of taxes and subsidies that will not have an adverse effect on the achievement of an optimal state (Arrow, 1963, p. 943, fn 2).

The problem identified in this footnote and the damage it does to the Second Theorem of Optimality ought not to be underestimated. The "adverse effects" whereof Arrow wrote became a major issue during the American health-reform debate in 1993-94, when the supply-side theorists among American economists warned policy makers about the adverse economic incentives inherent in a program that necessarily taxes families in the upper half or so of the nation's income distribution to subsidize the health insurance for the families in the lower third. Drawing on simulations at the National Bureau of Economic Research which he directs, Martin Feldstein (1994) warned policy makers and the public in an editorial entitled "Income-Based Subsidies Won't Work" that, in the end, it would cost $18,000 to insure a currently uninsured family of three (whose policy itself might cost less than a quarter as much).

There is an extraordinary analytic elegance to the Second Theorem of Optimality. Alas, when the rubber hits the road in the arena of truly applied policy analysis and politics, the fabled Theorem quickly loses its relevance. If one group of economists specializes in normative rules that advocate a free market for health care, assuming that the political process will put in place an ethically defensible distribution of purchasing power, and another group of economists specializes in alarming the political process over the loss of efficiency inherent in such redistributions, then jointly the profession merely demonstrates that the conceptual separation of equity and efficiency implied by the Second Theorem of Optimality is just that, a theorem.

Now it may be argued that, in a democracy, the *status quo* distribution of income *is* the ethically most defensible distribution, for otherwise the democracy would not tolerate that distribution.[10] On that assumption, it may be argued, one need not worry about the separation of equity and efficiency, because the willingness and ability to pay by different members of society interacting in a free market can legitimately be taken as the relevant measure of "social value" in normative economic analysis. This approach would also take care of Baumol's earlier critique that economists using the Kaldorian criterion duck the basic problem of interpersonal utility comparison by their tacit assumption that "the *status quo* distribution [of ability to pay] is a measure of the relative strength of feeling of two individuals" (Baumol, 1977). The argument would be that in a democracy willingness and *ability* to pay *is* the socially relevant measure of strength of feeling.

This argument cannot be dismissed out of hand; but one may point to its

---

[10] See Reinhardt, 1996c, pp. 63-99, especially p. 70.

weakness. For one, a lively debate can be had over the question whether modern democracies do, indeed, function so as to beget the distribution of income even a mere majority of the citizenry would accept as ethically defensible. One may test this hypothesis by asking the following question: Would the American public, or citizens elsewhere, be content to accept the currently prevailing distribution of general purchasing power as an ethically adequate platform for the auctioning off of, say, transplantable organs to the highest bidders?

As Arrow observed on this point: "The taste for improving the health of others appears to be stronger than for improving other aspects of their welfare" (Arrow, 1963). In other words there probably is not one initial distribution of general purchasing power that can satisfy the distributional ethic society wishes to impose on particular commodities within the set of all goods and services. It can explain the reliance worldwide on redistribution of specific benefits in kind.

The Alleged Inefficiency of Benefits in Kind

Arrow's oblique reference to the distribution of benefits in kind would be obvious to a general public that routinely countenances huge public expenditures on health care for the poor, but would be likely to reject quite vehemently a proposal to distribute a corresponding amount of cash instead. Many economists pretend to be deeply puzzled by that attitude. In one of the more triumphant applications of the indifference-curve apparatus that so often makes common sense needlessly difficult for undergraduates, every year thousands of economics professors persuade hundreds of thousands of American undergraduates that distributing benefits in kind to the poor is less "efficient" than simply transferring to them cash in an amount equal to the cost of the benefits in kind. In the words of Victor Fuchs:

> While elementary justice seems to require greater equality in the distribution of medical care, the question is complicated by the fact that the poor suffer deprivation in many directions. Economic theory suggests it might be better to redistribute income and allow the poor to decide which additional goods and services they wish to buy (Fuchs, 1983).

Ever on to the real world, however, Fuchs is quick to add:

> As a practical matter, however, it may be easier to achieve greater equality through a redistribution of services (such as medical care) than through a redistribution of money income (Fuchs, 1983)

By "practicality" Fuchs may have in mind merely the political process that governs the redistribution of income in a democracy. The distribution of benefits in kind inevitably feeds horses to feed the birds, so to speak. Out of pure self-interest, and under almost any form of government, the horses (the producers of benefits in kind) can be counted on to become strong political allies of the targets of society's compassion. In the process, they can stretch that compassion far beyond the level that could be justified, if one knew the true valuation donors and recipients jointly attach to some of the benefits taxpayers will be forced to finance. One objective of benefit-cost analysis is, of course, precisely to uncover these value deficits and to curb that venality.

But there may be more to the "practicality" of benefits in kind than the feeding of hungry horses. Taxpayers themselves may not be impressed by the economist's dictum. That dictum is driven by the assumption that taxpayers maximize their utility when the recipients of tax-financed transfers are allowed to maximize their own happiness, per dollar of taxes borne by the taxpayers. As Pauly puts it in passing, in his exploration of the willingness-to-pay approach for tax-financed benefit-in-kind programs:

> If we want to provide benefit to low-income people, a more efficient approach would be to use the money that would have been spent on the program to make a direct money transfer to them, since the money will benefit low-income people more than the program would. In this case, providing the program, as opposed to making a direct money transfer, is worse for both lower-income people and the rest of the community. If the community decides not to make the money income transfer, it must not have attached high value either to low-income persons' health or to their overall welfare (Pauly, 1995).

Is there actually persuasive empirical evidence that the typical taxpayer's utility function conforms to the economist's imagination? Perhaps a more realistic assumption would be that taxpaying voters typically exhibit a more parental form of altruism towards their poor fellow citizens. Taxpayers would like poor families to use a select few basic commodities (for example, health care and education) in adequate amounts, but specifically *not* use tax-financed subsidies to purchase whatever goods and services the poor fancy. The preference among voters for bestowing on the poor benefits in kind rather than cash transfers -- apparently so puzzling to economists who write textbooks -- may well rest in good part on that characteristic of the donors' utility function.

If that hypothesis is valid, then it would seem hopeless that we shall ever find a single, politically acceptable distribution of generalized purchasing power that will distribute through the free market all commodities among members of society in a fashion that the general public will accept as just. Furthermore, if that is so then economists would actually be misusing the word "efficiency" in this context. They would be misusing it, because they would be recommending the maximization of the wrong maximand.

"EFFICIENCY" AND HEALTH-SYSTEMS COMPARISONS

If one sought to travel by car from New York City to Seattle, Washington in the least amount of time, the American Automobile Association (AAA) surely could identify the route that meets these requirements. It would be the most *efficient* route, relative to these particular requirements. The most efficient route might not be quite the same, if one sought to minimize not only the time cost, but also the cost of fuel, for one might then have to trade off the monetary value of travel time against the monetary cost of fuel. The most efficient route might yet be different, if one also wanted to take in some beautiful sights along the route, and so on.

In any event, given a precise set of specifications, one could identify the most efficient route to Seattle and many less efficient ones. One could do the same with San Diego, California as the destination. And if San Diego were the destination, the most efficient route to Seattle would almost surely not be as desirable as a less efficient route to San Diego. In fact, of only two alternative routes -- the efficient route to Seattle (if that be the desired destination) and an inefficient one to San Diego (if that be the desired destination) -- the inefficient route to San Diego would be the relatively most efficient one, if to San Diego one wanted to go.

This is unavoidably so in road travel. It has been the central thrust of the preceding sections that it is so also in the practical affairs of health policy, the purely theoretical Second Optimality Theorem of welfare economics notwithstanding. The word "efficiency" in health economics has meaning only against a well-defined set of social goals. In abstraction from such goals, the term usually is meaningless. A policy that may be considered efficient in one country, for example, may be woefully inefficient in another country, because it deviates from a well articulated social goal, such as strict observance of the *Principle of Solidarity*. The term "economic efficiency" is just that brittle.

This conclusion is not meant to be nihilistic. There is plenty of useful work for health economists to do, even without sloppy use of the word "efficiency." There is the whole field of *positive* economic analysis, scrupulously applied. There is also room for *normative* economic analysis, if it is performed with the proper humility and scrupulous identification of the ethical foundation for that analysis. It also means that in formulating their normative recommendations, economists ought not to abstract from the distributional impact of their recommendations. That impact should be forthrightly identified.

But, in this author's view, there is no basis for the assertion that a market allocation of health care resources (say, on the emerging American model) is more efficient than an alternative model (say, the Canadian approach or that adopted in the United Kingdom) or, for that matter, *vice versa*. In fact, it is not even possible to judge the relative efficiency of the American health care system now and a decade ago, because the benefits and costs of the system are being redistributed in ways that are poorly understand and, moreover, there is no discernible consensus as yet among the American people about what ethical principles the allocation of health-care resources in the United States ought to obey.

Americans, in particular, ought to be more mindful than they sometimes are, as they strut about the globe seeking to export American ideas on how to run a health care system. An illuminating case in point is a recent report on the productivity of health care systems by McKinsey & Company (Dorsey, 1996). With the assistance of a distinguished panel of clinicians and economists, the authors undertook an in-depth cross-national comparison of the treatment of four diseases in the United States, the United Kingdom and Germany during the late 1980s. It was found that

> The US's higher *per capita* spending [on health care] was *not* due to low productivity; in fact it was more productive than Germany in all cases and than the UK in the treatment of lung cancer and gallstones. ... Germany was less productive because it used less outpatient care and kept patients in the hospital longer (Dorsey, 1996. p.125).

Evidently the study was an ambitious endeavor whose findings ought to raise interesting questions among clinicians who probably do have much to teach one another about the most cost-effective way of responding to particular illnesses. One ought not to be surprised if, in this international commerce of ideas at the purely clinical level, the United States turned out to be a net exporter. The value of the McKinsey study is the catalytic role it may play in this commerce of ideas.

But the overall tone of the McKinsey report, particularly its remarks on *systems* productivity, takes much too broad a sweep and, therefore, comes across as an arrogant rush to judgement. The authors offer the summary judgement that

> the US and the UK appear to be moving in the direction of productive change in their health care systems, with each adopting some of the other's beneficial characteristics. But given the questionable impact of German reforms to date, it is likely that the productivity gap between

Germany and the US -- and possibly between Germany and the UK -- is widening (Dorsey, 1996, p. 131).

One might forgive Germans and anyone familiar with cross-national comparisons of health care systems for being puzzled by this assessment. In fact, it may be asked why any German policy maker, faced with the entire palette of data presented in the McKinsey study, would want to rush into copying American health-systems reforms.

As the McKinsey report points out, in 1990 average health-spending per capita was in Germany was $1,473. In the United States, it was $2,439, roughly $1,000 higher. Yet in 1990 only about 12.6% of the American population was aged 65 while 14.9% of Germans were over the age of 65 (Organization for Economic Cooperation and Development, 1996). As the McKinsey report mentions, there are no overall differences in life expectancy between the two countries.

One must ask at what price Americans purchase their allegedly higher clinical productivity. Extrapolating from the four case studies to the whole health care system, the McKinsey team estimates that Americans in 1990 spent $390 less *per capita* on medical inputs than did Germans. On the other hand, according to the study, Americans spent $360 more *per capita* on administrative overhead, which wipes out almost the entire cost advantage on the clinical side. On top of the steep extra charge for administrative overhead, however, Americans reportedly also spent yet another $259 more per capita on items lumped by the McKinsey team together under the heading "Other." Finally, according to the McKinsey study, American patients paid the providers of care an extra $737 more *per capita* in the form purely of higher prices than did Germans.

For starters, in formulating their summary judgement on entire health care system_s_, the McKinsey team ought to have thought more about hard-nosed economics -- about a possible tradeoff between clinical productivity and administrative expense. After all, the enhanced price-competition among rival health insurance plans in the United States, and the vigilant reductions in the use of medical inputs through managed-care techniques do not come free of charge. They tend to absorb anywhere between 20 to 30% of the premiums collected by the competing, care managing private health insurance plans. There is no reason to expect that a diversion of real resources from direct patient care to administrative overhead would enhance patient satisfaction in Germany, yet high patient satisfaction surely must be one of the major goals of a health care system. Here it may be noted that, while already as many as 58% of German respondents in the previously cited survey felt that their "health care system involves too much bureaucracy," 83% of the American respondents felt that way (Blendon, 1995). Furthermore, while 15% of American respondents declared that they had to wait more than a week to see a doctor, only 6% of Germans responded likewise (Blendon, 1995).

American policy analysts are obsessed with the average length of hospital stay as a yardstick for the health care system's economic performance, and so is the McKinsey team. But one ought not to use that yardstick without reference to price. The average cost of a hospital day in Germany in 1990 was about DM 400 (about $270) (Deutsche Krankenhausgesellschaft, 1996). That figure includes the cost of all inpatient physician services, because these services are rendered by physicians in the hospitals' employ. The comparable American figure was a multiple of this average, probably in the neighborhood of $1,000. German hospital costs per day are so low partly because the average length of stay in German hospitals is about twice the American figure (Deutsche Krankenhausgesellschaft, 1996). But that cost is low also because administrative costs in German hospitals are lower than they are in American hospitals. According to the law of demand, when things are relatively cheaper, people buy relatively more of them, which may partly explain the higher average length of stay in German hospitals. Furthermore, one may debate whether, at the margin, all forms of outpatient care really are a more cost-effective substitute for inpatient care. It is not at all clear, for example, that the American enthusiasm for home infusion and intensive convalescent care at sites other than the hospital has reduced real-resource costs, at the margin (Reinhardt, 1996a).

The preceding critique focused only on the most tangible economics: costs. There remains the issue of the social goals of a health care system. Data on consumer satisfaction, such as they are, ought to be of more than passing interest to economists who treat "utility" as their ultimate output measure and to systems analysts who seek to improve the "efficiency" of health care systems. As the previously cited cross-national opinion surveys suggest, for all the criticism Germans may have about their own health care system, they nevertheless appear to be noticeably more satisfied with their system than Americans declare themselves to be with theirs (Blendon, 1995). For one, in Germany there are not public outcries over the drive-through deliveries and mastectomies and other manifestations of the "productivity" the McKinsey report extols. Rightly or wrongly, these manifestations do exercise the American public and lead even conservative politicians to write protective, clinical practice guidelines in legislation. Furthermore, unlike the United States, which at any time leaves some 17% of its population without any health insurance whatsoever, Germany has simple, comprehensive and universal health insurance coverage. A family's bankruptcy over medical bills is not uncommon in the United States. It would be the exception in Germany.

In extolling American health reform measures as a role model for Germany, the McKinsey team offers not a word about the impact these reforms have had on the social contract between rich and poor and between healthy and sick Americans. As Fuchs (1997) has pointed out, greater price-competition among private insurance carriers has had the effect of segmenting the private insurance market more and more by risk class, thereby shifting more of the financial burden of ill health from the shoulders of the healthy to the shoulders of the sick. Furthermore, it is generally thought that, in the near future, the financial pressures that these reforms might put on the providers of health care will make life much more difficult -- and literally more painful -- for the uninsured in their search for charity care.

These aspects of social equity may not matter as much to American policy makers as they do to German policy makers. They evidently did not loom at all on the radar screen of the McKinsey team, for they are not even mentioned in the team's paper. But these aspects of a health care system do give meaning to the terms "productivity" and "efficiency." Given their distinct social ethic -- that is, given the overall social goals Germans seek to achieve with their health care system -- there is no reason at all why they would regard the American notion of "efficiency" in health care as relevant to Germany. In particular, there is no reason why Germans ought to look upon the American health care system as more "productive" than theirs, anymore than someone who wants to travel to San Diego would consider the fastest route to Seattle an "efficient" way to San Diego.

CONCLUDING OBSERVATION

Finally, we return to the concept of "value," which is often mouthed in the current health reforms worldwide, but which has remained troublesome at the level of analysis. As nations everywhere seek to limit the fraction of GDP that is ceded to the providers of health care, it is inevitable that someone must put relative values on the wares being offered by these providers, to determine what is worth buying and what is not. That valuation, in turn, will depend on the outcomes achieved with the use of these goods and services, which ultimately requires someone to put relative values on alternative outcomes as well. One of the more fascinating and potentially fruitful lines of research among health-services researchers -- health economists prominent among them -- is the identification of the relevant relative values.

In that endeavor, it seems a sensible idea to base these relative values on the relevant persons' *willingness to pay* for the underlying health-care goods and services or, alternatively, for different health outcomes. Unfortunately, that approach will not be able to escape from the same conceptual and methodological issues raised throughout this essay.

First, in the face of income inequality, whose willingness to pay should be reflected in the valuation of health care goods and services and outcome? Should that valuation be immunized from contamination by the recipients' ability to pay? Practically, this could be achieved by basing all valuations on willingness to pay among middle-income groups.

Next, how should the added values inherent in the externalities of consumption in health care (*e.g.*, altruism) be incorporated in the valuation of particular health services or outcomes? This is less a conceptual than a practical problem. To illustrate, whose willingness-to-pay should be reflected in putting a value on, say, the use of an effective pharmaceutical product for a low-income person afflicted with AIDS? Practically, how should the willingness to pay of those who actually do pay the premium, or taxpayers, be factored into the valuation?

Third, in the absence of a normal market for health care, how is one to elicit from the relevant persons *credible* information on their willingness to pay for particular health-care goods and services or outcomes -- information that can be validated?

Health economists and health-services researchers in general will undoubtedly find answers of sorts to these conceptual and practical problems, for the simple reason that they must find answers. More than likely, these answers ultimately will lead to a set of *Generally Accepted Valuation Rules* agreed upon by some standard-setting body, just as there is a set of *Generally Accepted Accounting Principles* (the *GAAP*). The *GAAP* help business accountants accomplish the measurements at the practical level that are easily critiqued at the conceptual level. Basically, they establish a tacit, intra-professional embargo on mutual criticism. These rules should and probably will lean as much as possible on what patients actually value in health care; but they will inevitably also incorporate a good many somewhat arbitrary and bureaucratic rules, as is the case in business accounting. It must be accepted as a fact of life that the practical valuation principles in health care accounting, as in regular business accounting, will always remain conceptually flawed.

In his previously cited, thought-provoking essay on valuing health care in money terms, Pauly suggests that "European countries who take the absolute view on equity, and decision makers who want to be paternalistic, will therefore not accept the willingness to pay approach" and "value health outcomes relative to each other and to other things people value in a way different from *the way people value them*" (Emphasis added) (Pauly, 1995, p. 123). It is not clear whether Pauly refers here to all willingness-to-pay approaches (including the experimental ones that actually are used in Europe) or merely to market-based willingness-to-pay measures.

Either way, his reference to "value" brings us back to the simple homework exercise on welfare economics in Section II. Here is the rub: precisely what do we mean by the phrase "the way people *value*" things? Much of Pauly's essay is concerned with that question. It was seen in the homework exercise that the wealthy Chens "valued" a third annual visit of their healthy baby with a physician much more highly than the poor Smith family "valued" a third visit of their sickly baby with a physician. That is how people "value" things in the market. Evidently, in proposing his ideal health-insurance policy for America, Nobel Laureate Milton Friedman found market values of this sort to be the proper foundation for health policy. Is it, then, to be the policy-relevant way "people value things"?

REFERENCES

American Academy of Actuaries (1995) *Medical Savings Accounts: Cost Implications and Design Issues*, Public Policy Monograph 1, May: p. ii.

Arrow, K.J. (1963) Uncertainty and the welfare economics of medical care. *American Economic Review* December: 942-73.

Bator, F.M. (1995a) The simple economics of welfare economics. *American Economic Review* (72): 351-79.

Bator, F.M. (1958b) The anatomy of market failure. *Quarterly Journal of Economics* 72: 351-379.

Baumol, W.J. (1969) *Welfare Economics and the Theory of the State*. Cambridge, MA: Harvard University Press.

Baumol, W.J. (1977)*Economic Theory and Operations Analysis*, Fourth Edition. Englewood Cliffs, N.J.: Prentice-Hall, Inc., p.561.

Blendon, R.J., Benson, J., Donelan, K., *et al.* (1995) Who has the best health care system? A second look. *Health Affairs* 14(4): 210-30.

Brown, M.L. *et al.* (1990) Is the supply of mammography machines outstripping demand? *Annals of Internal Medicine* 547: 547-52.

Browning, E.K. and Browning, J.M. (1986) *Microeconomic Theory and Applications*, Second Edition, Boston, MA: Little, Brown and Co., p. 148.

Buchanan, J. and Tullock, G. (1962) *Calculus of Consent*. Ann Arbor, MI: University of Michigan Press, p. 122.

Cohn, V. (1989) *News & Numbers*. Ames, Iowa: Iowa State University Press. p.25.

Council for Affordable Health Insurance (1993) *Medical Savings Account Putting People First in Health Care*, February.

Deutsche Krankenhausgesellschaft (1996)   *Zahlen, Daten, Fakten '96*. Duesseldorf, Germany: Deutsche Krankenhausgesellchaft, July, 1996: 61.

Dorsey, L., Ferrari, B.T., Gengos, A., *et al.* (1996) The productivity of health care systems. *The McKinsey Quarterly* 4: 120-131.

Enterline, P.E., Salter, V., McDonald, A.D., and McDonald, J.C. (1973)The distribution of medical services before and after "free" medicare care -- the Quebec experience. *New England Journal of Medicine* 289(22): 1174-1178.

Feldstein, M. (1994) Income-based subsidies won't work. *The Wall Street Journal* June 17: A14.

Fuchs, V.R. (1983) *Who Shall Live? Health, Economics and Social Choice*. New York: Basic Books, pp. 148-9.

Fuchs, V.R. (1996) Economics, values and health care reform. *American Economic Review* 86(1): 1-24.

Fuchs, V.R. (1997) Managed care and merger mania. *Journal of the American Medical Association* 277(11): 920-921.

Greenberg, W. (1988) Introduction. *Journal of Health Politics, Policy and Law* Summer: 223-224.

Kaldor, N. (1939) Welfare propositions of economists and interpersonal comparison of utility. *Economic Journal* September: 549-52.

Krueger, A.B. and Reinhardt, U.E. (1994) The economics of employer versus individual mandates. *Health Affairs* Spring(II): 34-53.

Landsburg, S.E. (1995) *Price Theory And Its Uses*, Third Edition Minneapolis/St. Paul, MN.: West Publishing Co., p. 258.

Moon, M., Nichols, L. W., and Wall, S. (1996) *Medical Savings Accounts: A Policy Analysis*, Washington, D.C. : The Urban Institute, # 06571-001, March, 1996; p. 23.

Organization for Economic Co-Operation and Development (1996) *Policy Implications of Ageing Populations* May 13: Table A-2.

Pallarito, K. Adding fizz to balance sheet. *Modern HealthCare* 27(10): 76.

Pareto, V. (1897) *Cours d'Economie Politique*. Lausanne, Switzerland: F. Rouge.

Pauly, M.V. (1994) *An Analysis of Medical Savings Accounts: Do Two Wrongs Make a Right?*, Washington, D.C.: American Enterprise Institute.

Pauly, M.V. (1995) Valuing health care benefits in money terms. In Frank A. Sloan, editor, *Valuing Health Care*. Cambridge, England: Cambridge University Press, p. 122.

Rawls, J. (1971) *A Theory of Justice*. Cambridge, MA: Belknap Press of Harvard University.

Reinhardt, U.E. (1996a) Spending more through cost control: our obsessive quest to gut the hospital. *Health Affairs* 15(2): 145-154.

Reinhardt, U.E. (1996b) A social contract for 21st century health care: three-tier health care with bounty hunting. *Health Economics* 5(6): 479-500.

Reinhardt, U.E. (1992) Reflections on the meaning of efficiency. *Yale Law & Policy Review* 10(2): 302-15.

Reinhardt, U.E. (1996c) Rationing health care: what it is, what it is not, and why we cannot avoid it. In Altman, S.A., and Reinhardt, U.E., editors, *Strategic Choices for a Changing Health Care System*, Chicago, IL.: Health Administration Press, pp. 63-99.

Stockman, A. (1996) *Introduction to Microeconomics*. New York: The Dryden Press.

Taylor, H. and Reinhardt, U.E. (1991) Does the system fit? *Health Management Quarterly* 13(3): 2-7.

Webster's New World Dictionary of the American Language, College Edition. (1966) New York: The World Publishing Company, p.1609.

APPENDIX

SUGGESTED ANSWERS TO THE HOMEWORK EXERCISE

a. Why, do you suppose, do the two families' demand curves for physician visits not coincide? Why do the Smiths seem to *value* visits less than do the Chens at visit rates up to X and why might they value visits more than do the Chens at visit rates above X? (Not a silly question; many seasoned adults seem to have trouble with this question).

> *SUGGESTED ANSWER: The relative position of the two "marginal-value" (demand) curves is driven by the difference in family income and the difference in the health status of the two babies. In the debate on health policy, many seasoned adults confuse differences in ability to pay and in health status with differences in "tastes." You should be forever on the lookout for this confusion and be ready to call seasoned adults on it.*

b. If these two families can procure physician visits in a freely competitive market, at a price of, say, $40 per visit, then the free-market allocation of physician visits to the two babies would be

>   ___5___ visits/year to healthy Baby Chen
>   ___3___ visits/year to sickly Baby Smith

c. Accept for the moment the normative proposition adopted by many practicing economists (evidently by Professor Friedman and his colleagues) and by the politicians they inspire that the "marginal-value" (demand) curves of individual consumers or households (which might alternatively be called their "willingness-to-pay" curves) also signal the marginal <u>social</u> value of commodities. [Not every economist and politician would subscribe to that proposition.] Also assume that the free-market price of $40 per visit reflects the social marginal cost of producing visits, including the opportunity cost of the physician's time. Then, would the free-market allocation of visits you have identified in Part (b) above be "economically efficient" as economists define that term? Explain.

> *SUGGESTED ANSWER: The allocation then would be judged economically efficient, because it would not be possible to reallocate visits in a way that would leave one of the two families happier and the other no less happy. Furthermore, in equilibrium, the marginal social value placed by each family on the last visit the family had "consumed" (the 5th for the Chens and the 3rd for the Smiths) was equal to the marginal social cost of that visit.*

d. Continue with the proposition and assumptions made in Part (c). Then the marginal social value of, say, the 3rd visit per year by a baby to the physician is

$_100___ if it is made by healthy Baby Chen
$_40____ if it is made by sickly Baby Smith

e. Suppose now that, for some reason, physician visits were not allocated through a free-market algorithm, but instead have been allocated to the two families by the government, under some administrative algorithm, and in a way that had allocated to the sickly Baby Smith 4 visits per year and to the healthy Baby Chen only 2 visits per year. Would such an allocation be Pareto efficient as your text defines that term?

> *SUGGESTED ANSWER: According to your text, a "situation is economically efficient -- or Pareto efficient -- if there is no **potentially Pareto-improving** change." The text defines a "potential Pareto improvement" as a change in the economy under which the gainers from the change **could** compensate (pay) the losers to accept that change, even if in fact that compensation is not made (p. 305). Because, in principle, the wealthy Chens (who value a third visit at $100) could bribe the poor Smiths (who value the fourth visit at only $25) to release one visit to the Chens, the original allocation would not be Pareto efficient.*

f. Would it be a **Pareto improvement** if, in the situation described in part (e), one visit were taken away from sickly Baby Smith and given instead to healthy Baby Chen? Explain, in a sentence or two.

> *SUGGESTED ANSWER: A Pareto improvement is a change in the economy under which at least one person actually gains and no one actually loses. In this case, the Smiths would lose a visit with the physician. Unless they were, in fact, sufficiently compensated for that loss to relinquish that visit voluntarily, the reallocation would not be a Pareto improvement.*

g. Would it be a **potential Pareto improvement** if, in the situation described in part (e), one visit were taken away from sickly Baby Smith and given instead to healthy Baby Chen? Explain, in a sentence or two.

> *SUGGESTED ANSWER: As noted under (e) above, the author of your text defines a potential Pareto improvement" as a change in the economy under which the gainers from the change **could** compensate (pay) the losers to accept that change, even if, in fact, that compensation is not made. In this case, such a compensation would be possible, because the Chens "value" the third visit they would gain at $100 while the Smiths "value" the fourth visit they would relinquish only at $25. Therefore, the*

reallocation of a physician visit from the sickly to the healthy child would be a Pareto improvement because, in principle, the Chens could compensate the Smiths for the loss of that visit (say, pay the Smiths $30).

h. Would the reallocation of one physician visit from sickly Baby Smith to healthy Baby Chen described in parts (e) represent an **increase in economic efficiency** as the author of your text defines that term? Explain, in a sentence or two. Be sure to define all of the terms you use in your answer, including "economic efficiency."

SUGGESTED ANSWER: The author of your text instructs you that "a change causes an **increase in economic efficiency** *if it is a Potential Pareto improvement" (p. 307). We have already established under (g) that the reallocation of a visit from the sickly Smith baby to the healthy Chen baby would be a potential Pareto improvement. Therefore that reallocation represents an increase in economic efficiency, as economists are wont to define that term. You will find a similar use of the term "efficiency" in other textbooks. For example, in his* Price Theory and Its Uses, 3rd ed. *(West Publishing Co.,1995), Steven E. Landsburg instructs students:*

> *The* **efficiency criterion** *is an alternative way to judge policies. According to the efficiency criterion, any change in policy that makes George $2 richer and Martha only $1 poorer is a good thing. Any change in policy that makes George $1 richer and Martha $2 poorer is a bad one. More generally, the efficiency criterion pronounces that between two policies, we should always prefer the one that yields the higher social gain. The preferred policy is said to be* **more efficient** *than its rival (p. 258).*

On this definition of efficiency, a policy that takes away from the sickly Smith baby a physician visit for which the relatively poor Smith family would have been willing to bid a maximum money price of only $25 and then bestows that visit on the healthy Chen baby, whose parents would be willing to bid a money price of as much as $100 for that additional visit would represent an **increase in economic efficiency**. *As his previously cited editorial suggests, Professor Friedman most probably would subscribe to that interpretation as well, as would many other economists.*

Note, in this connection, Professor Landsburg's definition of "social gain," one that is widely shared among professional economists. It is simply the algebraic sum of the monetary value of the gain reaped by the gainers from a policy minus the monetary value of the loss suffered by the losers from that policy, regardless of who these gainers or losers are, or how wealthy or poor they are. It is a standard definition of "social gain" or "enhancement of social welfare," as economists typically use those terms in their textbooks and in their policy analyses. Quite commonly, in the benefit-cost analyses for particular policies, a policy that yields a "social gain" (increases "social economic welfare") in this sense is styled by

> economists as a "good thing" and one that causes a "social loss" is styled
> as a "bad thing."

i. Would the reallocation of one visit from sickly Baby Smith to healthy Baby Chen described in part (e) be a **better** allocation of resources? Would the author of your text say so? Explain, in a sentence or two.

> *SUGGESTED ANSWER: On this point, even economists would have divergent views. As textbook author Alan Stockman properly warns you on this point:*

>> *"Someone who does not care about the distribution of wealth among people would say all potential Pareto improvements [increases in economic efficiency] are good. Someone who cares about the distribution of wealth would say many potential Pareto improvements are good, but some are not...because [they] can be unfair to the losers" (p. 309).*

> *The previously cited textbook author Landsburg also points out that*

>> *"Many economists regard the efficiency criterion [as he had defined it earlier] as a good rough guide to policy choices, though few would defend it as the sole basis on which to make such decisions" (p. 259).*

j. Could the government-administered allocation of physician visits described in part (e) above be properly described as "rationing"?

> *SUGGESTED ANSWER: Yes, it would be. Rationing is simply the allocation of scarce resources among competing ends. The government-administered algorithm described in Part (d) above is one such algorithm. Stockman, the author of your text, calls it "non-price rationing" (pp. 194-5).*

k. Could the rationing of physician visits in this case be avoided if the government refrained from intervening in the market for physician visits and instead let free market forces determine their allocation? (Not a silly question; many seasoned adults seem to have trouble with it.)

> *SUGGESTED ANSWER: One of the most popular fallacies among seasoned adults is that the allocation of resources through the free market is an alternative to rationing. It was a commonplace during the recent debate on health policy. In fact, allocations of resources through markets is but one form of rationing, namely, rationing on the basis of money prices and ability to pay. In using the word "non-price rationing," the author of your text (pp. 194-5) implicitly acknowledges that fact,*

although he never comes out clearly to declare that markets ration scarce resources. Most other introductory textbooks in economics do not address the issue at all. A refreshing exception are Michael L. Katz and Harvey S.Rosen who write forthrightly in their Microeconomics (Irwin, 1991) that "prices ration scarce resources" (p.15). Using the economist's definition of "efficiency," however, it is easy to show that non-price rationing typically is less efficient than price-rationing.

l. Start with the free-market solution under Part (b) as the initial position. Suppose now the government used general tax revenues to grant the low-income Smith family a subsidy of $30 per visit and that the market price of $40 per visit reflects the marginal social cost per visit. Economists would impute a "welfare loss" (alias "deadweight loss) to such a policy. In a properly executed graph, show the size of this "welfare loss." In your own view, is this really a "welfare loss"? Defend your conclusion as best you can.

SUGGESTED ANSWER: Prior to the implementation of this subsidy, the Smith family demanded 3 visits and paid $40 per visit. The Smith family now pays only $10 out of pocket per visit. At that price, it will demand 6.5 visits per years (a rate equivalent to 13 visits every two years). Your properly executed graph will show that the marginal monetary value the mith family would assign to the extra 3.5 visits per year will be lower than the cost of those incremental visits to the government (i.e., taxpayers). The difference is the so-called "deadweight loss" (or "social loss" in Landsburg's jargon or simply "social welfare loss" as it is commonly called in economics.) This narrowly calculated loss of "social welfare," however, excludes from consideration that other members of society might derive satisfaction from the knowledge that poor children, like the Smiths' baby, have adequate health care. In the jargon of economists, there may be positive externalities in consumption. The value to the rest of societies of these externalities may exceed the narrowly calculated "deadweight loss." In addition, of course, there may also be externalities in the production of good health. In plainer English, it may be of great benefit to the rest of society to prevent Baby Smith from contracting a contagious disease or simply from growing up sickly. In short, the narrowly calculated "deadweight loss" is not the sole criterion on which such policies should be judged.

m. Finally, in the light of the preceding exercise, comment briefly on the following statement: "Freely competitive markets allocate scarce resources to those who value them the most."

SUGGESTED ANSWER: In the context of economic analysis, the verb "to value" means "to be willing and able to pay the most money prices." It does not mean "to appreciate."

2

Disadvantaged Populations, Equity, and the Determinants of Health: Lessons from Down Under

DAVID MAYSTON

Department of Economics and Related Studies
University of York
Heslington, York, United Kingdom

ABSTRACT

The paper examines the determinants of health status, and the extent to which equity is being achieved in the distribution of health care finance, in the context of one substantially disadvantaged population that exists within an otherwise affluent society, namely that of the Aboriginal population of the Northern Territory of Australia.

Health, Health Care and Health Economics: Perspectives on Distribution
Edited by Morris L. Barer, Thomas E. Getzen, and Greg L. Stoddart
Copyright 1998 Wiley & Sons, Ltd.

The paper argues that the analysis of Evans and others of the link between an individual's status in an occupational hierarchy, their stress level, and the individual's health state needs widening to include considerations of social and economic stress on entire disadvantaged groups within the wider population, and of the role of positional goods in influencing health outcomes. Acute levels of social and economic stress in the past have induced forms of both social and economic hysteresis, and associated low health status. Overcoming these hysteresis effects now requires greater, and more carefully targeted, public expenditures on health and environmental services for such disadvantaged groups.

INTRODUCTION

Disadvantaged populations highlight the importance of risk factors and determinants of health status other than simply health care expenditures. At the same time, the distribution of health care financing to disadvantaged populations raises important questions regarding whether or not equity is being achieved in health care policy. The Aboriginal population of the Northern Territory of Australia provides an example of a disadvantaged population where many of these issues are encountered in acute form, and from which wider lessons may be learned.

UNEQUAL HEALTH OUTCOMES

That the Aboriginal population of the Northern Territory of Australia is significantly disadvantaged in terms of health outcomes can be seen firstly from Figure 1. This compares the Life Expectancy at Birth of Aboriginal males and females in the Northern Territory (NT) with that for other indigenous populations in developed countries, and with the national averages for Australia, Canada, and India. At some 51.6 years, the life expectancy at birth for Aboriginal males in the NT is not only 22.9 years less than the 74.5 years for the male Australian population as a whole. It is also significantly shorter than the life expectancy for the indigenous populations of other developed countries; it falls short of the male life expectancy at birth of United States Indians and Alaskan natives by 21.5 years, of the corresponding figure for the New Zealand Maori population by 14.0 years and is 12.8 years shorter than that for Canadian Indians. Life expectancy at birth for Aboriginal males in the NT is also some 3.8 years less than that for males in India.

Except for India (where female life expectancy at birth is 4.2 years less than for NT Aboriginal females), there are similar disparities in the corresponding figures for females (Hogg, 1992, p. 336; UN, 1995).

There is, moreover, evidence of a *reduction* in the life expectancy of Aboriginal adults during the past 20 years (Thomson, 1991a) compared to the improvements in life expectancy enjoyed elsewhere over this period. As emphasized by Bhatia and Anderson (1995, p.3): "During recent decades, the indigenous populations of other Westernised nations have made large strides in the improvement of their health. Their infant and maternal mortality rates have declined substantially and there has been a noticeable decrease in adult mortality. By comparison, Aboriginal populations have lagged considerably. Not only has the decline in infant and maternal mortality slowed down in the past few years, but a concomitant increase

FIGURE 1 Life Expectancy at Birth
Sources: Hogg (1992), UN (1995)

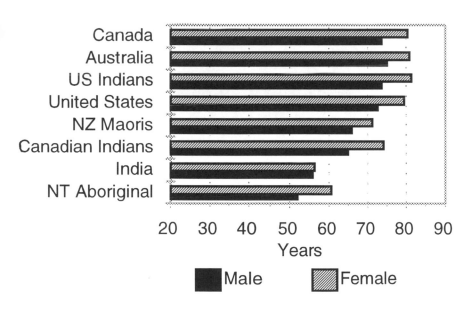

in young-middle adult mortality, particularly among males, has led to stagnancy in health trends.

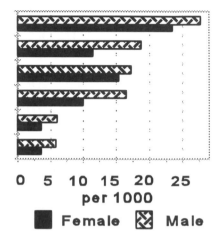

Ab. East Arnhem

Ab. Alice Springs

Ab. NT Average

Ab. Darwin Urban

Aus Average

Canadian

0 5 10 15 20 25
per 1000

■ Female ⧄ Male

Figure 2 Age-Standardized Mortality Rates
Source: Plant, Condon and Durling (1995)

The result is very high levels of age-standardised mortality amongst the Aboriginal population of the Northern Territory, as illustrated in Figure 2. Based on a three-year moving average in 1991, the age-standardised mortality rate of the male Aboriginal population of the NT from all causes of death was 17.17 per 1,000 population, compared to 6.80 per 1,000 for the non-Aboriginal population of the Northern Territory and 5.82 per 1,000 for the Australian population as a whole. The corresponding figures for females were 15.29 for the NT Aboriginal population, 2.85 for the NT non-Aboriginal population, and 3.58 for the overall Australian female population as a whole (see Plant, Condon and Durling, 1995, p. 12).

Substantial inequality of health outcomes for the Aboriginal population of the NT, however, prevails not only in international and national comparisons, but also within the Aboriginal population of the Northern Territory itself. The Aboriginal male age-standardised mortality rate from all causes of death for 1985 - 91 in Figure 2 varies from 16.26 per 1,000 population for the Darwin Urban district of the NT to 18.57 for the Alice Springs rural district, and 27.50 for the East Arnhem district of the NT, where the latter mortality rate is 4.44 times that for Australia as a whole. For Aboriginal females, the corresponding figures are 9.83 for the Darwin Urban district, 11.23 for the Alice Springs Rural district, and 23.24 for the East Arnhem district, where the latter is 6.21 times the corresponding figure for Australia as a whole (see Plant, Condon, and Durling, 1995, pp. 12, 46). In addition, while Aboriginal babies account for only 38% of all births in the NT, they account for 73% of all infant deaths (Bhatia and Anderson, 1995, p. 12).

Unequal health outcomes are reflected not only in the above mortality statistics but also in the relative morbidity of the Aboriginal and non-Aboriginal populations of the Northern Territory. Age-adjusted rates of End Stage Renal Disease (ESRD) have been found to be on average 17.4 times higher for the Aboriginal population of the Northern Territory than for its non-Aboriginal population over the period 1988-93, with this multiple rising to 59.6 within the Tiwi Island Aboriginal population in the Northern Territory (Hoy, Mathews, and Pugsley, 1995a). Guest and O'Dea (1992) report diabetes to be prevalent in up to 23% of the NT Aboriginal population over the age of 35 in remote communities, compared to approximately 4% for non-Aboriginal populations in Australia as a whole. The high relative incidence of birth defects in the infants of Aboriginal female diabetics, compared to both the non-Aboriginal population with diabetes (other than non-insulin-dependent diabetes) and the Aboriginal population without diabetes, is reported by Bower *et al.* (1992). Smith, Spargo, Hunter, *et al* (1992) report prevalence rates for ischaemic heart disease and hypertension for Aboriginal populations in remote Australia to be more than twice those of the Australian population as a whole.

The relative incidence of different diseases, expressed as a ratio of the incidence of each disease category for the Aboriginal population of the NT to that for the non-Aboriginal population of the NT, is shown in Table 1. The relative incidence is particularly high for Infectious and Parasitic Diseases; Endocrine, Nutritional and Metabolic Diseases; Diseases of the Blood, Nervous System and the Respiratory System; and Diseases of the Skin. The associated high cost of "excess morbidity" (costed at A$320 a day variable cost for NT acute care beds) is shown in the last column of Table 1.

The substantial variations in morbidity that also occur *within* the Aboriginal population of the Northern Territory are reflected in a recent study of the Maningrida region of the NT. This reports that: "Infectious diseases are very common amongst Aboriginal people in the Maningrida region. For example, rheumatic heart disease has a prevalence of 0.6/1000 in the general Australian population compared with 5.3/1000 in Aborigines of the Top-End (of the Northern Territory), 6.9/1000 in Soweto and 44/1000 in the Maningrida region....Other diseases that are otherwise rare in Australia are common. There has been a low grade Tuberculosis epidemic since 1967. Incidence rates for TB are over 500 times the Australian rate and over 7 times the NT Aboriginal rate. There are currently 71 past leprosy patients in the Maningrida region" (Menzies School of Health Research, 1995, pp. 1-2).

TABLE 1 The Relative Incidence of Aboriginal/Non-Aboriginal Disease
in the Northern Territory

Disease Category	Relative Incidence	Cost of Excess Morbidity
		A$m
Infectious and Parasitic Diseases	8.8	4.066
Neoplasms	0.6	(0.003)
Endocrine Nutritional & Metabolic Diseases	4.7	0.711
Diseases of the Blood	5.3	0.339
Mental Disorders	0.9	(0.243)
Diseases of the Nervous System	2.7	1.164
Diseases of the Circulatory System	1.8	0.897
Diseases of the Respiratory System	4.0	3.037
Diseases of the Digestive System	0.8	0.288
Diseases of the Genitourinary System	1.4	1.157
Complications of Pregnancy and Childbirth	1.5	2.741
Diseases of the Skin	3.3	1.359
Diseases of the Musculoskeletal System	0.6	0.393
Congenital Anomalies	1.7	0.300
Perinatal Conditions	1.4	0.805
Symptoms, Signs and Ill-Defined Conditions	2.4	1.829
Injury and Poisoning	1.9	2.112
V Codes excluding live births (outcomes)	2.5	1.160
Total	2.0	22.113

(Source: Cresap, 1991)

THE DETERMINANTS OF ABORIGINAL
POPULATION HEALTH

Before assessing the importance of the distribution of health care financing on the provision of Aboriginal health care and health outcomes, several of the suggested main determinants of the above adverse pattern of health outcomes for Aboriginal communities within Australia will be examined. Like many other disadvantaged communities (see *e.g.*, Townsend and Davidson, 1982), there are both *life-style* and inter-acting *socioeconomic factors* at work as influences on health outcomes. In addition, the low relative position of the Aboriginal population in the income distribution of Australia, combined with their low relative health status, would seem to reinforce the proposition advanced in Evans (1994, 1996) and Wilkinson (1992) that it is the *relative* position of different population groups in the distribution of income that is a major determinant of their health status. For those aged 15 years or more who provided details of their income in the 1986 Census, for example, only 11.5% of Aborigines had individual income of more than $15,000 compared to 51% for the non-indigenous population of the Northern Territory. In addition, only 29.6% of Aboriginal families had income of more than $22,000, compared to 70.8% of non-Aboriginal families in the NT (see Thomson and Briscoe, 1991, p.9).

However, we will argue that Aboriginal health illustrates the importance for a disadvantaged group also of changes in the *absolute levels* of a wide range of variables affecting health. The role of their *relative* position in the distribution of income and wealth is here predominantly one of influencing their command over the absolute levels of key *positional goods*. As noted by Hirsch (1977, p. 34-35), one key positional good is that of land. Hirsch argues that:

> An individual can improve his capacity to acquire scenic property by improving his position in the income and wealth distribution, that is, by getting richer *vis-à-vis* his fellows. The same result will not be achieved if he gets richer along with his fellows, that is, if his income and wealth rise in line with a general increase in average income and wealth in the community. Indeed, as the general level of income rises, acquisition of scenic or other property for leisure use, at the rising relative price, entails progressively increasing sacrifice of other goods. Thus for the early rich, who acquired an effective demand for such property when it was economically a free good, the sacrifice was zero.....Positional goods come first into the hands of the early rich.

Within Australia, before the first European settlement in 1788, the indigenous Aboriginal population was in the position of "the early rich," both in terms of its control over large areas of land, and probably also in terms of its health status. As noted by Thomson (1984, p. 939):

> While it is impossible to be precise, it is likely that the Aborigines in 1788 were physically, socially and emotionally healthier than most Europeans at that time... Evidence for this conclusion, and for the likely presence or absence of certain diseases comes from a combination of historical sources, palaeopathology and an understanding of the nature of individual diseases in human populations.

Similarly, as noted by Saggers and Gray (1991, p. 37):

> Although information about the pre-contact health of Aborigines is based upon impressionistic observations of the early explorers, brief historical references, and studies among people who have had minimal contact with Europeans, what evidence there is suggests a much healthier population. The physical isolation of the island continent and small scattered groups had led to a relative absence of vector-borne diseases and animal diseases (zoonoses) (Moodie, 1973, p. 29). Unencumbered with the disease-inducing lifestyle of their invaders, the Aborigines in the eighteenth century were described by many early observers as fit and healthy.... Governor Phillip was so impressed with the physique and presentation of Aborigines he met he named Manly Bay in the colony of New South Wales after them (Stone, 1974, p. 20). Eyre described the tribes of the River Murray area as 'almost free from diseases and well-shaped in body and limb' (in Cleland, 1928)...... According to Daisy Bates (White, 1985, p. 290) the Aborigines enjoyed long lives prior to contact with Europeans, with many reaching in excess of eighty years of age.

Such a health status for the Aboriginal population in the period before extensive European contact is likely to be associated with their relatively successful adaption to their natural environment. This environment included, in particular, an abundant supply of land that at the time was essentially a free good for the Aboriginal population as a whole. In response to such a low effective price of land, they developed a land-intensive nomadic life-style and associated hunter-gatherer production process. A key input into this land-intensive production process was their accumulated *human capital*, of appropriate specialised technological knowledge that was well-adapted to hunter-gatherer production, together with a form of social organisation that was capable of transforming the available inputs into a sustainable and healthy diet without excessive environmental degradation. As noted by the Australian historian Geoffrey Blainey (1980, p. 62-63):

> The Aboriginals had lived in the continent for at least forty thousand years... They lived on a wide variety of roots, greens, seeds, nuts, berries and other vegetables and fruits as well as meat and fish. Their diet in 1800 was probably more diverse than that of the London rich, but they hoarded virtually nothing for a hungry day. By skillfully moving in small groups from place to place and using their knowledge of botany and zoology they usually lived in relative

plenty, so long as the population in each region remained low. Their medicines were mainly herbal and psychological; their food-finding tools and hunting and fishing implements were simple but supplemented by physical dexterity, a minute knowledge of the seasonal ways of plants and animals, and the ability to observe with eyes, ears and nose. They could not read a book, but they read nature superbly.

However, with the coming of the British settlers and a boom in the newly established Australian wool industry in the 1820s, land was no longer a free good. Instead "the sheep-owners and the Aboriginals were competing for the same grassland, and neither was willing to retreat" (*ibid*, p. 72). The relatively low level of their military technology, and the small individual group sizes of the indigenous population, compared to those of the invading European settlers, put the Aboriginal population in a poor competitive position for maintaining their control over the increasingly scarce resource of land. The resultant loss of their effective property rights over large parts of their original terrain meant that they were no longer in a position to enjoy the "cumulative advantage" which "priority in historical sequence of access" (Hirsch, 1977, p. 36) might otherwise confer on the "early rich" from their initial holdings of land. Instead the fall in their *absolute* level of control over the prime positional good of land resources, that resulted from their greatly diminished *relative* position of power within Australia, had numerous other adverse effects on the *absolute* level of other key variables that have directly or indirectly affected their health status.

These variables include their *exposure to externally introduced diseases and to the spread of infectious diseases* within the Aboriginal population, the level of *physical violence* which they suffered, the *hygienic state of their water supply and sanitary arrangements*, their *dietary intake* of healthy and unhealthy substances, their level of *exercise and engagement in meaningful physical and mental activity*, their *social support* and *group authority* structures, and their *psychological and spiritual motivation*.

The externally introduced diseases that had a strongly adverse impact on Aboriginal health include smallpox, influenza, measles, and venereal disease. There remains some uncertainty over whether such diseases were accidentally introduced into the Aboriginal population by European contact or were instead part of a deliberate attempt to weaken their ability to resist the loss of their effective property rights over their land (Franklin and White, 1991. p. 5). As noted by Gray *et al.* (1991, p. 89):

Even the most extravagant reconstructions of the effects of introduced diseases cannot refute the contention that the rate of depopulation was proportionately much greater within the frontier of European settlement than beyond it. The presence of European settlers directly attacked the economic basis of Aboriginal society. In most parts of Australia, Aboriginal people were forewarned of the approach of Europeans, because they knew about the expeditions and settlers in other areas, they had encountered feral animals and they were already familiar with many introduced implements, and with the use of iron and glass. What they did not expect, and everywhere resisted, was forced dispossession of their homelands, and the introduction of grazing animals that fouled water resources, destroyed the habitats of native animals and changed the vegetation so much that traditional gathered foods could no longer be found. Aboriginals resisted, and often there was open warfare. It has been estimated that at least 20000 Aborigines died as a result of conflict, about 10 times the number of Europeans that died (Reynolds, 1981). Massacres of Aborigines continued right through to the 1920s and 1930s, and ended only when the entire country was effectively under white domination.

The loss of their previously well-adjusted nomadic life-style in small Aboriginal family groups was frequently accompanied by their relocation in larger Aboriginal settlements into which they were forced, or encouraged, by external missions or by the availability of free rations. The larger and more concentrated settlements themselves posed new problems of sanitation and clean water supply, as well as the more rapid spread of infectious diseases through overcrowding and a less dispersed distribution of the Aboriginal population. Problems of overcrowding in Aboriginal communities in the Northern Territory still persist. The 1991 Australian Census (ABS, 1994, pp. 5-6) found an average of 5.7 indigenous people per occupied private dwelling in the Northern Territory, more than double that of for the non-indigenous population of the NT, with 34.3% of the NT's indigenous population living in multi-family households, with an average household size of 10.7 people. This contrasts with only 1% of the non-indigenous population of the NT living in multi-family households, which themselves had an average household size of 5.5 persons. At 12.0%, the percentage of the indigenous population of the NT living in improvised dwellings is 20 times that for the NT's non-indigenous population.

The move to Aboriginal settlements also involved important changes in the *absolute* levels of their consumption of different items of food and other substances within their consumption vector, in response to changes in their *relative* availability and their implicit *relative* prices, as well in the *absolute* level of physical exercise needed to obtain their consumption vector. As noted by Franklin and White (*op. cit*, p. 11):

With the change to settlement life, major alterations in food habits were introduced. One reason for herding Aborigines onto settlements and reserves was to prevent hunting and gathering on land that had been taken over for stock-raising and agriculture. This meant the abandonment of the traditional healthy mixed diet and the substitution of rations, which needed to be cheap, portable and non-perishable. The rations consisted mainly of white flour, sugar, tea, rice, tinned meat and salt beef (Taylor, 1977, p. 154). In the 1950s when stores were opened on the settlements and Aborigines began to use money, they found the ration-type foods cheap and available. Some settlement dwellers were able to supplement their diet by hunting or fishing, but there was a serious shortage of fruit and vegetables. Even when available, fruit and vegetables were expensive. Moreover, Aborigines were also spending money on alcohol and tobacco, which had become available by that time.

There is evidence of continuing high levels of alcoholism (Weeramanthri *et al.*, 1994), sexually transmitted diseases (Thomson, 1991b, p. 63), smoking (Guest *et al.*, 1992) and of other substance abuse (Bryce *et al.*, 1992) within Aboriginal communities. In addition to their adverse direct effects on health, the associated relatively high levels of expenditure on alcohol and cigarettes continue to have a negative economic impact on the available local budget for an improved diet (Hoy *et al.*, 1995).

The adverse impact on Aboriginal health of the above dietary changes is likely to be substantial, particularly if one accepts the *"thrifty" genotype* hypothesis of Neel (1962; 1982) that Aboriginal metabolism had become genetically well-adapted to the traditional Aboriginal hunter-gatherer life-style, but is now much less well-adapted to the new life-style of Aboriginal communities. Thus O'Dea (1991, p. 258) argues that:

> The traditional hunter-gatherer lifestyle of Australian Aborigines, characterised by high physical activity and a diet of low energy density (low fat, high fibre), promoted the maintenance of a very lean body weight and minimised insulin resistance. In contrast, for most Aborigines a Western lifestyle is characterised by reduced physical activity and an energy-dense diet (high in refined carbohydrate and fat) which promotes obesity and maximised insulin resistance. When they make the transition from their traditional hunter-gatherer lifestyle to a westernised lifestyle, Aborigines develop high prevalence rates for obesity (with an android pattern of fat distribution), non-insulin dependent diabetes, impaired glucose tolerance, hypertriglyceridaemia, hypertension and hyperinsulinaemia.

with associated risks of premature corony heart disease.

A reduction in the absolute level of physical exercise in Aboriginal communities following European contact is noted by Altman (1987, p. 94) even for communities where the hunter-gatherer life-style is partially retained. In communities where it is not retained, the reduction in physical activity is compounded by the high rates of unemployment in alternative occupations which most Aboriginal communities now face. The unemployment rate for the indigenous population of the Northern

Territory for those aged 15 years and over is both high in absolute terms, at 25.8%, and relative to the corresponding rate of 9.5% for the non-indigenous population (ABS, 1994, p. 11).

The indigenous population of the NT is predominantly Aboriginal in origin. Thus of the total indigenous population of the NT of 39,910 individuals recorded by the 1991 Australian Census (ABS, 1994), 98.4% identified themselves as Aboriginal, with 1.6% identifying themselves as of Torres Strait Island descent. However, because of the difficulties in counting the indigenous population, the overall size of the indigenous population is estimated by the Australian Bureau of Statistics (1994) to be some 8.4% higher than the 1991 Census count, at 43,273 individuals in total.

Over a quarter of the indigenous population of rural Australia aged 15 years or over are unemployed, with around 13% having been unemployed for 12 months or more (ABS, 1995, p. 53). Such long-term unemployment is itself reinforced by the relatively high percentage (72.5%) of the indigenous population of the NT who were found in the 1991 Census to have no educational qualification, compared to 50.7% for the non-indigenous population (ABS, 1994, p. 10). In addition, 30.6% of the indigenous population of the Northern Territory aged 13 to 17 years do not attend any educational institution, compared to 16.2% for the non-indigenous population of the NT (ABS, 1994, p. 9).

Associated with such high rates of Aboriginal unemployment is a high level of dependency on government payments for the indigenous population. Indeed, 54.9% of the indigenous population of Australia depend upon government payments as their main source of income (ABS, 1995, p. 55). These payments include unemployment and social security payments, as well as payments through Community Development Employment Projects that Aboriginal communities can finance from the community income that would otherwise would have been paid directly as unemployment benefits. An additional 10.7% of the indigenous population are reported as having no source of monetary income at all, with only 24.1% having a main source of income from earned income other than Community Development Employment Projects (ABS, 1995, p.55).

The above changes in diet, sanitation, housing conditions, increased exposure to infectious diseases, alcoholism, and smoking are likely to produce a *multiple compounding* of risk factors for a wide range of adverse medical conditions. Thus in the case of tuberculosis, Plant *et al* (1995, p.487-489) emphasize that:

Tuberculosis is essentially a social disease. It occurs mostly in people who live in poverty and overcrowding ... Aborigines already have high rates of infection and disease from tuberculosis. They suffer from social disadvantage which in turn exposes them to the risks of poverty, underweight, homelessness, overcrowding and poor nutrition. As well, they have a higher than average prevalence of risk factors for tuberculosis, such as diabetes mellitus, renal failure, alcohol abuse and smoking. Although as yet largely untouched by HIV-AIDS, Aborigines are in considerable danger of being affected by the AIDS epidemic given their high rates of sexually transmissible diseases. If HIV spreads to Aboriginal people, it follows that the tuberculosis-HIV interface will become a major public health problem.

In the case of diabetes, Phillips, Patel and Weeramanthri (1995, p. 485) emphasize that:

Diabetes is most usefully understood as a disease that arises from a web of underlying social and economic determinants. It then acts as an independent predictor of premature mortality, as well as amplifying the effects of its fellow travelers of rapid social change: hypertension, obesity and hyperlipidaemia. Its own effects on mortality are in turn amplified by particular community factors, such as high rates of infectious disease, and treatment factors, such as the availability and acceptability of renal dialysis and transplantation.

The above vector of adverse circumstances is also likely to produce high rates of *co-morbidity*, of several adverse health conditions occurring together in the same individuals, with associated complications and reinforcement effects. Thus Hoy, Mathews, and Pugsley (1995a, p. 307) note that: "Many Aboriginals with ESRD had serious comordibities, especially chronic infections and alcohol abuse; these frequently precluded transplant and were often the ultimate cause of death." Similarly, Phillips, Patel and Weeramanthri (1995, p. 482) stress that the high prevalence of diabetes in the Australian Aboriginal population "amplifies the effect of the community prevalence of infection and renal disease," with Guest and O'Dea (1992, p. 340) noting that: "diabetes contributes to circulatory disease which is, for Aboriginal males and females, the leading cause of death. In Aboriginal adults, deaths due to circulatory disease occur up to ten times more than in the rest of the population."

The above adverse circumstances are also likely to have major lagged effects over time through their adverse impact also on infant health. As noted by the Menzies School of Health Research (1995, p. 2) in their recent detailed study of an NT Aboriginal community:

Even in infancy, the children of the Maningrida region suffer high levels of morbidity. Almost one in three babies born in 1994 to Maningrida mothers needed treatment in the special care nursery or neonatal intensive care. In 1994, on average, each child under two was admitted nearly 1.4 times per year. Half had diarrhoeal disease, 35% were underweight or malnourished, 50% were anaemic, 25% had diagnosed ear infections, urine infections and/or chest infections. Furthermore, hospital admissions for 0-4 year olds from Maningrida in 1994 were more frequent than for 1976 - 1985.

As in Barker *et al.* (1986, 1987, 1989) and Evans (1996, p. 59), the effects of such infant malnutrition and ill-health may well be high levels of premature adult mortality in years to come.

SOCIAL STRESS AND HEALTH

There are interesting parallels between the experience of the Aboriginal population of Australia and the proposition that the levels of stress induced by an occupational group's hierarchical position have a significant influence on its members' health status (Evans, 1994, 1996; Marmot *et al.*, 1978). The physical and psychological traumas suffered in past years by many Aboriginal communities, in their downgrading to a low ranking in the effective hierarchy of Australian society, clearly have been accompanied by impairments in their health status. There is a sense in which the associated past major stresses have now resulted in whole communities that are in many respects "bent out of shape" (Evans, 1994, p. 21). The magnitude of these past stresses is illustrated by estimates of the dramatic fall by 1933 in the size of the Australian Aboriginal population following European settlement, to a mere 10 to 23.5% of its pre-contact size (Saggers and Gray, 1991, p. 66-7). The disruption of, and stress upon, family groups and social hierarchies that this process has induced is in turn complicated by the abnormally large numbers of under 25 year olds in the age distribution of the present Aboriginal population. This abnormal age distribution itself results from a relatively small initial population size of the Aboriginal population in the 1930s, high subsequent rates of premature mortality and a high birth rate under later, relatively more settled, times.

The fact that physical violence, or even many other milder forms of direct contact, between Aboriginal communities and the increasingly urbanised non-indigenous population of Australia is currently at a much lower level than previously does not in itself overcome the *hysteresis* that may continue to persist in the partially buckled social structures and psychological predispositions of many Aboriginal communities following the earlier adverse contacts. Just as early environmental influences in the *history* of an individual (Evans, 1994, p. 18) may have profound effects on their physical and psychological condition in later life, so too may earlier historical stresses from the external environment still impair the current ability of whole communities to restore themselves to physical and psychological health.

In the case of Aboriginal communities, these past stresses have severely disrupted the key inter-relationships among land, belief-systems, social structures, and economic productivity. As noted by Reid and Lumpton (1991, p. xii):

> Much of the suffering of communities today can be traced back to the alienation of Aboriginal lands. This alienation was wrought by the violence of guerilla warfare, massacres and rape, the deadly stealth of epidemic disease, malnutrition and poverty, and the good intentions of government agencies and missions which confined Aborigines to 'civilise' them, seized children of dual ancestry and stifled the religious and cultural expressions of Aboriginal people.... the appropriation of lands that sustained Aborigines and shaped their theology, social lives and economic activities had traumatising effects on families and local groups, effects that ramified through generations.

It is clearly possible to argue that substance abuse is in large part *endogenous* to this process, while at the same time tending to reinforce it. Thus Gray *et al.* (1995) argue that "Alcohol misuse is both a consequence and cause of many of the social and health problems Aboriginal people face, and is exacerbated by the continuing legacy of dispossession, disadvantage and discrimination." Such endogeneity makes more difficult any simple distinction between "the deserving sick" and "the undeserving sick," such as is implicit in *The Economist* (1994).

Alcohol misuse here forms part of a wider self-reinforcing syndrome of ill-health, substance abuse, unemployment, and welfare dependency for the disadvantaged Aboriginal population, with Daly and Hawke (1994, p. 81) noting that:

> The relatively high level of Aboriginal welfare dependence also reflects their poor health status compared with other Australians. Poor health also has implications for the ability of an individual to take up and retain employment, so poor health status will have implications for both the numbers on sickness and invalid pensions and the numbers in receipt of employment-related benefits.

Poor health status is then one of the links in the chain that ties together the above *social hysteresis* with an *economic hysteresis*. The economic hysteresis results from the major impairment in the value of the traditional human capital, and of the associated stock of technological skills possessed by Aboriginal communities, once the hunter-gatherer process of production becomes economically and technologically obsolete as an efficient means of producing food. Poor health and the specialised nature of these traditional skills in turn reduce the *adaptability* of

Aboriginal communities to the new wider Australian economy, thereby lengthening the process of economic hysteresis.

THE DISTRIBUTION OF HEALTH CARE FINANCING

It is instructive to compare the distribution of health care financing to the disadvantaged Aboriginal population with several of the criteria of *equity* discussed in Mooney (1983). The first of these is that of:

EQUALITY OF EXPENDITURE *PER CAPITA*

The concept of *weighted population* that is used to determine the NT's Base Hospital Funding Grant under the Australian Medicare Agreement (Australian Government Solicitor, 1993) applies age and sex specific *national average* hospital cost weights to the *local population* age and sex distribution. These national average hospital cost weights give relatively little for those in middle and younger age groups, and substantially more for those aged 65 years and above. Those aged over 74 years yield 18.4 times for males, and 15.5 times for females, the amounts credited for members of the local population in the under 15 year age group.

However, one principal feature of the Aboriginal population of the NT is its younger average age than that of the general Australian population. Some 40.7% of the male indigenous population of NT, and 37.9% of the female indigenous population of NT, are aged 14 years or less (ABS, 1994). In addition, 62.2% of the male indigenous population and 59.8% of the female indigenous population are aged 24 years or less. Only 2.3% of the male indigenous population of the NT, and only 2.6% of the female indigenous, are aged 65 years or over. Less than 1% of the NT indigenous population is more than 74 years of age. Thus, rather than achieving *equality* of expenditure per capital, the result of the above computation of weighted population in determining the NT's Base Hospital Funding Grant is a *regressive* one, of *less* funding per capita from the Base Hospital Funding Grant for the NT's indigenous population than for the Australian population as a whole, despite their much greater health problems.

However, there are two additional features of the Australian hospital funding mechanism that add to the complexity of the overall funding system, and tend to offset the above regressive effect. The first is the Bonus Pool for hospital funding under the Australian Medicare Agreement, which is based upon *historical shares* and mitigates the transition to funding based upon *weighted population*. Because the NT has historically higher *per capita* funding than other Australian States/Territories, its high share of Bonus Pool funding helps to offset the regressive impact of allocation according to weighted population. The size of the Bonus Pool, however, is under political pressure from other Australian States whose overall allocations have suffered as a result of its creation. In addition, the use of past historical patterns of hospital expenditure to determine its allocation does not guarantee that the available finance will be allocated according to health care need.

A second offsetting factor is provided by the *fiscal equalisation* recommendations of the Commonwealth Grants Commission (1994a,b; 1995). These determine the level of additional untied revenue funding for the NT, although there is no requirement that this additional funding is used for hospital funding in general or for Aboriginal patients in particular. Nevertheless, the actual pattern of *hospital utilisation* that these additional sources of funding help to support is one of higher (age standardised) rates of hospital separation (*i.e.*, discharges or deaths) for the Aboriginal population of the NT compared to its non-Aboriginal populations, and of higher lengths of stay, as we discuss below.

This unequal level of expenditure *per capita* in favour of the Aboriginal population does not continue, however, when one moves from hospital care to primary care. The *per capita* level of funding through the Medical Benefits Scheme (MBS) component of Australian Medicare that reimburses primary care expenditure on private GPs on a fee-for-service basis, for example, was only some $5 *per capita* in the NT Aboriginal communities of Ngukurr, Port Keats and Angurugu in 1994-5, compared to the Australian and NT averages of $290 and $168 *per capita* respectively. The more affluent city areas of Sydney and Melbourne Ports attract private GPs much more readily than more remote areas of Australia. In these city areas, Medical Benefits funding of primary care is in excess of $400 *per capita*, some 80 times that received by several of the NT Aboriginal communities, despite major differences in health status in the converse direction.

While this dramatic inequality in Medical Benefits funding is to some extent offset by the direct funding by the NT Government of primary care through local community health centres, the overall level of provision of primary care *per capita* to NT Aboriginal communities is still substantially less than that for Australia as a whole. A recent study (Wright, 1995) of one NT Aboriginal community found a doctor:patient ratio of 1:3,050 compared to the Australia average ratio of 1:771. The Menzies School of Health Research (1995, p. 2) reports one District Medical Officer visiting the local community health center two days per week for an Aboriginal population of 2,100 at Maningrida, attempting to service 26,500 patient presentations a year, assisted by a temporary staffing level of seven nursing staff and four Aboriginal Health Workers.

EQUALITY OF ACCESS FOR EQUAL NEED

While the indigenous population accounts for approximately 24% of the total population of the Northern Territory, it accounts for 40% of hospital admissions and 53% of hospital bed-days (Plant, Condon, and Durling, 1995). The 76% of the NT population who are non-indigenous then account for only 47% of bed days. The bed-days utilisation *per capita* of the indigenous population is, therefore, 3.57 times that for the non-indigenous population of the NT. This is marginally greater than the ratio of 3.28 of the age-standardised mortality rates of the two populations. However, while the related concept of the Standardised Mortality Rate (SMR) was used as a proxy for *morbidity* and acute health care *need* for many years in the UK National Health Service (DHSS, 1976), the desirability of supplementing such mortality data by wider considerations of health care need is now recognised (Carr-Hill *et al.*, 1994). The Commonwealth Grants Commission (1994, a, b; 1995) uses only existing Aboriginal and non-Aboriginal separation and bed-days rates to determine its recommendations for fiscal equalisation revenue grants. This approach clearly suffers from being concerned only with existing Aboriginal hospital utilisation rates, rather than any more independent measure of health care need, including currently unmet need.

The unequal level of funding of primary care for Aboriginal communities, compared to non-Aboriginal communities, is compounded by the problem of uncertainty over whether the total primary and community care resources currently used in Aboriginal communities are themselves allocated according to need across different Aboriginal communities within the NT. As noted by Munoz *et al.*, (1992a,b), there are considerable variations in socio-environmental conditions and health status across different Aboriginal communities within the NT. However, a recent detailed study by Warchivker (1996) reports great difficulty in identifying with any precision the detailed pattern of health care expenditure in the different Aboriginal communities within the Alice Springs Rural District of the NT, largely because of the multiplicity of different funding programmes and agencies involved, and a lack of adequate accounting records on a community basis.

EQUALITY OF HEALTH OUTCOME

As noted above, equality of health outcomes is clearly not currently being achieved across Australia, within the Northern Territory, or within its Aboriginal population. In view of the socio-environmental conditions affecting Aboriginal health status that have been identified above, any such equality of health outcomes either across different Aboriginal communities, or between the indigenous and non-indigenous populations of the NT, would involve not only substantial increases in health care expenditure for the disadvantaged Aboriginal population, but also a substantial increase in expenditure to improve housing conditions and employment opportunities.

The declared aim of the Australian National Health Policy (Health Ministers' Forum, 1994) has been "to raise the health status of Australians to equal the best in the world." However, overcoming the hysteresis effects on *current* and *future* levels of health of *past* and *present* social and environmental stresses in the Aboriginal communities would require sustained improvements in their physical and economic environment, as well as in the resourcing of their primary and community health care.

As noted by Altman and Daly (1995, p. 72), "The future employment opportunities of indigenous Australians look bleak, with the need for rapid improvement in education status and work experience being essential for enhanced economic status." The importance of achieving culturally-appropriate improvements in housing conditions is emphasised by Reid and Lumpton (1991, p. xvii), who argue that:

> Compounding the absolute poverty of the dwellings of many communities is the inappropriateness of many houses that have been designed on the basis of the values and cultural assumptions about the concept of a 'home' held by white bureaucrats, social planners and architectural firms.... Many Aborigines do not value the isolation and privacy offered by the standard European house; they value human relationships, open living areas and space in which to be able to communicate freely with others and honour their obligations to offer accommodation to family and friends.

Such reciprocity can lead to high occupancy rates, plumbing becoming blocked, difficulty in keeping conventional houses clean and well-repaired, generators running out of fuel, and a reliance upon hardware that is difficult to repair locally.

The scope for providing culturally more appropriate housing designs for Aboriginal communities is discussed in Pholeros *et al.* (1993). Both the cultural and the physical distance between Aboriginal communities in remote Australia and many of the urban administrators making public expenditure decisions intended to improve Aboriginal welfare is emphasised in a study by Rowse (1993), entitled *Remote Possibilities*. A recent example of such a divide is provided by government spending of A$1 million on the construction at the remote Aboriginal community of Milakapiti in the Northern Territory of an old people's home that now stands empty after the intended elderly Aboriginal inhabitants have fled its confines back to their own families in the community. The fortress-like structure of the Royal Darwin Hospital (RDH), that forms the largest hospital facility in the Northern Territory, is itself based upon an architectural design that was originally intended for Edmonton, Alberta, where the climatic conditions are significantly different from those in Darwin, Australia. The resulting feelings of imprisonment of Aboriginal patients have led some Aboriginal mothers to flee from RDH with their newborn babies immediately after birth.

The growing outstation movement of recent years (see, for example, Reid and Trompf, 1991, p. 98) involves the indigenous development of smaller remote Aboriginal communities that are more akin to traditional lifesyles, together with some economic benefits. Thus Altman (1987, p. 227) notes that:

> The economic tradeoff between life at outstations or at Maningrida is today fairly clear. At Maningrida, life is marginal, particularly for groups from outlying regions. There [are] limited employment prospects, limited access to subsistence resources, and a limited supply of raw materials to manufacture artefacts. At outstations in north-central Arnhem Land on the other hand, the subsistence economy is viable and artefact manufacture is unimpeded by raw material supply constraints.

While there may be some compensating health benefits from an improved life-style at outstations, their increased dispersion and smaller size raise significantly the public expenditure costs that would be involved in seeking to provide education and health care services to a comparable level to those enjoyed by non-indigenous communities in the NT. This in turn widens further the substantial gap that currently exists between the prevailing levels of educational and health care provision and those which would be required for *equality* in educational and health status between the indigenous and non-indigenous populations of the NT. As noted by the Menzies School of Health Research (1995, p. 2) in their recent report on the NT Aboriginal community of Maningrida, "Because of time constraints medical officers never visit outstations", with resultant likely unmet health care need from the current relatively low levels of provision of primary health care to such Aboriginal communities and their outstations.

EQUALITY OF MARGINAL MET NEED

The existing inequality in health outcomes across different Aboriginal communities within the NT, and the associated scope for positive Aboriginal health gains through community-based programmes, are confirmed by Munoz *et al.*, (1992b), who conclude that:

> Our studies are encouraging, firstly because they show that the health outcomes in some Aboriginal communities can be much better than in others, and secondly because it is plausible, on the basis of the associations reported here, that improvements in social, behavioural and environmental conditions in Aboriginal communities will be followed by improvements in childhood health outcomes..... Our cross-sectional findings strongly support the rationale for accelerated social action and community development because of the improved health outcome that will almost certainly follow.

A greater emphasis on community-based programmes would also be consistent with the earlier recommendations of the CRESAP (1991) Review of Health and Community Services in the Northern Territory. This review argued in favour of a "shift from the largely reactive demand-driven system of health and welfare delivery which exists at present to a more strategically focused, planned and *managed* system - a system responsive to demands but which assesses community needs, prioritises its services and better directs its energies towards achieving sustainable improvements in measurable outcomes against performance targets" (*op. cit.*, p. 47). In pursuit of its goal that "the principal strategic imperative of the Department must be to achieve major sustainable improvements in the health status of the Aboriginal population," the Review argued that "there needs to be a strengthened commitment to contain the growth in the acute care hospital sector in favour of those sectors which offer greater opportunity to decrease morbidity. This can be achieved as a result of greater emphasis being placed on preventive health and community care....Health centres within the community are the logical starting point from which extensions to the current range and/or intensity of services can be made" (*ibid*, p. 50-51). However, in the years since the CRESAP (1991) Review was published, hospital costs in the NT have continued to rise significantly, with other areas of the NT health care budget, such as primary and community care, squeezed as a result of hospital cost over-runs.

The associated imbalance between inadequately funded primary and community care and the urban hospital sector absorbing a large proportion of the available health care resources is consistent with a similar international pattern discussed in the World Development Report (1993, p. 134). This notes that:

> Nearly all countries face the same fundamental problems with human resources in the health sector. There are not enough primary care providers and too many specialists. Health workers are concentrated in urban areas. Training in public health, health policy, and health management have been relatively neglected.... A central role in delivery of most cost-effective health interventions belongs to primary care providers (ibid, p. 139).

The inequality of marginal met needs that is fostered by the current imbalance between the financing of the NT's urban hospital sector and the financing of primary and community care for remote communities within the NT is similarly consistent with the World Development Report's (1993, p. 8) finding that: "The health gain per dollar spent varies enormously across the range of interventions currently financed by governments." The recent construction of a spacious new marble-clad legislative building for the Northern Territory in Darwin, at a cost of some A$160 million, suggests that inequality of marginal unmet need may apply not just to health care expenditure, but also to public expenditure more generally.

CONCLUSIONS

The problems of Aboriginal health within the Northern Territory of Australia illustrate in acute form many of the lessons that need to be taken into account in determining the distribution of health care financing to disadvantaged populations. These lessons relate particularly to (*i*) the importance of factors other than health care as major determinants of population health; (*ii*) the importance of adequate attention and resources being given to culturally appropriate ways of addressing these other factors if health care expenditures are themselves to have lasting effect; (*iii*) the importance of improved primary and community care for disadvantaged communities; and (*iv*) the need to view current health problems within a wider historical context of a process of hysteresis resulting from past high levels of social and economic stress on entire communities.

We have argued that the analysis of Evans and others of the link between an individual's status in an occupational hierarchy, their stress level and the individual's health state needs widening to include considerations of social and economic stress on entire disadvantaged groups within the wider population, and of the role of positional goods in influencing health outcomes in this context. Acute levels of social and economic stress in the past have induced forms of both social and economic hysteresis, and associated low current health status for these disadvantaged groups. Overcoming these hysteresis effects now requires greater, and more carefully targeted, public expenditure on health and environmental services for such disadvantaged groups.

The experience of Aboriginal health within Australia illustrates the major inequalities that continue to exist in health outcomes across different communities. The process of dispossession and impairment of human and social capital that underlies much of the process of hysteresis has parallels not only with the experiences of other indigenous communities, in North America and elsewhere, but also with the process of de-industrialisation and long-term unemployment that has affected disadvantaged groups in many urban inner city areas. However, these are clearly subjects for a later paper.

REFERENCES

Altman, J. (1987) *Hunter-Gatherers Today: An Aboriginal Economy in North Australia.* Australian Institute of Aboriginal Studies, Canberra: ACT, Australia.

Altman, J. and Daly, A. (1995), Indigenous Australians in the Labour Market: Historical Trends and Future Prospects. *Economic Papers,* Economic Society of Australia 14(4): 64-73.

Australian Bureau of Statistics. (1991) 1991 Census of Population and Housing: Aboriginal Community Profile (ABS 2722.7) - Maningrida, Canberra, ACT.

Australian Bureau of Statistics (1994) *Northern Territory's Indigenous People: 1991 Census of Population and Housing.* Darwin, NT, Australia.

Australian Bureau of Statistics (1995) *National Aboriginal and Torres Strait Islander Survey 1994,* Canberra, ACT, Australia.

Australian Government Solicitor (1993) *Agreement between the Commonwealth of Australia and the Northern Territory in Relation to the Provision of Public Hospital Services.* Barton, ACT, Australia.

Barker, D. and Osmond, C. (1986) Infant mortality, childhood nutrition and ischaemic heart disease in England and Wales. *The Lancet i*:1077-81.

Barker, D. and Osmond, C. (1987) Inequalities in health in Britain: specific explanations in three Lancashire towns. *British Medical Journal* 294:749-752.

Barker, D., Winter, P., Osmond, C., *et al.* (1989) Weight in infancy and death from ischaemic heart disease. *The Lancet, ii*: 577-80.

Bhatia, K. and Anderson, P. (1995) *An Overview of Aboriginal and Torres Strait Islander Health: Present Status and Future Trends.* Australian Institute of Health and Welfare: Canberra, ACT, Australia.

Blainey, G. (1980) *A Land Half Won.* Macmillan Company of Australia: South Melbourne, Australia.

Bower, C., Stanley, F., Connell, A., *et al.* (1992) Birth defects in the infants of Aboriginal and non-Aboriginal mothers with diabetes in Western Australia. *Medical Journal of Australia* 156:520-523.

Bryce, S., Rowse, T., and Scrimgeour, D. (1992) Evaluating the petrol-sniffing prevention programmes of the healthy Aboriginal life team. *Australian Journal of Public Health* 16(4):387-396.

Carr-Hill, R.,Hardman, G., Martin, S., *et al.* (1994) *A Formula for Distributing NHS Revenues Based on Small Area Use of Hospital Beds* Centre for Health Economics, University of York, York, UK.

Commonwealth Grants Commission (1994a), *Report on General Revenue Grant Relativities 1994 Update.* Canberra, ACT, Australia.

Commonwealth Grants Commission (1994b) *Report on General Revenue Grant Relativities 1994 Update,* Volume 2. Canberra, ACT, Australia.

Commonwealth Grants Commission (1995) *Report on General Revenue Grant Relativities 1995 Update.* Working Papers: Dispersion Factors, Canberra, ACT, Australia.

CRESAP (1991) *Final Report of Review of Health and Community Services Northern Territory.* Darwin, NT, Australia.

Daly, A. and Hawke, A. (1994) How important is the welfare system as a source of income for indigenous Australians? *Economic Papers.* Economic Society of Australia 13(3):74-83.

Department of Health and Social Security (1976) *Sharing Resources for Health in England - Report of the Resource Allocation Working Party.* HMSO: London, UK.

Evans, R.G. (1994) *Introduction.* In Evans, R.G., Barer, M.L., and Marmor,T.R. editors, *Why Are Some People Healthy and Others Not? The Determinants of Health of Populations.* New York: Aldine De Gruyter, pp. 3-26.

Evans, R.G. (1996) Health, hierarchy and hominids - biological correlates of the socioeconomic gradients in health, Chapter 3. In Culyer, A. and Wagstaff, A., editors, *Reforming Health Care Systems: Experiments with the NHS.* Cheltenham, UK:Edward Elgar, pp. 35-64.

Evans, R.G., Barer, M.L., and Marmor, T.R. (eds.) (1994) *Why Are Some People*

Healthy and Others Not? The Determinants of Health of Populations. New York:Aldine De Gruyter.

Franklin, M.A. and White, I. (1991) The history and politics of Aboriginal health, Chapter 1. In Reid J. and Trompf, P., editors, *The Health of Aboriginal Australia.* Sydney Australia: Harcourt, Brace, Jovanovich, pp. 1-36.

Gray, A., Trompf, P. and Houston S. (1991) The decline and rise of Aboriginal families, Chapter 3. In Reid J. and Trompf, P., editors, *The Health of Aboriginal Australia.* Sydney Australia: Harcourt, Brace, Jovanovich, pp. 80 - 122.

Gray, D., Drandlich, M., Moore, L., *et al.* (1995) Aboriginal wellbeing and liquor licensing legislation in western Australia. *Australian Journal of Public Health,* 19:(2):177-185.

Guest, C.S. and O'Dea, K. (1992) Diabetes in Aborigines and other Australian populations. *Australian Journal of Public Health* 16(4):340-349.

Guest, C., O'Dea, K., Carlin, J. and Larkins, R. (1992) Smoking in Aborigines and persons of European descent in southeastern Australia: prevalence and associations with food habits, body fat distribution and other cardiovascular risk factors. *Australian Journal of Public Health* 16 (4):397-402.

Health Ministers' Forum (1994) *The Development of the National Health Policy.* Canberra, ACT, Australia.

Hirsch, F. (1977) *Social Limits To Growth* . London: Routledge and Kegan Paul.

Hogg, R.S. (1992) Indigenous mortality: placing Australian Aboriginal mortality within a broader context. *Social Science and Medicine* 35(3):335-346.

Hoy, W., Mathews, J., and Pugsley, D. (1995a) Treatment of Australian Aboriginals with end-stage renal disease in the top end of the Northern Territory: 1978-93. *Nephrology* 1:307-313.

Hoy, W., Mathews, J., and Pugsley ,D. (1995b) A brief health profile of adults in a northern territory Aboriginal community, with an emphasis on preventable morbidities, mimeo. submitted to *Australian Journal of Public Health.*

Marmot, M. G., Rose, G., Shipley, M., and Hamilton, P. (1978) Employment grade and coronary heart disease in British civil servants, *Journal of Epidemiological and Community Health* 32: 244 -249.

Menzies School of Health Research (1995) *Feasibility Study and Service Plan of Health Services at Maningrida.* Final Report. Darwin, NT, Australia.

Moodie, P.M. (1973) *Aboriginal Health.* Australian National University Press: Canberra, ACT, Australia.

Mooney, G. (1983) Equity in health care: confronting the confusion. *Effective*

Health Care 1:179-85.

Munoz, E., Powers, J., and Mathews, J.D. (1992a) Hospitalisation patterns in children from 10 Aboriginal Communities in the Northern Territory. *Medical Journal of Australia* 156: 524-528.

Munoz, E., Powers, J., Nienhuys, T., and Mathews, J.D. (1992b) Social and environmental factors in 10 Aboriginal communities in the Northern Territory: relationship to hospital admissions of children. *Medical Journal of Australia* 156:529-533.

Neel, J.V. (1962) Diabetes mellitus: a thrifty genotype rendered detrimental by "Progress"? *American Journal of Human Genetics* 13:353-362.

Neel, J. V. (1982) The thrifty genotype revisited. In Kobberling, J. and Tattersall, R., editors, *The Genetics of Diabetes Mellitus* London: Academic Press, UK, pp. 283-293.

O'Dea, K. (1991) Westernisation, insulin resistance and diabetes in Australian Aborigines. *Medical Journal of Australia* 155:258-264.

Phillips, C., Patel, M., and Weeramanthri, T. (1995) High mortality from renal disease and infection in Aboriginal central Australians with diabetes. *Australian Journal of Public Health* 19(5):482-491.

Pholeros, P., Rainow, S., and Torzillo, P. (1993) *Housing for Health*, HealtHabitat, Newport Beach, NSW, Australia.

Plant, A., Condon, J., and Durling, G. (1995) *Northern Territory Health Outcomes: Morbidity and Mortality, 1979 - 1991.* NT Department of Health and Community Services: Casuarina, NT, Australia.

Plant, A., Krause, V., Condon, J., and Kerr, C. (1995) Aborigines and tuberculosis: why they are at risk. *Australian Journal of Public Health* 19(5):487-491.

Reid, J. and Lupton, D. (1991) Introduction. In Reid, J. and Trompf, P., editors, *The Health of Aboriginal Australia*, pp. xi - xxii.

Reid, J. and Trompf, P. (eds.) (1991) *The Health of Aboriginal Australia.* Sydney, Australia: Harcourt Brace Jovanovich.

Reynolds, H. (1981) *The Other Side of the Frontier: An Interpretation of the Aboriginal Response to the Invasion and Settlement of Australia,* Townsville, Queensland, Australia: James Cook University.

Rowse, T. (1993) *Remote Possibilities.* Canberra, ACT, Australia: Aboriginal Studies Press.

Saggers, S. and Gray, D. (1991) *Aboriginal Health and Society,* Sydney, NSW, Australia: Allen and Unwin.

Smith, R., Spargo, R., Hunter, E., *et al.* (1992) Prevalence of hypertension in Kimberley Aborigines and its relationship to ischaemic heart disease *Medical Journal of Australia* 156:557-562.

Stone, S.N. editor (1974) *Aborigines in White Australia.* Melbourne, Australia: Heinemann.

Taylor, J.C. (1977) Diet, health and economy: some consequences of planned social change in an Aboriginal community. In Berndt, R.M., editor, *Aborigines and Change: Australia in the 70s.* Canberra, ACT, Australia: Australian Institute of Aboriginal Studies, pp. 147-158.

The Economist (1994) The Unhealthy Poor, 4th June, pp. 27-28.

Thomson, N. (1984) Australian Aboriginal health and health care. *Social Science and Medicine* 18:939-948.

Thomson, N.(1991a) Recent trends in Aboriginal mortality. *Medical Journal of Australia* 154:235-239.

Thomson, N. (1991b) A review of Aboriginal health status, Chapter 2. In Reid, J. and Trompf, P., editors, *The Health of Aboriginal Australia*, Sydney, Australia: Harcourt, Brace, Jovanovich, pp. 37-79.

Thomson, N. and Briscoe, N. (1991) *Overview of Aboriginal Health Status in the Northern Territory*, Canberra, ACT, Australia:Australian Institute of Health.

Townsend, P. and Davidson, N., editors. (1982*) Inequalities in Health: the Black Report.* Harmondsworth, UK: Penguin.

United Nations (1995) *Demographic Yearbook 1993.* New York: UN Department for Economic and Social Information and Policy Analysis.

Warchivker, I. (1996) Variations in Health care expenditure in the Alice Springs Rural District in 1993-94. *Australian and New Zealand Journal of Public Health* 20(1):11-13.

Weeramanthri, T., D'Abbs, P., and Mathews, J.D. (1994) Towards a direct definition of an alcohol-related death: an analysis of Aboriginal adults. *Australian Journal of Public Health,* 18(1):71-78.

White, I., editor (1985) *Daisy Bates: The Native Tribes of Western Australia.* Canberra, ACT: Australia: National Library of Australia.

Wilkinson, R.G. (1992) Income distribution and life expectancy. *British Medical Journal* 304:165-168.

World Development Report (1993) *Investing in Health.* New York: Oxford University Press for the World Bank.

Wright, J. (1995) *Aboriginal Health Needs Pilot Project: Community X.* Casuarina, NT, Australia: NT Department of Health and Community Services.

3

Parents' Schooling and Investments in the Health Capital of Children - Multisample Estimates from Bangladesh and The Philippines

DAVID M. BISHAI
The Johns Hopkins University
School of Hygiene and Public Health
Baltimore, MD

ABSTRACT

A child health production function is developed based on a dynamic stochastic version of Grossman's model of health capital. The model indicates that because health has the properties of a durable good, even when the effects of health on future earnings are neglected, investments in health capital will have

Health, Health Care and Health Economics: Perspectives on Distribution
Edited by Morris L. Barer, Thomas E. Getzen, and Greg L. Stoddart
Copyright 1998 John Wiley & Sons, Ltd.

a financial payoff in terms of lower shadow prices for health in the future. In the empirical implementation the key feature is an interaction term between a caregiver's schooling and their exposure time to the child. I estimate the production function using a 2SLS fixed effects model with lagged child care time, resource allocation, and child health as instruments for the first differences of these same endogenous variables. The 1978 Intrafamily Food Distribution and Feeding Practices Survey dataset from Bangladesh is used together with census data for one set of estimates. The 1984 Philippines Cash Cropping Survey data set is used for another. The production function estimates indicate that part of the salutary effect of parents' education on child health requires that the child actually be exposed to the educated parent. Younger caregiver age and male caregiver sex enhanced the productivity of child care time. Given the demographic makeup of the Bangladesh study sample teenage brothers and fathers would have the highest marginal productivity for child health and mothers and grandmothers the least. The robustness of the model across the two samples was tested with an LM test that supported the hypothesis that the effect of quality time was the same in the two samples. If economic opportunity draws mothers away from child care, the presence of other household members with higher schooling levels offers the potential for an improvement in the overall quality of child care time. In the present study the households failed to set the marginal labor product of child health for each of the caregivers equal. In an environment where there is little variation in wages for household members this would indicate that the quality of child care may not be the household's sole concern in determining time allocation.

INTRODUCTION

This paper adapts the standard Grossman model of health capital to a dynamic stochastic framework wherein parents invest in the health capital of children. Within this framework I focus on how parental schooling influences child survival. The goal is to determine whether the extensively documented association between parents' schooling and child health (See Hobcraft, 1993 for a review) is influenced by the time spent in child care by the schooled parent. There has been some evidence to suggest that the effect of parents' schooling on child health might operate completely through the effect of a familial hereditable endowment (Behrman & Wolfe, 1987). The demonstration of a significant interaction between time spent and parents' schooling would argue strongly that schooling actually influences the child health productivity of the parents. A related goal is to ask whether the health production technology which ought to represent a stable biological process is robust across disparate populations.

The null hypothesis for this study is that the salutary effect of a parent's schooling on her child's health is unaffected by the time spent by the parent in direct child care.

THEORETICAL MODEL

For the generic household with J children indexed by j, K adults indexed by k and I persons indexed by i, define the following vectors (vectors are depicted in bold):

$$\mathbf{H}_t = \left(H_{1t}, \ldots H_{jt}, \ldots H_{Jt} \right)$$

$$\mathbf{Z}_t = \left(z_{1t}, \ldots z_{it}, \ldots z_{It} \right)$$

$$\mathbf{M}_t = \left(M_{1t}, \ldots M_{jt}, \ldots M_{Jt} \right)$$

$$\mathbf{TH}_t = \left(TH_{11t}, \ldots TH_{1Kt}, \ \ldots \ TH_{j1t}, \ldots TH_{jKt}, \ \ldots \ TH_{J1t}, \ldots TH_{JKt} \right)$$

where
H_{jt} is the health stock of the jth child at time t
z_{it} is the consumption of non health-related goods by the ith household member at time t
M_{jt} is the consumption of health-related goods by the jth child at time t
TH_{jkt} is the childcare time allocated to the jth child by the kth adult at time t.

The problem at hand can be cast as a stochastic control problem where for each period the household seeks to select $\mathbf{Z}_t$, $\mathbf{TH}_t$, and $\mathbf{M}_t$ to maximize:

[1] $E_s \sum_{t=s}^{\tau} \beta^t \, U(\mathbf{H}_t, \mathbf{Z}_t)$

subject to the intertemporal budget constraint and health production function whose equations are:

[2] $A_{t+1} = (1 + r_t)[A_t - \mathbf{Z}_t \mathbf{P}_t - \mathbf{M}_t \mathbf{V}_t - \mathbf{TH}_t \mathbf{w}_t + \Omega \omega_t]$

[3] $H_{jt+1} = I(M_{jt}, TH_{j1t}, \ldots TH_{jKt}, \tilde{X}_{jt}, H_{jt}) + \delta(\tilde{X}_{jt}, a_{jt}) H_{jt}$

E_s represents expectations taken at time s
β represents the rate of time preference
A_t denotes assets at the beginning of period t.
P_t is the real price vector for non health-related goods
V_t is the real price vector for health-related goods
$w_t = (\underset{\sim J}{1} \otimes \omega_t)$ where ω_t is the real wage K- vector for the K adult household members over time
Ω is the full endowment of time vector for the K adult household members
H_{jt} denotes health stock at the beginning of period t.
$I_t(\ )$ is the investment in health stock of the j_{th} child at time t.
a_{jt} is the age of child j at time t
$\tilde{X}_{jt}$ is a stochastic influence of exogenous environmental factors such as injury and illness.
δ_t is the durability of the health stock: $\delta_t = 1$-depreciation. (Stochastic variables are denoted with ~.)

I assume $\tilde{X}_{jt}$ becomes known only at the end of period t, after decisions about z_{it}, M_{jt} , and TH_{jkt} have been made. $\tilde{X}_{jt}$ is governed by a first-order Markov process, with transitions governed by

[4] $\text{prob}\{X_{jt} \leq X' \mid X_{jt-1} = X\} = F(X', X)$

For a household with J children a vector of health shocks can be defined as
$\tilde{\mathbf{X}}_t = \left(\tilde{X}_{1t} \ldots \tilde{X}_{jt}, \ldots \tilde{X}_{Jt} \right)$

Equation [3] is different from the standard health capital model of

Grossman. In particular the net return to health investment is assumed to depend on the current health state as well as on stochastic shocks. In reality, stochastic factors such as illness, injury, and current health capital do alter the net return to health investment. However, as will be seen, imposing this condition severely lessens tractability. I will revert to the conventional Grossman specification below after illustrating the difficulties of a more realistic model.

The timing in the model is such that when time t decisions must be made, the household knows H_t and $\tilde{X}_t$, $\tilde{X}_{t-1}$,...

State

Define the state as vector $\chi_t = (A_t, H_t, \tilde{X}_{t-1})$ which can be partitioned as $(\gamma_t, \tilde{X}_{t-1})$ with nonstochastic component vector $\gamma_t = (A_t, H_t)$.

Control

The control is defined as vector $\hat{u}_t = (M_t, TH_t, Z_t)$.

Equations of motion for the State

The transition equation for the nonstochastic portion of the state γ_t is given by $(A_{t+1}, H_{t+1}) = g(A_t, H_t, \hat{u}_t)$

[5] $\qquad A_{t+1} = (1 + r_t)[A_t - Z_t P_t - M_t V_t - TH_t w_t + \Omega \omega_t]$

[6] $\qquad H_{jt+1} = I(M_{jt}, TH_{j1t}, ... TH_{jKt}, \tilde{X}_{jt}, H_{jt}) + \delta(\tilde{X}_{jt}, a_{jt}) H_{jt}$

The transition equation for $\tilde{X}_{t-1}$ is implicitly defined by F(X',X).

Return

The return function is $U(\mathbf{H}_t, \mathbf{Z}_t)$

Bellman's Equation

Then Bellman's functional equation is

[7] $W(\chi_t) = \underset{\hat{a}_t}{Max}\{U(\chi_t, \hat{a}_t) + \beta\ E_t\ (W[g(\chi_t, \hat{a}_t)])\}$

where E_t represents the expectations operation taking place at time t.

First Order Conditions

The first-order necessary conditions for the problem can be presented after substituting in the following:

$$\frac{\partial\ A_{t+1}}{\partial\ TH_t} = -w_t(1 + r_t) \qquad\qquad \frac{\partial\ H_{t+1}}{\partial\ TH_t} = \tilde{I}_{TH_t}$$

$$\frac{\partial\ A_{t+1}}{\partial\ Z_t} = -P_t(1 + r_t) \qquad\qquad \frac{\partial\ H_{t+1}}{\partial\ Z_t} = 0$$

$$\frac{\partial\ A_{t+1}}{\partial\ M_t} = -V_t(1 + r_t) \qquad\qquad \frac{\partial\ H_{t+1}}{\partial\ M_t} = \tilde{I}_{M_t}$$

to yield

[8] $TH : -w_t(1 + r_t)\beta\ E_t\left(\dfrac{\partial\ W}{\partial\ A_{t+1}}\right) + \beta\ E_t\left(\dfrac{\partial\ W}{\partial\ H_{t+1}}\tilde{I}_{TH_t}\right) = 0$

[9] $Z : \dfrac{\partial\ U}{\partial\ Z_t} - P_t(1 + r_t)\beta\ E_t\left(\dfrac{\partial\ W}{\partial\ A_{t+1}}\right) = 0$

[10] $M : -V_t(1+r_t)\beta \ E_t\left(\dfrac{\partial \ W}{\partial \ A_{t+1}}\right) + \beta \ E_t\left(\dfrac{\partial \ W}{\partial \ H_{t+1}}\tilde{I}_{M_t}\right) = 0$

Benveniste-Scheinkman (Envelope) Equation

[11] $\dfrac{\partial \ W}{\partial \ A_t} = \dfrac{\partial \ U}{\partial \ A_t} + \beta \ E_t\left(\dfrac{\partial \ W}{\partial \ A_{t+1}}\dfrac{\partial \ A_{t+1}}{\partial \ A_t}\right) = \beta(1+r_t)E_t\left(\dfrac{\partial \ W}{\partial \ A_{t+1}}\right)$

[12] $\dfrac{\partial \ W}{\partial \ H_t} = \dfrac{\partial \ U}{\partial \ H_t} + \beta \ E_t\left(\dfrac{\partial \ W}{\partial \ H_{t+1}}\dfrac{\partial \ H_{t+1}}{\partial \ H_t}\right)$

$= \dfrac{\partial \ U}{\partial \ H_t} + \beta \ E_t\left(\dfrac{\partial \ W}{\partial \ H_{t+1}}(\tilde{I}_{H_t} + \delta_t)\right)$

Equation [9] offers an expression for $\beta \ E_t\left(\dfrac{\partial \ W}{\partial \ A_{t+1}}\right)$ as follows:

[13] $\beta \ E_t\left(\dfrac{\partial \ W}{\partial \ A_{t+1}}\right) = \dfrac{P_t^{-1}}{(1+r_t)}\dfrac{\partial \ U}{\partial \ Z_t}$

which can be substituted in Equation [11] yielding

[14] $\dfrac{\partial \ W}{\partial \ A_t} = P_t^{-1}\dfrac{\partial \ U}{\partial \ Z_t}$

with its updated version

$\dfrac{\partial \ W}{\partial \ A_{t+1}} = P_{t+1}^{-1}\dfrac{\partial \ U}{\partial \ Z_{t+1}}$

Euler Equation for Commodities

The updated expression can be substituted back into [9] to provide an Euler equation governing the intertemporal progress of the marginal utility of commodity consumption.

$$[15] \qquad \frac{\partial U}{\partial Z_t} = \beta(1+r_t)E_t\left(\frac{\partial U}{\partial Z_{t+1}}\right)$$

Euler Equation for Health

I turn my attention now to Equation [8] and attempt to eliminate the terms involving W. First I apply equation [13] to the first term of [8] to produce:

$$[16] \qquad -w_t P_t^{-1}\frac{\partial U}{\partial Z_t} + \beta E_t\left(\frac{\partial W}{\partial H_{t+1}}\tilde{I}_{TH_t}\right) = 0$$

I note that due to the timing of the expectations,

$$E_t\left(\frac{\partial W}{\partial H_{t+1}}\tilde{I}_{TH_t}\right) = E_t\left(\frac{\partial W}{\partial H_{t+1}}\right)\tilde{I}_{TH_t}$$

After some algebra [16] yields an expression for $\beta E_t\left(\dfrac{\partial W}{\partial H_{t+1}}\right)$ as follows:

$$[17] \qquad \beta E_t\left(\frac{\partial W}{\partial H_{t+1}}\right) = w_t P_t^{-1}\frac{\partial U}{\partial Z_t}\tilde{I}_{TH_t}^{-1}$$

This result can now be substituted into [12] to yield:

$$[18] \qquad \frac{\partial W}{\partial H_t} = \frac{\partial U}{\partial H_t} + w_t P_t^{-1}\frac{\partial U}{\partial Z_t}\tilde{I}_{TH_t}^{-1}(\tilde{I}_{H_t} + \tilde{\delta}_t)$$

which can be updated to yield :

$$\frac{\partial W}{\partial H_{t+1}} = \frac{\partial U}{\partial H_{t+1}} + w_{t+1}P_{t+1}^{-1}\frac{\partial U}{\partial Z_{t+1}}\tilde{I}_{TH_{t+1}}^{-1}(\tilde{I}_{H_{t+1}} + \tilde{\delta}_{t+1})$$

Finally [18] can be transformed into

$$[19] \quad \beta E_t \left(\frac{\partial W}{\partial H_{t+1}} \right) = \beta E_t \left(\frac{\partial U}{\partial H_{t+1}} \right) + \beta E_t \left(w_{t+1} P_{t+1}^{-1} \frac{\partial U}{\partial Z_{t+1}} \tilde{I}_{TH_{t+1}}^{-1} (\tilde{I}_{H_{t+1}} + \tilde{\delta}_{t+1}) \right)$$

then combined with [17] to produce:

$$[20] \quad w_t P_t^{-1} \left(\frac{\partial U}{\partial Z_t} \right) \tilde{I}_{TH_t}^{-1} = \beta E_t \left(\frac{\partial U}{\partial H_{t+1}} \right) + \beta E_t \left(w_{t+1} P_{t+1}^{-1} \frac{\partial U}{\partial Z_{t+1}} \tilde{I}_{TH_{t+1}}^{-1} (\tilde{I}_{H_{t+1}} + \tilde{\delta}_{t+1}) \right)$$

At this point the model's treatment of returns to health investment as stochastic impedes tractability. The model can be greatly simplified if at this point I relax that assumption to permit perfect foresight regarding future realizations of I_{TH}, I_H, w, P, V, and r.

$$[21] \quad w_t P_t^{-1} \left(\frac{\partial U}{\partial Z_t} \right) \tilde{I}_{TH_t}^{-1} = E_t \left(\frac{\partial U}{\partial H_{t+1}} \right) + w_{t+1} P_{t+1}^{-1} E_t \left(\frac{\partial U}{\partial Z_{t+1}} \right) \tilde{I}_{TH_{t+1}}^{-1} (\tilde{I}_{H_{t+1}} + \tilde{\delta}_{t+1})$$

Applying [15] and making the approximation that $w_{t+1} \cong w_t$, $P_{t+1} \cong P_t$, and that the marginal product vector of childcare time I_{TH} is constant yields:

$$[22] \quad w_t P_t^{-1} (1 + r - (\tilde{I}_{H_{t+1}} + \tilde{\delta}_{t+1})) \tilde{I}_{TH_t}^{-1} \left(\frac{\partial U}{\partial Z_{t+1}} \right) = E_t \left(\frac{\partial U}{\partial H_{t+1}} \right)$$

Defining π_t, the shadow prices of children's health capital as follows:

$$[23] \quad \pi_{t+1} = w_t P_t^{-1} (1 + r - (\tilde{I}_{H_{t+1}} + \tilde{\delta}_{t+1})) \tilde{I}_{TH}^{-1}$$

or taking Z as numeraire and setting $P = 1$

$$\pi_{t+1} = w_t (1 + r - (\tilde{I}_{H_{t+2}} + \tilde{\delta}_{t+1})) \tilde{I}_{TH}^{-1}$$

and again applying [15] to [22] and a date t version of [22] produces the familiar Euler equation.

$$[24] \quad \frac{\partial U}{\partial H_t} \pi_t^{-1} = \beta (1+r) E_t \left(\frac{\partial U}{\partial H_{t+1}} \right) \pi_{t+1}^{-1}$$

The most notable feature of the price of health capital here is the result that an increase in the health stock at any time has investment implications in that it makes it easier to achieve any given health stock subsequently. Considering the formula for π_{t+1} above reveals that the shadow price of the health capital gained at time t+1 through an increment in period t health production time offers a discount below the conventional effective price of wI_{TH}^{-1}. The discount is proportional to the marginal product of the period t+1 health stock in facilitating future health gains. The discount increases with the durability of health capital.

Investing in health today makes future investments in health less costly. As a durable good health has quasi-investment properties. One can desire health as a pure consumption good but health expenditure today pays a financial dividend in the form of less costly health purchases in the future. The durable goods nature of health capital is implicit in Grossman's model of health capital (Grossman, 1972a, 1972b). Foster uses epsilon delta arguments to derive a rental price of health capital and an Euler equation very similar to the one presented here (Foster, 1995). The dynamic analytic approach to this result which I have presented here is new.

BANGLADESH DATA

The most extensive data used to estimate the model come from the Intrafamily Food Distribution and Feeding Practices Survey conducted in Matlab, Bangladesh in 1978 under the direction of Dr. Lincoln Chen. The primary focus of the study was to collect micro level data on nutrition, work activities, anthropometric outcomes, and morbidity. Baseline data on 882 children under 5 years of age from six villages was obtained in February and

March of 1978 from which a sampling frame was constructed. Inclusion criteria were twofold: presence of one or more children under 5 and accessibility from the field research station (Chen, Huq, *et al.*, 1981). Sample selection was thus not fully random. This narrowed the sample to 207 children in 130 different households. All of the families were Muslim. Data collection commenced in June-August and continued bimonthly for 12 months.

The dataset includes total calories, total protein, and breastfeeding status measured every 2 months assayed by direct observation of meals and apportionment. Of special interest for our study, the data set includes the observed total number of hours spent per day by each household adult and older sibling in child care measured every 2 months. Household assets and land holdings were also delineated, and various forms of household expenditure are tallied. Unfortunately, the first round observations on child care time allocations for all but 34 of the children are missing and this round was therefore discarded. As indicated in Table 1, missing variables were encountered for some of the other entries, further shrinking the dataset. This leaves 5 total rounds of information, but only 4 rounds of lagged information to regress upon, thus the maximum number of complete observations is 4 x 207 = 828. Regressions employing differenced data naturally use up one of the rounds in the differencing and can only hope to employ 621 observations. My estimation method calls for the inclusion of lagged, differenced, health capital $\Delta H_{j,t-1}$, as an independent variable. Heeding this call would use up still another round of information.

Juxtaposed against the household survey data is the 1982 census data for the region which includes education type, years of schooling, and source of drinking water. Table 1 displays the sample means of the variables of interest. Starred items enter the model after having been transformed by $\log(x+1)$. Because some of these items include zero for many households, direct logarithms would have artificially scored much of the data as missing. Anthropometric data were normalized using Z-scores relative to the reference population of the National Center for Health Statistics and CDC Center for Disease Control (1994). I confine my analysis to weight for height as the most sensitive indicator of short term health effects such as wasting (Waterlow, 1973). Because the standard population to which these Z-scores refer is an

Table 1 Description of Variables from Bangladesh

Variable	Mean	Std. Dev.	Obs
Weight for Height 5Percentile	12.8769	23.9075	1035
Weight for Height Z-Score**	-1.5631	1.0066	1035
Illness Days*	26.4406	21.4859	1035
Bed Days*	1.2937	4.2196	1035
Calories per Day*	796.132	496.4114	1035
Cereal Protein per Day*	153.1814	92.3229	1035
Non Cereal Protein per Day*	77.9474	92.9895	1035
Age in Months	28.8792	16.6389	207
Sex of Child (0=Male)	0.4541	0.4991	207
Mother's Age in Year	29.8317	6.7027	202
Father's Age in Years	40.3005	8.7959	193
Avg. Age of Brothers in Years	10.3709	4.8735	152
Avg. Age of Sisters in Years	9.5524	3.8952	131
Avg. Age of Uncles in Years	30.2261	13.4002	69
Avg. Age of Aunts in Years	24.4143	12.6896	70
Grandmother's Age in Years	61.2371	11.428	97
Grandfather's Age in Years	66.3429	9.2956	35
Mother's Education in Years*	1.7723	2.3239	202
Father's Education in Years*	3.1503	3.2183	193
Avg. Education of Brothers in Years*	2.0696	2.1795	152
Avg. Education of Sisters in Years*	1.3308	1.5644	131
Avg. Education of Uncles in Years*	3.8618	3.3479	69
Avg. Education of Aunts in Years*	1.8214	2.3181	70
Grandmother's Education in Years*	0.4845	1.3159	97
Grandfather's Education in Years*	2.0857	2.7048	35
Mother's Child Care Time Fraction Whole Sample	0.5217	0.2439	1035
Father's Child Care Time Fraction Whole Sample	0.0261	0.0616	1035
Brother's Child Care Time Fraction Whole Sample	0.0737	0.1137	1035
Sister's Child Care Time Fraction Whole Sample	0.1345	0.1716	1035
Uncle's Child Care Time Fraction Whole Sample	0.0119	0.0517	1035
Aunt's Child Care Time Fraction Whole Sample	0.0054	0.0312	1035
Grandmother's Child Care Time Fraction Whole Sample	0.0536	0.1101	1035
Grandfather's Child Care Time Fraction Whole Sample	0.0051	0.0272	1035
Mother's Child Care Time Fraction Where Mother Exists	0.5715	0.1917	939
Father's Child Care Time Fraction where Father Exists	0.0291	0.0634	901
Brother's Child Care Time Fraction Where Brother Exists	0.0988	0.1261	710
Sister's Child Care Time Fraction Where Sister Exists	0.2169	0.1778	604
Uncle's Child Care Time Fraction where Uncle Exists	0.0109	0.0425	311
Aunt's Child Care Time Fraction Where Aunt Exists	0.027	0.0743	323
Grandmother's Child Care Time Fraction Where She Exists	0.1134	0.141	428
Grandfather's Child Care Time Fraction Where He Exists	0.0321	0.0627	155

*Indicates that variable will be transformed by log(X+1) prior to regression

**Indicates that variable will be transformed by log (X+10) prior to regression

American one, I am also   taking advantage of the documented racial insensitivity of weight for height norms (Waterlow, 1973). Since Z-scores naturally range below zero they are transformed by $\log(x+10)$.

The dataset suffers from the absence of reliable information about wages. Self-reported wages were elicited but were coded as zero or missing for over half of the respondents.

PHILIPPINES DATA

The Philippine Cash Cropping Project collected data from a stratified random panel of 448 farming households including 673 children in Bukidnon, Philippines.   Respondents from each household were interviewed in four rounds at four month intervals in 1984-85.   The data was collected under the aegis of the International Food Policy Research Institute by Bouis and Haddad (Bouis and Haddad, 1990).   Barrios (villages) were first separated into three classifications based on the predominant crop type.   Within these strata, households and barrios were selected randomly.   There is information in each round on weight, height, and calorie intake for each household member. Baseline demographic data includes age, education , and land owned. The most significant drawback of the dataset is that child care time allocation information is available only for mothers.   Thus when I compute education-weighted child care time it can only be a partial account of the child's exposure to educated caregivers except for cases (unknown to me) in which the mother delivered 100% of the child care.

Table 2 shows the descriptive statistics for the sample children used for analysis.   The most stunning feature of this dataset is that the mean education of the mothers exceeds that for fathers.   This result holds true even when I exclude all mothers with more than 10 years of education to control for any possible outliers.

Table 2 Description of Variables from Philippines

Variable	Mean	Std. Dev.	Obs
Weight for Height Percentile	36.82594	20.68558	2594
Weight for Height Z-Score**	-0.55469	0.870972	2594
Illness Days*	1.748421	3.443796	2691
Calories per Day*	1694.848	860.9325	2256
Cereal Protein per Day*	37.00091	19.45587	2256
Age in Months	38.18868	16.18733	636
Sex of Child (0=Male)	0.462264	0.498672	636
Father's Education in Years*	5.625557	3.031273	637
Mother's Education in Years*	6.251863	2.729837	671
Mother's Child Care Time Fraction	87.7533	115.2448	2644
Mother's Age in Years	32.27156	6.8547	673

*Indicates that variable will be transformed by log(X+1) prior to regression
**Indicates that variable will be transformed by log(X+10) prior to regression

The sample of children from the Philippines, although impoverished, is better off in many ways than the children from Bangladesh. In making this comparison it bears note that the Filipino children are on average 10 months older than the Bangladeshi children and have a full 25 percentile points greater weight for height. Their mean calorie intake is nearly double that of the Bangladeshi children -- a difference that is not fully accounted for by the difference in age.

EMPIRICAL IMPLEMENTATION

Taking logs of [24] and rearranging yields:

$$[25] \quad \Delta \log\left(\frac{\partial U}{\partial H_t}\right) = \Delta \log(\pi_t) - \log(\beta(1+r)) + \log(e_t) + \log(\mu_t)$$

where Δx denotes $x_{t+1} - x_t$ and where μ_t denotes an error term that is assumed independent and identically distributed and has zero mean.

I now subsume $\beta(1+r)$ in a constant term denoted C and impose a Cobb-

Douglas functional form for utility and impose the definition for π_t with the approximation that r and δ are roughly constant across the short (2 month) time frame of the dataset and that I_H is small; $\log(1+r-I_H - \delta) = \log(1-I_H) \approx 0.5(r-I_H-\delta)$, to derive the following:

[26] $\quad \Delta \log H_{jt} = C + \gamma_w \Delta \log w_{jt} + \gamma_{MP} \Delta \log\left(I_{TH\,jt} \right) + \gamma_{MP} \Delta (I_{H_g}) + \log(\mu_t)$

Referring back to [3] suggests that appropriate control for I_H and I_{TH} would include measures of health-altering goods, childcare times of all caregivers, age, lagged health stock, and the unobserved health endowment, e.

[27] $\quad \Delta \log H_{jt} = C + \gamma_w \Delta \log w_{jt} + \gamma_M \Delta \log\left(M_{jt} \right) + \gamma_{TH} \Delta \log(TH_{jt}) + \gamma_a \Delta \log(a_{jt}) +$
$\qquad \gamma_H \Delta \log(H_{jt-1}) + \log(e_j) + \log(\mu_t)$

Quality Adjusted Time Inputs

The K-vector γ_{TH}, of returns to childcare time of each of the K child care givers is the focus of this investigation. If the fundamental determinant of the quality of child care time were thought to be the nature of the caregiver's kinship tie to the child I could simply estimate the model using relationship-specific dummies to denote time provided by mother, father, sister, brother, etc. However I believe it is more fruitful to investigate the notion that quality is determined by educational attainments of the caregivers as suggested by a vast accumulation of literature on maternal education and child health. Because education is correlated with age and gender, which may exert independent effects on childcare quality, these will need to be controlled for.

To incorporate the notion that there is variation in the quality of care provided by the child care givers I will introduce a productivity measure denoted PTY_k for each of the K caregivers. I propose to estimate the parameter for the interaction between $TH_k * PTY_k$. I assume that child care quality depends log-linearly on the education, E_k, age, a_k, and gender, G_k of the caregiver. Given the luxury of an enormous dataset, it might be fruitful to explore the parameters for age, gender, and education separately for mother, father, sister, brother, etc. Unfortunately this exercise is extremely taxing for more modest data sets. I therefore make the assumption that the parameters for returns to education-adjusted childcare time, age-adjusted childcare time, and gender-adjusted childcare time are the same for all caregivers. I can now sum the interaction terms across child care providers to produce:

$$\text{education-adjusted childcare hours} = \sum_{k=1}^{K} TH_k \log(E_k)$$

$$\text{age-adjusted childcare hours} = \sum_{k=1}^{K} TH_k \log(a_k)$$

$$\text{and gender-adjusted childcare hours} = \sum_{k=1}^{K} TH_k G_k \cdot$$

In each of these constructions I normalize TH_k such that $\sum_{k=1}^{K} TH_k = 1$.

There is some variation in the total number of childcare hours received per child per week. In my opinion most of this variation is determined by the child's sleep-wake cycle and may, through this means, be correlated with health outcomes. Essentially I am imposing a production process that provides no return to providing child care hours in excess of the total number of waking hours of the child. Since the data collection was structured such that each child had only as many child care hours as waking hours, I gain no understanding of returns to hours by not normalizing. Thus normalized time provides a unitless measure of the "dose" of childcare quality delivered to the child. The issue is returns to the quality-mediating factors -- not returns to time itself. I note that in terms of available variables M_i turns out to be calories and protein. At this juncture the health production function has the following form:

[28]

$$\Delta \log H_{jt} = C + \gamma_w \Delta \log w_{jt} + \gamma_{CAL} \Delta \log\left(CAL_{jt}\right) + \gamma_{PRO} \Delta \log\left(PRO_{jt}\right) + \gamma_{ETH} \Delta \sum_{k=1}^{K} TH_{kt} \log(E_k) +$$

$$\gamma_{aTH} \Delta \sum_{k=1}^{K} TH_{kt} \log(a_k) + \gamma_{GTH} \Delta \sum_{k=1}^{K} TH_{kt} G + \gamma_a \Delta \log(a_{jt}) +$$

$$\gamma_H \Delta \log(H_{jt-1}) + \Delta \log(e_j) + \log(\mu_t)$$

Controlling for Fixed Effects Bias in Production Function Estimates

In my specification of [28] I have indicated that the independent variable is correlated with the unobservable (to the researcher) familial and individual fixed effects denoted above as e_j. The household may very well garner information about these fixed effects and adjust for them in its allocations of resources and child care time. Thus were [28] to be estimated using levels data it would contain bias from correlation between the regressors and the fixed effect which is subsumed in the error term. Because these individual fixed effects are assumed constant, it turns out that as specified in [28] $\Delta\log(e_j) = 0$. The differenced specification controls for the unobservable fixed effects.

Because the input variables are measured with error it would be helpful to adopt an instrumental variables approach provided that instruments for M and TH can be had. Following Rosenzweig and Wolpin (Rosenzweig, 1988) I use measurements of the lagged level variables of health inputs and health measures as instruments for the differences which enter the right hand side of [28]. In essence this requires the assumptions that 1) Allocations to child j at time t are uncorrelated with any unforeseen period specific stochastic shock to child j's health at a more remote future time, and 2) Health capital is AR(1). Naturally, allocations to child j at time t are correlated with past health disturbances of longer duration, but I am assuming that the effects of these disturbances never skip periods. The effect of a stochastic health shock at time t-2 cannot disappear at time t-1, then reappear at time t. Most physiological and cultural processes that would transmit a signal between inputs at time t and future stochastic shocks to the health outcome or vice versa would tend to endure across several time periods *e.g.*, the development of chronic disease or the introduction of a social service institution.

BANGLADESH RESULTS

Different measures used to approximate the children's health capital can be expected to vary in their reliability and suitability. Reporting bias which varies systematically with the socioeconomic status of the household can be anticipated in the reports of recalled bed days and illness days (Sindelar and Thomas, 1991; Foster, 1994). Given that a bed day includes an observable change in behavior (albeit one that is itself mediated by choice as well as pathology) it may be somewhat more robust to reporting bias and recall bias. The anthropometric measures will be least prone to reporting bias and *a priori* ought to yield the best indication of health production. This is a region where disease incidence is bound tightly to nutritional status. (Kielman, DeSweemer *et al.*, 1983; Martorell and Ho, 1984). Although height for age is known to reflect long-term nutritional processes such as stunting, weight for height is preferred here because it is a more appropriate indicator for wasting processes which might occur over the space of 2-6 months (Waterlow, 1973).

Table 3 shows the results of estimating the health production function for weight for height Z-score using not only the preferred Lagged Instrument Fixed Effect (LIFE) technique but also by OLS, and a Fixed Effects method (FE) which amounts to applying OLS on differenced data.

TESTS FOR HETEROSKEDASTICITY

The Goldfeld-Quandt test indicates heteroskedasticity which is not surprising given a panel dataset comprised of multiple observations on the same individuals. Thus the covariance matrix of estimated coefficient $\hat{\beta}$ which equals $(X'X)^{-1} [X'(\sigma^2\Omega)X] (X'X)^{-1}$ employs a matrix Ω which is in this case not the identity matrix. Some methods of adjusting for heteroskedasticity rely on producing a consistent estimate of $\sigma^2\Omega$ as in two-step GLS or maximum likelihood. However a consistent estimate of $\sigma^2 X'\Omega X = \sum_i \sigma_i^2 x_i x_i'$ would also be an adequate starting point. White's method is based on his proof (White, 1980) that with very general assumptions $S = \sum_i e_i^2 x_i x_i'$ (where e_i is the ith least squares residual) is a consistent estimate of $\sigma^2 X'\Omega X$. Consequently, all of the standard errors are adjusted for heteroskedasticity by White's method. The estimated variance of $\hat{\beta}$ is computed as

[29] $\hat{\beta} = (X'X)^{-1} S(X'X)^{-1}$.

The White's standard errors were neither consistently larger nor smaller than the OLS standard errors in the analyses presented.   Since the White's standard errors are robust both to the presence of heteroskedasticity and to distributional assumptions they are preferred.

TESTS FOR EXOGENEITY

Given the assumption that the instrumental variables are exogenous, the Hausmann test can be used to assess the exogeneity of the independent variables. Under the null that the independent variables are weakly exogenous for the dependent variable and OLS is consistent, the Hausmann test statistics shown in Table 3 would be observed with probability given by a chi squared distribution. The Hausmann test in Column IV was computed as $(\beta_{FE}-\beta_{LIFE})'$ $(V_{FE}-V_{LIFE})^{-1} (\beta_{FE}-\beta_{LIFE})$ (Hausmann, 1978; Ruud, 1984; Smith and Blundell, 1986).   The test results favor rejection of the null of exogeneity for the LIFE estimates for Weight for Height.

The robustness of the LIFE estimates to dropping various subsets of the set of instruments was tested. The estimates and their precision were negligibly affected when the instrument set excluded lagged prices, excluded lagged child behaviors, excluded lagged nutrient inputs, or excluded lagged child care inputs.

What Inputs Make Children Healthy?

The first three columns of Table 3 all present regression models that are susceptible to the fixed effect and endogeneity biases discussed above. The fourth (LIFE) column shows the theoretically preferred estimate with lagged child body size excluded to preserve data. Column V includes lagged child weight for height, but as a consequence suffers a reduction in sample size. Columns I - III are presented to provide some intuition for the magnitude of the respective biases. Comparing the OLS coefficients in columns I and II to the FE and LIFE estimates in columns III and IV indicates that failure to account for fixed effects understates the coefficients by as much as a factor of 10. Endogeneity which is not controlled for in the results of column III, appears to also lead to understating the coefficients relative to column IV but to a lesser degree.

Column II is presented to give irremediably flawed measures of the importance of fixed household features that would otherwise be lost to the differencing procedure. These results, contaminated as they are by fixed effects bias, indicate in Table 3 a surprisingly insignificant (and negative) effect of maximal household education. I already know that the fixed effects bias in these estimates is biasing all of the other coefficients towards zero so perhaps the result is not unexpected. Nevertheless, previous studies have found a strong salutary effect of household education on child health and this is not showing up in Table 3. Although I am reluctant to search for meaning in estimates that I know are flawed, a speculative explanation for the insignificant results of Table 3 column II may be that for economic reasons families with a lower propensity to have increased body size (a familial fixed effect) devote more attention to educational attainment. A similar inverse relationship between body mass index and parents' education has been documented for adult US white women and adult African American males -- the mechanism for this remains unclear (Greenlund, Liu, *et al.*, 1996). In any case, the results of column II indicate that fixed effects interfere profoundly with inference.

The preferred estimates of the health production model are presented in the fourth and fifth columns of Table 3. The inclusion of lagged child body size in Column V does not appear to alter the magnitude of the coefficients but it does reduce precision noticeably. The significant t-test on the level of lagged body size in Columns I and II provides statistical support for its inclusion in the model. The specification in Column IV is purely *ad hoc* and defensible on the grounds that omitting lagged body size preserves data and does not appear to lead to coefficient estimates that greatly differ from those in Column V. Furthermore, the Hausmann Test in Column V suggest that the inputs are not

Table 3 Bangladesh Child Body Size Production Estimates

Variable	Weight for Height Score				
	I	II	III	IV	V
	OLS	OLS	FE	LIFE	LIFE
N	828	766	621	566	365
AdjR^2	0.5273	0.5306	0.0102		
Cons	0.7185	0.7271	0.0056	0.0068	0.0003
	(5.8918)	(5.6102)	(2.5739)	(2.8681)	(0.0416)
Education Weighted Childcare Hours	0.0023	0.0076	0.03310	0.03580	0.0544
	(0.5365)	(1.1997)	(1.6316)	(2.2663)	(1.5691)
Age Weighted Childcare Hours	0.0013	0	-0.0074	-0.0095	-0.02265
	(0.5435)	(-0.0106)	(-1.1469)	(-1.9923)	(-1.8629)
Childcare Hours by Males	0.0111	0.0127	0.0092	0.0628	-0.052
	(0.7727)	(0.7977)	(0.6088)	(1.4709)	(-0.7534)
Calories	0.0036	0.0042	0.0156	0.0479	0.0453
	(0.4767)	(0.5481)	(2.2027)	(3.5981)	(1.5057)
Cereal Protein	0.0002	0.0001	-0.0136	-0.0351	-0.0393
	(0.0313)	(0.0205)	(-2.4848)	(-4.1716)	(-1.7069)
Non-Cereal Protein	0.0008	-0.0006	-0.0009	-0.004	-0.0019
	(0.3956)	(-0.2568)	(-0.4452)	(-1.3306)	(-0.2528)
Lagged Weight for Height	0.6503	0.6485			-0.3241
	(11.7196)	(11.1557)			(-1.9744)
Age		0			
		(0.0862)			
Sex of Child (0=Male)		0.0003			
		(0.063)			
Household Wealth		0			
		(-0.9039)			
Maximum Household Education		-0.0055			
		(-1.2558)			
Number of Children		0			
		(-0.0811)			
Total Household Size		0.0011			
		(0.8716)			
Hausmann Test			7511.9	14.49	25.98
Probability for Hausmann			0	0.043	0.0005
Goldfeld-Quandt Test		1.512			
Probability for Goldfeld-Quandt		0.0003			

LIFE denotes Lagged Instruments Fixed Effects Model; FE denotes OLS Fixed Effects Model; Instruments for LIFE estimates are observed at lag2, lag3, and lag 4 of levels of: log calories, log protein, log cereal

All independent variables except age, sex, wealth, max. Educ., number of children and household size are lagged by one period (2 months) relative to the dependent variable; t-statistics in parentheses adjusted for heteroskedasticity by Huber's (White's) method and adjusted (in column IV and V) for IV method exogenous even when lagged child body size is included as an independent variable. The coefficient on differenced lagged body size is significant and negative in the LIFE estimates of Column V, whereas in the OLS estimates in level in columns I and II the coefficient is positive. I believe that the reason for this difference is the difference in how homeostasis relates to the intertemporal correlation of body size (positively correlated) and the intertemporal correlation of body growth (negatively correlated -- negative growth followed by positive growth).

Confident that the more precise estimates of Column IV do not harbor a gross misspecification from excluding lagged child body size I will proceed to discuss them in detail. The estimates of Table 3 column IV (and with less significance column V) demonstrate that there is a worker competence effect in the production of child health. The coefficient on education-weighted child care hours in the production of weight for height is significant and positive. The negative coefficient on Age-Weighted Child Care hours suggests that more exposure to elderly caregivers decreases the child's weight for height. This suggests that the older household members are applying a less efficient technology or that the requisite sensory and cognitive skills for effective child care are prey to senescence. The coefficient on male-supplied child care hours is positive but not significant. This fails to support the folk belief that women are superior in supplying child care. An alternate explanation for this gender-related finding is that higher male-supplied child care hours are simply correlated with a tendency for fathers to have health figure more highly in the utility function. These doting fathers may be using their time in child care to improve their children's health outcome in a manner related to intensity of preferences rather than sheer skill.

Table 4 displays the production elasticities computed from the LIFE estimates in Table 3. Column I expresses these elasticities as %Δ weight for height Z score/ %Δ input. Column II expresses them as the change in weight for height percentile that would accompany a 10% upward shift in input. The elasticity for years of schooling and age are the product of the estimated coefficient times the child care time of respective caregiver times an adjustment for the use of the $\log(x+1)$ specification. Thus, because mothers spend the most time in child care, the elasticity on shifts in their years of schooling and age is

Table 4 Bangladesh Child Body Size: Derived Elasticities

	Weight for Height	
	I	II
Variable	**Z-Score***	**Percentile****
Mother's Years of Schooling	0.068	1.1858
Father's Years of Schooling	0.003	0.0871
Sister's Years of Schooling	0.0537	0.5128
Brother's Years of Schooling	0.0137	0.2933
Uncle's Years of Schooling	0.0026	0.0416
Aunt's Years of Schooling	0.0049	0.0721
Grandmother's Years of Schooling	0.0053	0.124
Grandfather's Years of Schooling	0.0034	0.0962
Mother's Age in Years	-0.0689	-0.9439
Father's Age in Years	-0.0019	-0.0487
Sister's Age in Years	-0.033	-0.3249
Brother's Age in Years	-0.0072	-0.1555
Uncle's Age in Years	-0.0012	-0.0175
Aunt's Age in Years	-0.0021	-0.0397
Grandmother's Age in Years	-0.0172	-0.1926
Grandfather's Age in Years	-0.0022	-0.0573
Mother's Childcare Time (Normalized))	-0.1012	-0.937
Father's Childcare Time (Normalized)	0.0119	0.3331
Brother's Childcare Time (Normalized)	0.0583	1.2798
Sister's Childcare Time (Normalized)	0.0038	0.1046
Uncle's Childcare Time (Normalized)	0.01	0.1485
Aunt's Childcare Time (Normalized)	0.0028	0.0036
Grandmother's Childcare Time (Norm)	-0.0606	-0.5526
Grandfather's Childcare Time (Norm)	0.0129	0.3502
Calories	0.6021	0.8627
Cereal Protein	-0.3705	-0.6224
Non Cereal Protein	-0.0467	-0.0642

*Column I displays sample mean %Δ WHZ / %ΔInput.
Value for each child calculated by applying estimated LIFE coefficients to child's existing caregivers
**Column II displays sample mean ΔWH Percentile Points accompanying a 10% upward shift in input.
Value for each child calculated by referring values from Column I to data on each child's Wt. for Ht.

greatest. A 10% increase in the mother's years of schooling at time t would be associated with a 1.858 point raise in the weight for height percentile of her child. Because these estimates are based on analysis of a short time series with effects occurring on the order of 2 months it would be impossible to surmise what the long run effects of such a change would be.

The elasticity for child care time turns out to be the calculated productivity of each caregiver times their child care time. As per Table 3 productivity is enhanced by education (significantly) and male gender (not significantly) and reduced by age (significantly). Thus, unschooled women in the sample will suffer from lower (even negative if they are old enough) productivity given this simplistic specification. This effect is magnified for mothers because of their high amount of child care time. This accounts for the negative elasticity on child care time provided by mothers and grandmothers. The parameters do turn out to be quite flattering to the household men -- particularly the brothers who take the prize for highest quality child care providers.

The negative sign for mother's time in Table 4 represents the marginal as opposed to average effect of mother's time. The result is highly dependent upon the functional form chosen to represent the determinants of productivity -- in assuming the Cobb-Douglas form I implicitly assumed equivalent treatment for age and schooling.

I also explicitly assumed that age, gender, and schooling gave a complete account of the determinants of schooling -- simply being *the child's mother* was not permitted to enhance productivity.

The results of Table 4 are not intended to demonstrate the point that the Bangladeshi mothers have reached a point at which their marginal hour of child care harms health. It is the negative coefficient on age (insufficiently made up for by schooling and gender effects) that is responsible for the negative elasticity on mother's time. The point is that giving serious attention to schooling as a key determinant of child care competence is bound to rank more schooled individuals more highly. If age truly has a negative effect on competence then the younger caregivers will be ranked higher, etc. Table 4 is one account of how such a ranking might turn out.

At the very least one might use the heterogeneity of the elasticities of child care time to defend the assertion that child health cannot be the sole consideration in determining time allocation. If it were, then optimizing households would have achieved a time allocation that led to some semblance of equalizing marginal products to shadow wages for the labor inputs.

PHILIPPINES RESULTS

What Inputs Make Children Healthy?

Table 5 shows the results of estimating child body size. The presentation is analogous to Table 3. The primary difference from the Bangladesh specification is that only the child care time of the mother is available. Once again the first three columns are estimates of the production function tainted by either endogeneity bias (Column III) or both fixed effects and endogeneity bias (Columns I and II). The Goldfeld-Quandt statistic is significant at less than 0.01, strongly suggesting heteroskedasticity in OLS estimates.

Accordingly standard errors were adjusted using White's method as was done for the Bangladesh analysis. The overall precision of the estimates leaves something to be desired and inhibits inference about the overall direction and magnitude of the fixed effects and endogeneity biases in Columns I-III.

Column II is augmented by age, sex, and maximal household education despite the suspicion that these variables are correlated to the residual in the undifferenced specification. Once again I fail to detect a significant effect of raw household education on child health.

The preferred estimate in Column IV shows that education weighted child care hours provided by the mother are a significant, but small positive determinant of child health. The other coefficients in Column IV, though imprecisely estimated have the same signs as those obtained from the Bangladesh analysis. Age weighted child care time is negative, calories positive, and protein intake negative.

Column V includes lagged differenced health as an independent variable and suffers a loss of precision due to the lower sample size. None of the parameters attain significance.

Table 5 Philippines Child Body Size Production Estimates

	Weight for Height Score				
	I	II	III	IV	V
Variable	OLS	OLS	FE	LIFE	LIFE
N	1862	1755	1240	1240	599
AdjR^2	0.2623	0.2555	0.0011		
Cons	1.0918	1.1368	0.006	0.0066	0.0148
	(12.003)	(12.1184)	(9.3406)	(7.4935)	(3.3679)
Education Weighted Childcare Hours	0	0	0	0.0001	0.0003
	(0.2797)	(1.7123)	(0.6222)	(1.9695)	(0.2918)
Age Weighted Childcare Hours	0	0	0	0	-0.0001
	(0.6032)	(2.0384)	(0.3179)	(1.4815)	(-0.1950)
Calories	0.0053	0.0048	0.0154	0.0052	-0.0312
	(0.6701)	(0.5963)	(1.8774)	(0.5574)	(-0.6195)
Protein	-0.0014	-0.0024	-0.0167	-0.008	0.0014
	(-0.1496)	(-0.2633)	(-1.5835)	(-0.5705)	(0.0329)
Lagged Weight for Height	0.4998	0.4723			-0.6022
	14.8768	13.522			(-2.6781)
Age		0.0045			
		(3.5469)			
Sex of Child (0=Male)		0.0057			
		(1.5678)			
Max Household Education		0.0006			
		(0.1924)			
Hausmann Test				3.17	28.93
Probability for Hausmann				0.013	0
Goldfeld-Quandt Test	1.22				
Probability for Goldfeld	0.005				

LIFE denotes Lagged Instruments Fixed Effects Model
FE denotes OLS Fixed Effects Model
Instruments for LIFE estimates are observations at lag 2 and lag 3 of levels of: log calories, log protein, log cereal protein, log health knowledge score * childcare hours, log education * caregiver hours, log age * caregiver hours, log unweighted childcare hours by each mother, weekly food expenditure, cleaning frequency

All independent variables except age, sex, wealth, max educ., number of children and hh size are lagged by one period (2 months) relative to the dependent variable t-statistics in parentheses adjusted for heteroskedasticity by Huber's (White's) method and (in column IV) for IV method

The imputed elasticities from Column IV are shown in Table 6. A 10% upward shift in mother's years of schooling input would be associated with a rise of 0.118 percentile points for weight for height. This imputed elasticity is remarkably similar to that obtained for Bangladesh. Because the coefficients upon which the other elasticities are based are estimated so imprecisely, I am hesitant to carry inferences from them.

Table 7 is included as an alternate to 5 and is distinguished by the inclusion of unweighted child care hours in addition to the interaction terms. With the addition of the unweighted hours the Column IV LIFE coefficient on Education Weighted Hours remains significant. The conventional explanation for this observation would be that it is not just the variation in the raw hours component of the education-hours interaction that is responsible for the significant coefficient in Table 5. The magnitudes and signs of the coefficients do not change with the addition of unweighted hours. Unlike the case of Bangladesh where time inputs could be normalized, the time inputs for the Filipina mothers only are reported in the data and there is no denominator with which to normalize them. Thus higher raw child care time inputs may represent more waking hours for the children and less total income due to less participation of adults in income generation.

Table 6 Philippines Child Body Size: Derived Elasticities

| | Weight for Height | |
| | I | II |
Variable	Z-Score*	Percentile**
Mother's Years of Schooling	0.249	0.1118
Mother's Age	-0.1147	-0.0522
Mother's Childcare Time	-0.0019	-0.0007
Calories	0.1449	0.0604
Protein	-0.2128	-0.0879

*Column I displays sample mean %Δ WHZ / %ΔInput.
Value for each child calculated by applying estimated LIFE coefficients to child specific data.
**Column II displays sample mean ΔWH Percentile Points accompanying a 10% upward shift in input.
Value for each child calculated by referring values from Column I to data on each child's Wt. for Ht.

Table 7 Philippines Child Body Size Production Estimates With Unweighted Hours

Variable	I OLS	II OLS	III FE	IV LIFE	V LIFE
			Weight for Height Score		
N	1862	1755	1240	1240	599
AdjR^2	0.2628	0.256	0.0003		
Cons	1.0972	1.1416	0.006	0.0066	0.012
	(12.4713)	(12.4355)	(10.5513)	(4.0933)	(2.0787)
Education Weighted Childcare Hours	0	0	0	0.0001	0.0005
	(0.2995)	(1.6446)	(0.631)	(2.3113)	(0.3707)
Age Weighted Childcare Hours	0	0	0	0	-0.0002
	(0.5672)	(1.9295)	(0.3082)	(0.5478)	(-0.2274)
Calories	0.0048	0.0043	0.0155	0.0058	-0.0153
	(0.64)	(0.5703)	(1.8345)	(0.5227)	(-0.2826)
Protein	-0.0008	-0.0018	-0.0168	-0.0117	-0.0014
	(-0.0941)	(-0.2135)	(-1.5547)	(-0.7134)	(-0.0241)
Unweighted Childcare Hours	0	0	0	-0.0002	-0.0002
	(1.2668)	(1.067)	(0.1344)	(1.7969)	(-1.3554)
Lagged Weight for Height	0.4988	0.4714			-0.5236
	15.1126	13.6517			(-1.5004)
Age	0.0044				
	(3.453)				
Sex of Child (0=Male)	0.006				
		(1.5978)			
Max Household Education		0.0005			
		(0.1759)			
Hausmann Test				4.32	12.33
Probability for Hausmann				0.0007	0.0000
Goldfeld-Quandt Test	1.22				
Probability for Goldfeld	0.005				

LIFE denotes Lagged Instruments Fixed Effects Model
FE denotes OLS Fixed Effects Model
Instruments for LIFE estimates are observations at lag 2 and lag 3 of levels of: log calories, log protein, log cereal protein, log health knowledge score weighted care hrs, log education weighted caregiver hours, log age weighted hours,log unweighted care hrs by each mother, weekly food expenditure, cleaning frequency

All independent variables except age, sex, wealth, max educ., number of children & hh siz eare lagged by one period (2 months) relative to the dependent variable t-statistics in parentheses adjusted for heteroskedasticity by Huber's (White's) method and (in column IV and V) for IV method

What Inputs Make Children Healthy?

Table 8 shows the results of estimating the production function for WHZ when the Bangladesh and Philippines datasets are combined.   The underlying assumptions here are:
- The health technology is the same in each country and
- The market forces that underlie the connection between the instrumental variables and the endogenous variables are the same.

In the next section I will formally test these assumptions by means of covariance estimation. For now let me comment on Table 8.   The LIFE estimates of Table 8 confirm the results of Table 3 and 5.   Calories and Education Weighted Child Care Time are positively associated with child health, Protein and Age Weighted Child Care Time are negatively associated with child health.

   Because the process of imputing elasticities relies heavily upon the measurements of each child's body size to produce child specific elasticities which are then averaged, it makes little sense to present an average of imputed elasticities when the two populations are demonstrably heterogeneous regarding their degree of deviation from international age adjusted norms. The presentation of population specific elasticities (as done in Table 4 and Table 6) is more appropriate and the coefficients from Table 8 column IV are accordingly used in Table 9 to provide separate elasticities for Bangladesh and Philippines. The coefficient on Education Weighted Child Care Time from the combined analysis is similar in magnitude to that from the Philippines analysis and smaller by a factor of 100 compared to the Bangladesh coefficient. The elasticities derived by imposing the coefficients of the joint estimation on each country are accordingly disparate for the two countries.

   To decide whether the parameters produced by estimating the production process jointly are a better characterization of the data generating process than the parameters from individual countries it is necessary to test the assumption that the production process is the same. Since the health production function estimated above relies heavily upon physiological events which ought to be the same in both Bangladesh and the Philippines the hypothesis is somewhat tenable.

Table 8 Joint Data Body Size Production Estimates

	Weight for Height Score			
	I	II	III	IV
Variable	OLS	OLS	FE	LIFE
N	2770	2614	1861	1861
AdjR2	0.277	0.239	-0.0005	
Cons	1.938	1.9399	0.0056	0.0066
	(71.7891)	(65.6922)	(3.7187)	(4.2011)
Education Weighted Childcare Hours	0.0001	0.0001	0	0.0002
	(1.6038)	(1.5844)	(0.6607)	(2.3449)
Age Weighted Childcare Hours	0	-0.0001	0	-0.0001
	(-1.7893)	(-1.9111)	(-0.3363)	(-1.7737)
Calories	0.0485	0.0439	0.0029	0.0594
	(13.4775)	(8.8054)	(0.5575)	(2.6385)
Protein	-0.0369	-0.0312	-0.0021	-0.0591
	(-13.8273)	(-6.2896)	(-0.4557)	(-2.7477)
Lagged Weight for Height	0.037	0.0379		
	(6.0145)	(5.9061)		
Age		-0.0002		
		(-0.4757)		
Sex of Child (0=Male)		0.0104		
		(2.0075)		
Household Wealth		0		
		(0.7262)		
Max Household Education		0.0029		
		(0.5201)		
Hausman Test				3.20
Probability for Hausman				0.0125

LIFE denotes Lagged Instruments Fixed Effects Model

FE demotes OLS applied to first differences=Fixed Effects Model

Instruments for LIFE estimates are observations at lag 2 and lag 3 of levels of log education weighted caaregiver hours, log age weighted hours, log unweighted childcare hours by each mother and log calories and log protein.

All independent variables except age, sex, wealth, max educ., number of children and hh size are lagged by one period (2 months) relative to the dependent variable.

T stats in parentheses adjusted for heteroskedasticity by Huber's (White's) method and adjusted (in Column IV) for IV method.

Table 9 Joint Data Child Body Size Production Elasticities

	Weight for Height			
	Bangladesh		Philippines	
	I	II	III	IV
Variable	Z-Score	*Percentile**	**Z-Score	*Percentile**
Mother's Years of Schooling	0.0004	0.0007	0.3875	0.1741
Mother's Age	-0.0007	-0.001	-0.2312	-0.1051
Mother's Childcare Time	-0.0009	-0.0015	-0.0066	-0.0026
Calories	0.7471	1.0705	1.6447	0.6855
Protein	-0.7347	-1.057	-1.5748	-0.6506

*Column I & III display sample mean %Δ WHZ / %ΔInput Value for each child calculated by applying estimated LIFE coefficients to child specific data.
**Column II & IV display sample mean ΔWH Percentile Points accompanying a 10% upward input shift.
Value for each child calculated by referring values from Column I to data on each child's Wt. for Ht.

MULTISAMPLE COVARIANCE STRUCTURE ANALYSIS PRESERVING LIFE FRAMEWORK

One way to test constraints on parameters across samples is to employ covariance structure analysis. The basic statistical theory behind this form of estimation is minimization of a fitting function given as:

[30] $Q = (s - \sigma(\chi))'W (s - \sigma(\chi))$

where s is a vector of data-the variances and covariances of the observed variables, σ is a model for the data taken to be a function of more basic parameters, χ that are to be estimated to minimize Q (Bentler, 1993). The matrix W is a weight matrix that can be specialized depending on the distributional assumptions-normal, elliptical, or arbitrary. To test between sample constraints on parameters c $(\chi)=0$, one can generalize [30] to form a multisample version of the fitting function in [30] as follows:

[31] $$T = \sum_{m=1}^{M} n_m (s_m - \sigma_m(\chi))' W_m (s_m - \sigma_m(\chi))$$

where there are M samples indexed by M and the between sample constraints have been incorporated into the M separate models, σ_m . Conditional upon selection of the weighting matrices, W_m , being selected in accordance with the actual sample distribution then at its minimum T is distributed asymptotically as a Chi Square (Bentler, 1993). This Chi Square property can be used to test the between sample constraints.

I propose to use the LIFE framework as the basis for the parameter model. The basic model structure imposed on s_m is as per equation [24]. To account for measurement error, an IV approach was again used where stage 1 was estimated separately. The estimation of s_m in the second stage relied upon the variance-covariance matrix of (ΔX_4 , ΔX_3, , ΔX_2 , $\Delta \hat{Y}_3$, $\Delta \hat{Y}_2$, $\Delta \hat{Y}_1$) where $\Delta \hat{Y}_t = Z_{t-1} \hat{\gamma}_{t-1}$ relies upon a first stage estimate of $\hat{\gamma}_{t-1}$ being obtained by OLS regression. The instruments, Z_{t-1} used for each sample were the same as those used in the LIFE estimates - see notes to Table 3 and Table 5.

STATISTICAL TESTS AND FIT INDEXES

Table 10 displays the results of this exercise as applied to each individual country. The Independence Chi-Square statistic is that obtained under a model that each variable is independent and uncorrelated with the other. If the restrictions imposed by my model fail to fit the data better than this then serious questions about my model would arise. The restricted Chi-Square is based on $T = n\hat{Q}$ where Q is given by [30]. Bentler argues against rigid acceptance or rejection of model fit based on T. A plethora of fit indices abounds to aid in model evaluation.

The simplest of these, called the Normed Fit Index is simply $(T_i - T_m)/T_i$. Under the normal distribution the Comparative Fit Index is designed to be robust at both large and small sample sizes and is accordingly displayed in Table 10 because the joint estimation required the assumption of normality.

RESULTS

Table 10 columns I and II shows the estimates of the model on the dataset from each separate country. The last three rows of the table indicate that the restrictions imposed by the model fit substantially better than the hypothesis of complete independence. Still, were I to judge model fit with rigid Chi-Square hypothesis testing, the probability of obtaining a Chi-Square of 409 for Bangladesh is less than 0.001, the same can be said for the Philippines Chi-square of 167. The respective fit indices of 0.821 and 0.978 suggest that the model depicted above is relatively adequate.

The coefficient estimates for the individual countries are similar in sign but do not attain significance at conventional levels. LM (Lagrange Multiplier) tests are displayed in Columns I and II which evaluate the appropriateness of the restriction that the coefficient within each country is the same from the first period to the last--a span of 3 periods = 6months in Bangladesh and 2 periods = 8 months in The Philippines. The LM tests support the hypothesis that the coefficients are the same across periods.

Does the Theoretical Model Hold up to Joint Estimation?

Table 10 Column III displays LM Test results for the restrictions that each of the structural parameters in question is the same in both samples. Each of the LM test results in Column III of Table 10 support the hypothesis that the corresponding coefficient is the same in both samples.

The bottom of Table 10 shows Likelihood Ratio tests of the sets of restrictions for the whole model. Imposing the restriction that all of the coefficients are the same across samples does not significantly raise the magnitude of the log likelihood function. The Chi-square statistic on the difference in the log likelihood between the restricted and unrestricted models is not significant. Thus I find support for the hypothesis that the whole model is the same in the two samples. This would accord with the intuition that a body size production function is in essence a biological process. At the same

Table 10 Stacked Child Body Size Production Estimates

		Weight for Height Score	
	I	II	III
Variable	Bangladesh	Philippines	JOINT
N	207	600	807
Education Weighted Childcare Hours*	0.017	0.066	0.043
t	(0.551)	(1.894)	(2.627)
LM Test for Null That Coefficient is Equal...			
...Across Periods	0.917	0.301	
...Across Samples			0.679
Probability of Observing this LM under Null	0.338	0.583	0.410
Age Weighted Childcare Hours*	-0.009	-0.025	-0.014
t	(-1.129)	(-1.336)	(-1.903)
LM Test for Null That Coefficient is Equal...			
...Across Periods	0.089	0.350	
...Across Samples			0.108
Probability of Observing this LM under Null	0.766	0.554	0.742
Calories	0.005	0.009	0.006
t	(0.406)	(0.664)	(0.618)
LM Test for Null That Coefficient is Equal...			
...Across Periods	0.086	0.538	
...Across Samples			0.594
Probability of Observing this LM under Null	0.77	0.463	0.441
Protein	0.0001	-0.011	-0.004
t	(0.014)	(-0.753)	(-0.411)
LM Test for Null That Coefficient is Equal...			
...Across Periods	0.374	0.009	
...Across Samples			0.882
Probability of Observing this LM under Null	0.541	0.922	0.348

Comparative Fit Index	0.821	0.978	0.942
A. Periods & Samples Equal Model Chi Square	409	167	578
B. Periods Equal Model Chi Square			576
C. Unrestricted Model Chi Square			562
LR test A vs. B (df=4) Test of null that each coefficient same across samples			2
Probability for LR (A vs. B)			Pr=0.72
LR test B vs. C (df=12) Test of null that each coefficient same across periods			14
Probability for LR (B vs.C)			Pr=0.29
LR test A vs. C (df=16) Test of null that coeffs unchanged across samples & periods			16
Probability for LR (A vs. C)			Pr=0.43

*Mothers only

time it is somewhat surprising that education which is not a biological process and might be very different in the two countries plays a similar role in mediating child body size in the two countries.

With the joint data sample more precise estimates of the parameters of the child body size production function can be had. These parameters indicate that education-weighted child care hours have a positive and significant relationship to child weight for height and that age-weighted child care hours have a negative and significant relationship to weight for height. The parameters for the nutrients are not estimated with precision.

CONCLUSION

Unlike some routine production processes where the skill of the laborer matters little, it appears that for child body size there is variation in productivity related to the characteristics of the caregivers. Thus were there such a thing as a foreman in the household exclusively responsible for improving output child health, the foreman would be ill-advised to attend exclusively to capital inputs and technology. Due to the presence of a worker effect, competence matters. In Bangladesh and The Philippines more education for a caregiver makes each hour spent with the child a more health-producing hour. This effect would be unlikely to be observed if education merely gave caregivers greater bargaining power. This observation also implies that not all of the effect of education can be carried to the child through inheritance of a family-specific endowment. Inheritance effects would have been unrelated to exposure time.

There has been concern that attempts to improve child health by improving the education of girls may fail because the girls would find higher returns to their schooling in endeavors other than child care. In previous work I have presented evidence that in the Bangladesh study population this effect did not occur (Bishai, 1996). There was no significant effect on childcare time of the education of mothers or sisters.

Some of the evidence here suggests that health production competence in Bangladesh and The Philippines is negatively related with age. This may be related to a generational adherence to a less efficient child health production technology or senescence or the fact that older caregivers are more likely to abound where competing small siblings abound. Male gender of the caregiver was associated (but not significantly) with increased productivity in Bangladesh.

The extensive data on child care time allocation in the Bangladeshi household permits comparison between the productivity of family members in the production of child health . This comparison is carried out under the premise that the relationship of the caregiver to the child plays no role in determining productivity. One could reasonably suggest that more distant relatives might be more likely to provide child care time jointly with other household activities. Since the data I use provide no information about what activities are being performed jointly with child care--my assumption that the propensity toward joint production is homogeneous is not testable. I have no data on when, where, and which caregivers might attempt to jointly produce child health and other goods. But I can say that if distractions due to performing multiple tasks along with child care harm child health the more educated and less aged caregivers are either more adept at juggling multiple tasks or more single-minded in their devotion to child care.

Given these caveats in comparing household members I find that mothers in Bangladesh suffer from a relative deficit of education and a surfeit of age relative to the household adolescents. The mothers in Bangladesh were old enough, unschooled enough, female enough and contributed enough to child care such that the marginal hour by an average Bangladeshi mother would lead to a net decrease in child health as reflected by body size. Grandmothers were prey to the same effect. In contrast the average teenage brother with male gender, higher education and lower age and lower contribution to child care time would be most productive at the margin. These wide differentials in productivity elasticities provide support for the hypothesis that child care time allocation is guided by other considerations in addition to child health. If household utility depended only on child health, then optimizing behavior would lead the household to an allocation which tended to equalize the marginal productivities of the caregivers.

In extrapolating the model across countries I find support for the hypothesis that the structural parameters relating the effect of a quality adjusted child care time factor on body size is the same in both Bangladesh and the Philippines.

ACKNOWLEDGMENTS

I am grateful for helpful comments from Andrew Foster, Mark Rosenzweig, Patricia Danzon, Alessandro Quandrini, Kevin Frick, and Eric Slade. All errors are my own.

REFERENCES

Behrman, J.R. and Wolfe, B.L. (1987) How does mother's schooling affect family health, nutrition, medical care usage, and household sanitation? *Journal of Econometrics* 36:185-204.

Bentler, P.M. (1993) *EQS Structural Equations Program Manual.* Los Angeles: BMDP Statistical Software.

Bishai, D. (1996) Quality time: how parents' schooling affects child health through its interaction with childcare time in Bangladesh. *Health Economics* 5:383-407.

Bouis, H.E. and Haddad, L.J. (1990) *Agricultural Commercialization, Nutrition, and the Rural Poor: A Study of Philippine Farm Households.* Boulder: Lynne Reinner Publishers.

Center for Disease Control (1994) *EPI Info.* Atlanta: CDC.

Chen, L.C., Huq, E., *et al.* (1981) Sex bias in the family allocation of food and health care in rural Bangladesh, *Population and Development Review* 7(1):55-71.

Foster, A. (1994) Poverty and illness in low-income areas. *American Economic Review* 84(2):216-220.

Foster, A.D. (1995) Prices, credit markets and child growth in low-income rural areas. *Economic Journal* 105(430):551-570.

Greenlund, K.J., Liu, K., *et al.* (1996) Body mass index in young adults: associations with parental body size and education in the CARDIA study.

American Journal of Public Health 86(4): 480-485.

Grossman, M. (1972) *The Demand for Health: A Theoretical and Empirical Investigation.* New York: Columbia University Press.

Grossman, M. (1972) On the concept of health capital and the demand for health. *Journal of Political Economy* 80:223-255.

Hausmann, J.A. (1978) Specification tests in econometrics. *Econometrica* 46(6):1251-1271.

Hobcraft, J. (1993)Women's education, child welfare and child survival: a review of the evidence. *Health Transition Review* 3(2):159-175.

Kielman, A., DeSweemer, C., *et al.* (1983) *Child and Maternal Health Services in Rural India: The Narangwal Experiment.* Baltimore: Johns Hopkins University Press.

Martorell, R. and Ho, T.J. (1984) Malnutrition, morbidity, and mortality. *Population and Development Review* 10(supp):49-68

Rosenzweig, M.R. and Wolpin, K.I. (1988) Heterogeneity, intrafmily distribution, and child health. *Journal of Human Resources* XXIII(4):437-461.

Rund, P.A. (1984) Tests of specification in econometrics. *Econometric Reviews* 3:2):211-242.

Sindelar, J. and Thomas, D. (1991) *Measurement of Child Health: Maternal Response Bias.* New Haven, Ct: Economic Growth Center, Yale University.

Smith, R.J. and Blundell, R.W. (1986) An exogeneity test for a simultaneous equation Tobit model with an application to labor supply. *Econometrica* 54(3):679-685.

Waterlow, J. (1973) Note on the assessment and classification of protein-energy malnutrition in children. *Lancet* 2:87-89.

White, H. (1980) A heteroskedasticity-consistent covariance matrix estimator and a direct test for heteroskedasticity. *Econometrica* 48(4):817-838.

4

Measuring Income-Related Health Inequalities in Sweden

ULF-G GERDTHAM[1] and GUN SUNDBERG[2]

[1] Centre for Health Economics
Stockholm School of Economics
Stockholm, Sweden
[2] Department of Economics
Uppsala, Sweden

ABSTRACT

In Sweden, health, measured as self-assessed health, is distributed fairly evenly in an international perspective. The purpose of this paper is to study whether specific disorders and diseases also are distributed fairly evenly. There are 44 diseases or disorders dealt with in this study, from a common cold or cough to serious diseases such as cancer and heart attack. All disorders and diseases are rated on a three-point scale. The data used are the Swedish Level of Living Survey from 1981 and 1991 (LNU81 and LNU91), where income data received from the National Tax Statistics have been linked to the LNU data. The method is the same as the one used by the EC-

Health, Health Care and Health Economics: Perspectives on Distribution
Edited by Morris L. Barer, Thomas E. Getzen, and Greg L. Stoddart
Copyright 1998 John Wiley & Sons, Ltd.

group on equity, where the different disorders and diseases are measured by concentration indices. All 44 illness conditions are age and sex standardized. The income measure is disposable household income per equivalent adult. The results show that even if there are no inequalities in health in Sweden, there are significant inequalities in diseases and disorders, as well as differences between the two periods 1980 and 1990.

INTRODUCTION

Good health affects several aspects of life and personal well-being. A healthy population will have a high work productivity, and thereby contribute to the country's living standards. A healthy population may also require less health care, which implies lower health expenditures for both the individual and the public sector. Furthermore, good health for the entire population is an important goal for the public health policy in Sweden (The Swedish Health Care Act, 1982). The Health Care Act (1982) states that people are to be treated equally, *i.e.*, people with equal need are to be treated in the same way, and that limited health care resources are to be distributed as equitably as possible in the population. However, it has also been argued that it is difficult to rationalize a concern about the distribution of health care other than in terms of a distribution of health in itself (Culyer, 1993). This explains why it is interesting to analyze the degree of inequality of health in the population.

Health is affected by medical and socioeconomic circumstances in which income plays an important role.[1] If income is low, for example, people may be required to work more hours and/or forced to work in more risky businesses to obtain higher incomes. In this sense, the health of people with low income is getting worse. On the other hand, poor health may make people unable to work full-time, and thus reduce their income level. This means that income affects health but income is also affected by the individual's health. By means of a simultaneous model, Sundberg (1996) found that the causality between health and wage may be bidirectional. Moreover, higher income implies increasing prosperity and standards of living, which have positively contributed to the decreasing mortality in the industrialized countries. However, although many countries have poor economic standards, they still have managed to

---

[1]See for example Townsend and Davidson (1982), Le Grand and Rabin (1986), Le Grand (1987, 1989), Blaxter (1989), Lundberg (1990, 1991), Lundberg and Fritzell (1994), Vågerö and Illsley (1995).

increase the life expectancy of the individual. This suggests that income differentials within the country also matter (Lundberg and Fritzell, 1994).

Health is an aggregate measure that in empirical work is primarily measured by self-assessed responses to questions concerning general health conditions. In many industrialized countries, income inequality is a strong determinant of self-assessed health and income-related inequalities in health exist that favor the better-off (van Doorslaer and Wagstaff *et al.*, 1996). However, the general health condition depends, to a large degree, on specific diseases and disorders. Although there are international studies on income-related self-assessed health, in which Sweden is included, (*i.e.*, van Doorslaer, Wagstaff, *et al.*, 1996), there are no studies on income-related specific diseases for Sweden.[2] It is important to analyze whether there are income-related inequalities for different diseases and disorders in the sense that these inequalities may be related to occupation. Further, if diseases are income-related, it may have equity consequences, because people with higher incomes are able to pay more to remain healthy. Such a situation may be regarded as being unfair to the poor section of society.

The purpose of the current study was twofold: First, to investigate income-related health inequalities in both aggregate self-assessed health and in different disorders and diseases. The second purpose was to compare potential changes between 1980 and 1990 in the distribution of disorders and diseases. The paper is organized into six sections describing the methodological background of previous studies; present data and incidence assumptions; methods used in the present study to measure inequalities in health; results; and, finally, a summary of our findings and presentation of our conclusions.

METHODOLOGICAL BACKGROUND

When measuring inequalities in health one approach is the class-based one used in the Black Report (Townsend and Davidson, 1982) and by Blaxter (1989), who focused on comparisons of mortality measures and morbidity patterns across socioeconomic groups. However, there are problems with the class-based approach

---

[2]Lundberg and Fritzell (1994) have examined the impact of income on health in Sweden. However, the health indicators included in this study are physical illness and psychological distress computed as additive indices from different items and not as specific disorders and diseases.

because it fails to reflect the relative size of the groups being compared and because the classification scheme of individuals in different groups is arbitrary. Most countries tend to change their classification schemes over time and different countries tend to define occupational groups differently.

Le Grand (1986, 1989) suggested an alternative to the class-based approach that involved Lorenz curves and Gini coefficients. In his empirical analyses, Le Grand used age-at-death as an indicator of health. The Lorenz curve for health plotted the cumulative proportions of the population (starting from the sickest, which is the one with the lowest age at death, to the healthiest individual, which is the one with the highest age at death) against the cumulative proportions of health, which is the cumulative proportion of age at death. If health is equally distributed in the population, the Lorenz curve would coincide with the diagonal and the corresponding Gini coefficient for health would equal zero.

However, Wilkinson (1986) argued that Le Grand's approach fails to address the issue that researchers are really interested in, namely if there are inequalities in health related to socio-economic status. Le Grand analyses inequalities in health *per se* by the argument that measures of inequalities in health should not implicitly incorporate any hypothesis of why they exist. However, Wilkinson's view is that what matters about inequalities in health is not that they exist, but that they may reflect inequalities in economic status.

Wagstaff *et al.* (1991a, 1991b) have suggested another approach, one that reduces the problems with the class-based approach and also meets Wilkinson's critique of Le Grand. In this approach, the individuals are ranked by their incomes from the poorest to the richest. The concentration curve for health plots the cumulative proportions of health against the cumulative proportions of the population ranked by income, and the estimated concentration index is a measure of inequality. The concentration index method has also been used by the EC-group on equity[3] (van Doorslaer *et al.*, 1993; van Doorslaer and Wagstaff, 1992; van Doorslaer and Wagstaff *et al.*, 1996). The study on inequalities in health by this group shows that in an international perspective, health is very evenly distributed in Sweden. Concentration indices have been calculated on grouped data for eight European countries[4] and the United States. In all countries the concentration indices are

---

[3] This group is called the ECuity-group. In this group there are people from Belgium, Denmark, England, Finland, France, Germany, Ireland, the Netherlands, Norway, Spain, Sweden, Switzerland, and United States with Adam Wagstaff (England) and Eddy van Doorslaer (the Netherlands) as project leaders.
[4] The European countries are Finland, East Germany, West Germany, the Netherlands, Spain, Sweden, Switzerland, and United Kingdom.

negative and significantly different from zero. Thus, in all these countries income-related inequalities in health exist favoring the better-off. Among those countries, the largest inequality was observed in the United States and smallest in Sweden.

DATA AND VARIABLE DEFINITIONS

The empirical analysis in the present study is based on data from probability samples of the Swedish population, the Level of Living Survey (LNU) from 1991 and 1981. The interviews were made during spring and summer, and the samples consist of about 7,000 individuals, in the ages 18-76 in 1991 (15-76 years in 1981). The response rate was about 80% in both samples. After correcting for missing values the sample consists of 5,185 in 1991 (5,487 in 1981) individuals. The surveys contain data on health status, illness conditions, use of medical care, socioeconomic variables, and family composition. LNU samples have been linked to national income tax statistics. Also available from this source are data on income, wages, and transfers, including non-taxable transfers. For further details, see Institutet för social forskning (1992) and Fritzell and Lundberg (1994). All figures about income, subsidies, and transfers refer to the year before the interviews, *i.e.*, 1990 and 1980.

In the survey from 1991 there is a question to the respondents concerning self-assessed health. People were asked how they judged their own present health condition, whether the condition is good, bad or something between. Both the 1981 and 1991 surveys supplied answers to questions on headache, cough, problems with seeing or hearing, chest pain, bronchitis, heart problems, gastric pain, and other illness conditions. The surveys included questions on 44 conditions, for which respondents were asked whether they had been suffering severely, mildly or not at all from the relevant illness conditions during 12 months preceding the surveys (*i.e.*, mainly in 1980 or 1990). This means that both health conditions and incomes refer to 1980 and 1990. Inequalities in health were also measured by the self-assessed health measure in the survey from 1991.

The income concept in this study was disposable household income per equivalent adult. The source of all income data was the National Income Tax Statistics, linked to the LNU data. The Swedish equivalence scale used was the one used by Jansson (1990): One adult equals 1, two adults equal 1.65, children younger or equal to 5 years equal 0.51, children 6 to 15 years equal 0.62 and children 16-18 years equal

0.65.[5] Another equivalent scale commonly used in studies of income distribution in Sweden was the one recommended by the National Board of Health and Welfare, and derivations from these recommendations. Some of those scales did not use different weights for children, and instead used different weights only for different number of persons in the household. This meant that a household with two adults received the same equivalent weight as a single person with one child, irrespective of the age of the child.[6] We argue that it is better to describe the economic burden in the household by using the above mentioned equivalence scale. The samples were separated into 10 equivalent disposable income deciles and four age groups in the ages 18 - 34, 35-44, 45-64, and 65+ years.

The distribution of the answers to the questions on health and different health conditions can be seen in Table 1. The general conclusions were that people on the whole are very healthy, and there are few people who experience severe suffering. However, for some of the diseases we saw that there were changes in the distribution between 1980 and 1990. For example, in 1990 a lower proportion of individuals in 1990 claimed that they had not been suffering from disorders such as lower back pain, painful shoulders, and headache, than the proportion of people in 1980.

METHODS

An inequality measure of health should reflect socioeconomic dimensions of inequalities in health for the entire population, and be sensitive to changes in the distribution of the population (Wagstaff *et al.*, 1991a). According to Wagstaff *et al.* (1991a), the concentration index approach fulfils these requirements. Here the individuals were ranked according to their incomes from the lowest to the highest. The concentration curve for health plots the cumulative proportions of the population (starting with the poorest) against the cumulative proportions of their health.[7] By means of the concentration index, we were able to measure the relative inequality in health because this index does not change if, for example, health is doubled for the entire population. In this study, the concentration curve for morbidity or illness was used instead of health. This meant that a measurable concept for illness had to be

---

[5]Jansson (1990) has equivalent weights for children 0 - 15 years only. We argue that children 16-18 years are the same burden in the family as the second adult.
[6]See, for example, Björklund et. al. (1995).
[7]We assume that we are supported with a continuous measure of health. See later in this section for a discussion of the assumption.

Table 1 Frequencies (in percent) of complaints for different illness conditions.

DISORDERS AND DISEASES	NO		MILD		SEVERE	
	1980	1990	1980	1990	1980	1990
Anaemia, low blood value	96.8	97.9	2.5	1.7	0.7	0.4
Arthritis/painful joints	76.9	74.8	14.3	15.8	8.8	9.4
Cancer	99.1	99.2	0.4	0.3	0.5	0.6
Chest pain	90.9	91.8	6.5	5.8	2.6	2.5
Chronic bronchitis	93.3	95.4	4.7	3.3	2.0	1.4
Common cold	31.1	28.8	49.8	54.5	19.1	16.7
Constipation	94.2	94.9	4.2	3.8	1.6	1.3
Cough	75.4	75.6	20.0	20.3	4.6	4.1
Diabetes	97.2	97.6	2.0	1.7	0.9	0.7
Diarrhoea	90.2	88.6	8.0	9.2	1.7	2.2
Difficulty breathing	93.2	93.4	4.7	4.6	2.2	2.0
Difficulty hearing	87.1	85.3	10.3	11.6	2.6	3.1
Difficulty seeing	92.3	93.2	5.0	4.4	2.7	2.4
Difficulty sleeping	86.9	87.3	9.0	9.2	4.1	3.5
Dizziness, vertigo	89.3	90.0	8.5	8.3	2.2	1.8
Elevated blood pressure	89.7	90.8	8.2	7.6	2.1	1.7
Feeling of sickness	88.1	86.8	9.9	10.6	2.0	2.5
Gall bladder	96.6	97.6	2.2	1.7	1.1	0.7
Gastric pain	77.7	77.9	16.2	16.6	6.1	5.5
Gastric ulcer, duodenal ulcer, dyspepsia	98.1	97.9	1.1	1.3	0.8	0.8
Goitre	98.5	98.0	1.3	1.6	0.3	0.4
Haemorrhoids	93.4	94.5	5.2	4.2	1.4	1.3
Headache	54.6	46.7	35.3	41.9	10.1	11.5
Heart attack, myocardial infarction	99.3	99.2	0.5	0.4	0.3	0.4
Heart failure	95.7	97.6	3.2	1.7	1.1	0.7
Hernia	98.4	98.6	1.1	1.0	0.4	0.4
Kidney disease	97.9	98.1	1.1	1.0	1.0	0.9
Lower back pain	68.8	64.0	18.2	22.9	13.0	13.1
Mental depression	94.1	94.1	3.8	3.8	2.1	2.1
Nervous problems	87.6	89.4	9.0	8.1	3.4	2.5
Neurological disorder	98.7	99.3	0.4	0.4	0.9	0.3
Over weight	88.6	87.0	9.7	10.6	1.7	2.4
Painful shoulders	77.7	68.7	14.1	20.6	8.3	10.7
Perspiration problems	93.5	93.8	4.8	4.7	1.7	1.6
Psychiatric disease	98.4	99.2	0.9	0.5	0.7	0.3
Rash, eczema, psoriasis	88.0	86.5	9.5	11.1	2.5	2.4
Strain, unsolved problems, stressful situation	94.8	93.5	4.0	5.5	1.1	1.0
Swelling of the legs	91.4	92.0	6.5	6.3	2.1	1.7
Tiredness, exhaustion, weakness	80.3	76.9	15.3	18.4	4.4	4.7

(Continued)

(Table 1 Continued)

DISORDERS AND DISEASES	NO		MILD		SEVERE	
	1980	1990	1980	1990	1980	1990
Tuberculosis	99.7	99.7	0.2	0.2	0.1	0.1
Varicose veins, leg ulcers	92.8	93.9	5.5	4.9	1.8	1.2
Voiding difficulties, prostate, lower urinary tract inf.	93.0	95.3	4.3	3.0	2.7	1.7
Vomiting	92.7	91.8	5.6	6.2	1.7	2.0
Weight loss	97.2	97.8	2.1	1.6	0.7	0.6
Ill health[8]		77.5		18.1		4.3

defined. In most empirical studies, illness is measured by self-assessed responses to questions about illnesses, where the different alternatives were rated on a scale. However, people value their illnesses differently, depending on differences in occupations, incomes or other socio-economic conditions, or depending on the normal situation in their group. What is known from the self-evaluated responses is the individual ranking; that is, that the rating "very bad" is worse than the rating "bad" for each individual.

The concentration curve for morbidity, $g^{ill}(y)$ shown in Figure 1, plots the cumulative proportions of the population (ranked by income) against the cumulative proportions of illness in the population. If morbidity is equally distributed over income, then the concentration curve will coincide with the diagonal. If morbidity in the population is concentrated to those with lower incomes, then the concentration curve will be located above the diagonal, as is the case in Figure 1. The concentration index for illness is defined as one minus twice the area under the concentration curve.[9] This is a measure of the degree of income related inequality in health. The index will be negative when illness is concentrated to the poor section of the population. The lowest value that the concentration index can take is -1. This occurs when the population's morbidity is concentrated to the poorest individual. The highest value that the concentration index can be is +1, which describes a situation in which the total illness of the population is concentrated to the richest.

This analysis of self-assessed ill health, diseases and disorders first standardized

---

[8]The question to the respondent is: "How do you value your own health conditions? Is it good, bad or something between?" There was no such question in 1980.
[9]Note that the concentration index is negative if the concentration curve lies above the diagonal.

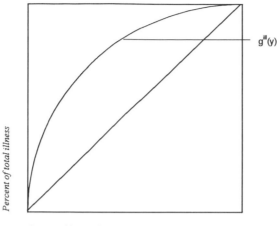

Figure 1 Concentration curve of illness

for age and sex in order to make the study internationally comparable.[10] The standardized number of persons in each morbidity category j, and income group t have been calculated as

$$N_{jt}^* = \sum_{i=1}^{n} (f_i / f_{it}) N_{ijt}$$

where N^*_{jt} is the standardized number of persons in income group t falling into morbidity category j, f_i the fraction of the sample in demographic group i, f_{it} the fraction of the sample in demographic group i, income group t and N_{ijt} is the number of persons in demographic group i, category j, income group t.[11]

---

[10]The reason for standardisation is that there are different age/sex distribution in the different income deciles. Thus, if we do not standardize we will have inequalities which depend on different age/sex distributions in different deciles (See Wagstaff *et al.* (1991b), p.178-182). By means of standardization we obtain the same age/sex distribution in each decile.

[11]For example, if we standardise for the demographic groups age and sex, the standardised number of persons in morbidity group 1, income group 1 equals [(number of women 18-34/total number of women)/(number of women 18-34 in income group 1/total number of women in income group 1)]*number of women in morbidity group 1, income group 1, 18-34 summarized for all age groups for women and for men.

In most health economic studies, health -- or ill health -- is measured as a categorical variable, for example good or bad health, rather than a continuous variable.[12] This paper will follow Wagstaff and van Doorslaer (1994) and assumes that there is a continuous latent variable representing the individual's self-assessed ill health, disorder or disease that underlies the categorical variable. Thus, instead of using the ordinal self-assessed indicator, the continuous latent variable is used in this analysis of inequalities. Suppose that the self-assessed ill health variable, H, has J categories, where 1 represents very bad health and J very good health. The latent ill health variable H^* is then related to H as follows:

$$H = 1 \ if - \infty < H^* \leq \alpha_1$$
$$H = 2 \ if \ \alpha_1 < H^* \leq \alpha_2$$
$$H = 3 \ if \ \alpha_2 < H^* \leq \alpha_3$$

.

$$H = J \ if \ \alpha_{J-1} < H^* \leq + \infty,$$

where α_J are thresholds. Assume first that health status (H^*) has a standard normal distribution. Then values of H^* can easily be computed for each individual. First, we estimate the $(J-1)$ thresholds as

$$\hat{\alpha}_j = \phi^{-1}\left(\sum_{i=1}^{j} N_j^* / N\right), j = 1,2,....j - 1,$$

where Φ^{-1} is the inverse standard normal cumulative density function, N_j^* the standardized number in category j and N the total number. In fact, the area under the standard normal distribution is divided into the proportion to the numbers in each category. The mean values in each interval were estimated as normal scores $\left(\hat{z}_j\right)$ using the formula:

$$\hat{Z}_j = \left(N / N_j^*\right)\left[\phi\left(\hat{\alpha}_{j-1}\right) - \phi\left(\hat{\alpha}_j\right)\right],$$

where $\Phi(\cdot)$ is the standard normal density function. These scores were the scores that

---

[12]When the morbidity indicators have more than two categories the indicators may be dichotomised. However, it has been shown [Wagstaff and van Doorslaer (1994)] that the estimated concentration indices are very sensitive to how the cut-off points are chosen and that the degree of inequality depends on the choice of cut-off points. This is the reason why we assume that there is a continuous latent variable underlying the categorical variable.

may be used when we calculate concentration indices. The most appropriate way to calculate the concentration index for ill health is by the covariance method proposed by Jenkins (1988). Here the concentration index is estimated by the formula $[(n^2 - 1)/6n](b/\bar{x})$, where $\bar{x}$ = mean for ill health, $b = cov(x,rx)/var(rx)$ and rx the rank variable for x. b is estimated by a regression of x on rx. This implies that $\bar{x}$ has to be non-zero. However, when the latent variable is constructed a standard normal distribution is assumed, that is, the mean value is zero. Moreover, most of the distributions concerning ill health were very skewed, in that there were few persons reporting severe illnesses while most report good health. Rather than assuming a standard normal distribution, we therefore assume a standard log-normal distribution. Hence, it is assumed that:

$$\hat{Z}_j = -\ln H^*, \text{ so that } H^* = \exp(-\hat{Z}_j).$$

The scores are calculated in the way described above, but interpreted as the negative logarithm of the corresponding latent ill health variable. The latent ill health variable is obtained by exponentiating the negatives of the normal scores. This latent variable is always positive. Hence, it is possible to use this variable when we construct the usual illness concentration curve and calculate the illness concentration index. The self-assessed ill health variable is only available in the data from 1990. The distribution of ill health and the value of the latent ill health variable can be seen in Table 2. Category 1 refers to poor health, category 2 to something between and category 3 to good health. Table 2 also shows the distribution of the unstandardized frequencies and latent health in the different categories.

Table 2. Calculation of latent ill health variable assuming a standard lognormal distribution

Category	Standardized for age and sex		Unstandardized for age and sex	
	Frequency (%)	Latent health	Frequency (%)	Latent health
1	4.2	8.4657	4.3	8.3417
2	18.2	3.1625	18.1	3.1432
3	77.6	0.6800	77.5	0.6794

To test whether the concentration indices were significantly different from zero, we have calculated standard errors for the concentration indices following Kakwani *et al.* (1996). The variance of the concentration index *(C)* has been calculated as

$$\text{var}(C) = 1/n\left[1/n\sum_{i=1}^{n} a_i^2 - (1+C)^2 \right],$$

where $a_i = (x_i/\mu)((2R_i - 1 - C) + 2 - q_{i-1} - q_i)$, x_i is the value of the latent variable for individual i, μ = mean value for the relevant latent variable, R_i the relative rank of individual i, and $q_i = (1/\mu)\sum_{r=1}^{i} x_r / n$. We also test for differences by pairwise comparisons of 1980 and 1990 by using the conventional t-test for groups.

RESULTS

The results from the estimations of disorders and diseases in 1980 and 1990 are shown in Table 3. The concentration indices are ranked in increasing order for 1990; that is, the first condition or disease is the one where the most income-related inequality in favor of the more wealthy was found. For 1980, the disorders and diseases were also ranked in the same order and a ranking number was put on the condition. We are thus able to study differences between the two periods. At the bottom of the table, the aggregate measure for 1990 is presented, which shows an almost even distribution of reported health status. Also calculated is a concentration index for self-assessed health that is not standardized for age and sex; the index changes only marginally to 0.00694.

From an international perspective, Sweden has small inequalities in health. In an earlier study (van Doorslaer, Wagstaff, *et al.*, 1996), in which concentration indices were calculated on grouped data for eight European countries and the United States, Sweden had the smallest inequality, although the concentration index was negative and significantly different from zero. The current study shows that the concentration index for the aggregate measure self-assessed health was close to zero, indicating that there were no income-related health inequalities in Sweden. However, when we disaggregate by looking at the different self-assessed diseases or disorders, the general pattern for 1990 was that several of the disorders or diseases had a distribution that is unfavorable to the poor section of the population; people with lower incomes report more diseases. Of the 44 conditions, 28 had a negative sign, of which 17 were significantly different from zero, indicating inequalities unfavorable to the poor. The conditions for which the concentration indices were positive in 1990 are close to zero, and only five conditions had concentration indices that were significantly different from zero. These disorders, which were reported more frequently by higher income groups, are cancer, overweight, elevated blood pressure, difficulty hearing, and perspiration problems. These conditions also had positive signs in 1980, although significant only for overweight, elevated blood pressure, and perspiration problems.

Table 3. Concentration indices for illness conditions.
(Standard errors are given in parentheses.)

DISORDERS AND DISEASES	CONCENTRATION INDEX 1990	RANK 1980	CONCENTRATION INDEX 1980	INDEX 1980-INDEX 1990 (T-VALUE)	RANK (1980-1990)
1. Feeling of sickness	-0.06495** (0.01003)	2	-0.03294*** (0.00954)	0.03201 (2.31)	2
2. Gastric pain	-0.04843*** (0.00910)	6	-0.02239*** (0.00876)	0.02604 (2.06)	3
3. Vomiting	-0.04535*** (0.01050)	3	-0.02854*** (0.01001)	0.01681 (1.16)	9
4. Headache	-0.03757*** (0.00786)	4	-0.02834*** (0.00778)	0.00923 (0.83)	17
5. Nervous problems	-0.03250*** (0.00911)	21	-0.00799 (0.00894)	0.02451 (1.92)	4
6. Rash, eczema, psoriasis	-0.02869*** (0.01008)	18	-0.00890 (0.01017)	0.01979 (1.38)	6
7. Gastric ulcer, duodenal, ulcer dyspepsia	-0.02700*** (0.01026)	36	0.00894 (0.00880)	0.03594 (2.66)	1
8. Tiredness, exhaustion, weakness	-0.02699*** (0.00899)	11	-0.01567* (0.00873)	0.01132 (0.90)	15
9. Common cold	-0.02599*** (0.00750)	5	-0.02325*** (0.00707)	0.00274 (0.26)	29
10. Mental depression	-0.02282*** (0.00959)	17	-0.00925 (0.00928)	0.01357 (1.02)	10
11. Cough	-0.02223** (0.00962)	1	-0.03748*** (0.00889)	-0.01525 (-1.16)	39
12. Difficulty breathing	-0.02105** (0.01002)	15	-0.01185 (0.00862)	0.00920 (0.70)	18
13. Psychiatric disease	-0.02004*** (0.00768)	20	-0.00860 (0.00819)	0.01144 (1.02)	14
14. Chronic bronchitis	-0.01909* (0.01002)	8	-0.01801* (0.00953)	0.00108 (0.08)	30
15. Diarrhoea	-0.01889* (0.01027)	28	0.00187 (0.00948)	0.02076 (1.49)	5
16. Tuberculosis	-0.01796** (0.00847)	26	-0.00010 (0.00755)	0.01786 (1.57)	8
17. Weight loss	-0.01771* (0.01002)	13	-0.01334 (0.00870)	0.00437 (0.33)	25
18. Varicose veins, leg ulcers	-0.01297 (0.00952)	16	-0.00953 (0.00906)	0.00344 (0.27)	28

(Continued)

(Table 3 continued)

DISORDERS AND DISEASES	CONCENTRATION INDEX 1990	RANK 1980	CONCENTRATION INDEX 1980	INDEX 1980-INDEX 1990 (T-VALUE)	RANK (1980-1990)
19. Strain, unsolved problems, stressful situation	-0.01238 (0.01092)	34	0.00731 (0.01030)	0.01969 (1.31)	7
20. Diabetes	-0.01198 (0.00895)	23	-0.00526 (0.00913)	0.00672 (0.52)	20
21. Anaemia, low blood value	-0.01132 (0.01036)	12	-0.01476* (0.00989)	-0.00344 (-0.24)	33
22. Constipation	-0.00793 (0.01057)	33	0.00540 (0.00936)	0.01333 (0.94)	11
23. Lower back pain	-0.00537 (0.00777)	30	0.00490 (0.00750)	0.01027 (0.95)	16
24. Goitre	-0.00499 (0.00998)	29	0.00260 (0.00931)	0.00759 (0.56)	19
25. Difficulty seeing	-0.00431 (0.00914)	14	-0.01214 (0.00936)	-0.00783 (-0.60)	36
26. Dizziness, vertigo	-0.00416 (0.00969)	27	-0.00003 (0.00938)	0.00413 (0.30)	26
27. Voiding difficulties, prostate, lower urinary tract infection	-0.00334 (0.00101)	37	0.00911 (0.00953)	0.01245 (0.90)	13
28. Chest pain	-0.00141 (0.00956)	24	-0.00362 (0.00872)	-0.00221 (-0.17)	32
29. Kidney disease	0.00283 (0.00989)	35	0.00861 (0.00996)	0.00578 (0.41)	22
30. Swelling of the legs	0.00367 (0.01021)	22	-0.00601 (0.00984)	-0.00968 (-0.68)	37
31. Arthritis/painful joints	0.00382 (0.00862)	19	-0.00861 (0.00818)	-0.01243 (-1.05)	38
32. Haemorrhoids	0.00562 (0.01013)	42	0.01895** (0.00928)	0.01333 (1.36)	12
33. Gall bladder	0.00611 (0.00987)	25	-0.00163 (0.00891)	-0.00774 (-0.58)	35

(Continued)

(Table 3 Continued)

DISORDERS AND DISEASES	CONCENTRATION INDEX 1990	RANK 1980	CONCENTRATION INDEX 1980	INDEX 1980-INDEX 1990 (T-VALUE)	RANK (1980-1990)
34. Heart attack, myocardial infarction	0.00659 (0.00892)	39	0.01222 (0.00870)	0.00563 (0.45)	24
35. Difficulty sleeping	0.00672 (0.00965)	31	0.00494 (0.00862)	-0.00178 (-0.13)	31
36. Painful shoulders	0.00963 (0.00812)	40	0.01344 (0.00806)	0.00381 (0.33)	27
37. Heart failure	0.01213 (0.00934)	8	-0.01830** (0.00895)	-0.03043 (-2.35)	43
38. Neurological disorder	0.01268 (0.00937)	10	-0.01674** (0.00807)	-0.02942 (-2.38)	42
39. Hernia	0.01522 (0.01056)	11	-0.01644* (0.00896)	-0.03166 (-2.29)	44
40. Cancer	0.01814** (0.00836)	38	0.01182 (0.00954)	-0.00632 (-0.50)	21
41. Overweight	0.02224*** (0.00863)	41	0.01657* (0.00968)	-0.00567 (-0.43)	34
42. Elevated blood pressure	0.02670*** (0.00974)	44	0.03247*** (0.00911)	0.00577 (0.43)	23
43. Difficulty hearing	0.03029*** (0.00886)	32	0.00535 (0.00859)	0.00535 (-2.02)	41
44. Perspiration problems	0.04645*** (0.01052)	43	0.03002*** (0.00937	-0.01643 (-1.17)	40
Ill health	0.00699 (0.00875)				

Notes: *** denotes significantly different from zero at the 1% level, ** at the 5% level and * at the 10% level. In the **RANK (1980-1990)**-column, conditions with rank numbers 1 - 4 are positive and significant and conditions with numbers 41 - 44 are negative and significant. The conditions with rank numbers 5 - 40 are conditions that are similarly distributed for the two periods.

In 1980, 27 conditions had negative signs, of which 12 were significantly different from zero. Thus, there were more conditions that were unfavorable to the poor section in 1990 than in 1980. Feeling of sickness, gastric pain, vomiting, headache, tiredness, common cold, cough, and chronic bronchitis were distributed towards the poor in both 1980 and 1990. Nervous problems, rash, mental depression, difficulties to breathe, psychiatric disease, tuberculosis and weight loss are diseases that were more commonly reported by the poor, although significant only in 1990. For gastric ulcer and diarrhoea there was a positive, though nonsignificant, index in 1980, and negative and significant index in 1990.

There were also interesting differences in the signs for heart failure, neurological disorder and hernia. In 1980, there were significant inequalities that adversely affected the poor, but, in 1990, there were no significant inequalities, although the concentration indices were positive. Overall, the indices were closer to zero in 1980 than in 1990; there were 22 diseases where the concentration indices were significantly different from zero in 1990 (17 negative and 5 positive), but only 16 were significantly different from zero in 1980 (12 negative and 4 positive). Moreover, the variation in the concentration index was greater in 1990 than in 1980; between -0.03748 (cough) and 0.03247 (elevated blood pressure) in 1980 and between -0.06495 (feeling of sickness) and 0.04645 (perspiration problems) in 1990. Thus, the diseases were in general more evenly distributed in 1980 than in 1990.

To test whether the differences in concentration indices between the two periods for different disorders and diseases were statistically significant t-tests of the differences in all conditions were performed. Significant differences were found for eight of the 44 diseases, of which four were positive. A positive significant difference between the two periods indicates either that the poor section of the population has been worse-off concerning that specific condition (the concentration indices were negative both in 1980 and 1990, but the absolute value was higher in 1990), or that the rich section is worse-off both in 1980 and 1990, but the absolute value of the concentration index is lower in 1990. A positive difference may also indicate that the rich section is worse-off in 1980 and the poor section in 1990. The conditions with a significant positive difference in concentration indices include feeling of sickness, gastric pain, nervous problems, and gastric ulcer. The distribution is unfavorable for the poor for both periods concerning feeling of sickness, gastric pain and nervous problems, thus indicating that the poor section of the population has been worse-off with respect to those diseases. Concerning gastric ulcer, the distribution was unfavorable regarding the rich section of the population in 1980, but the poor section in 1990, and thus making the poor section worse-off.

A negative sign on the difference between the concentration indices indicates either that the rich section was worse-off, that the poor section was still worse-off, but to a lesser degree, or that the poor section was worse-off in 1980 and the rich section in 1990. The four conditions for which the difference is negatively significantly different from zero include heart failure, neurological disorder, hernia, and difficulty hearing. In our study, the poor section was worse-off in 1980 and the rich section in 1990 concerning heart failure, neurological disorder and hernia, whereas the rich section was worse-off regarding difficulties to hear.

The ranking numbers shown in the last column refer to the differences between concentration indices for 1980 and 1990. We have ranked the differences between the two periods to study those conditions that have changed most dramatically. The diseases with a low rank number are those that have changed most between the two periods, and are unfavorable to the less well-off; a high rank number indicates diseases that have changed most in disfavor to the well-off.

CONCLUSION AND DISCUSSION

This study compared inequalities in health in Sweden in 1980 and 1990 for 44 disorders and diseases and investigated overall health inequalities in 1990. The general measure for self-reported ill health showed that health was not income-related in 1990.[13] However, the conclusion reached concerning the 44 diseases and disorders was that, in 1990, half of the 44 diseases and disorders were distributed unevenly and that the inequalities were mostly unfavorable to the poor. In general, the inequalities in the diseases and disorders were less obvious in 1980 than in 1990, even if the aggregate measure in 1990 showed an almost even distribution. The reason may be that people in general answer that they feel fit regarding their own general health condition, although they may have actually been suffering from one or more specific diseases during the last twelve months. These afflictions could have occurred many months in the past, but they are healthy at the time of interview and thus answer that they are in good health.

When changes between the two periods were compared, age and sex were standardized for, as is a customary procedure in other studies. We could also have controlled for other variables (*e.g.*, nationality) because there are reasons to believe that some of the inequalities found in this study may depend on variables other than income. Tuberculosis, for example, which afflicts the poor more than the rich in 1990, is more common among immigrants.

Some inequalities could also be explained by information and how that information

---

[13]Remember that our measure does not tell us anything about the direction of the causality; it only tells us that there may or may not be a relation between income and health or the specific disease or disorder. It does not say whether income affects or is affected by health or the specific disease or disorder.

was used in different income groups.[14] Gastric ulcer, for example, which afflicts the poor more than the rich in 1990, may depend on more effective use of information in higher income groups in that they visit doctors and receive effective medicine at an early stage in their gastric pain. Better use of information may also be an explanation when we study the changes in the distribution between the two periods. Feeling of sickness, gastric pain, nervous problems and gastric ulcer are all diseases where there have been changes resulting in the poor section of the population being worse-off, and which may depend on information. Also, elevated blood pressure, which is a disadvantage to the rich, may depend on information; higher income groups visit doctors more frequently than lower income groups to control their blood pressure. In this way, the rich become aware of the potential disorder. Further, cancer may depend on better use of information by higher income groups, because these groups are more aware about the risks and visit doctors earlier. Thus, there is a greater likelihood of revealing the disease at an earlier time.

Most of the diseases and disorders were distributed similarly in 1980 as in 1990, although sometimes the distribution is uneven for both periods. Overweight and perspiration problems, for example, were unfavorable to the rich for both periods. However, this may not necessarily mean that higher income groups weigh more and have more perspiration problems, because higher income groups may define normal weight and perspiration differently than low income groups.

In this study, concentration indices for different self-assessed conditions in 1980 and in 1990 were calculated and compared with one another. This calculation may not reveal fully the truth about the distribution of health, in that people in different income groups may have disparate evaluations about normal health status. Instead of using self-assessed measures in studies on health inequalities, it is possible to use so-called medical models and functional models. In these models, health conditions were assessed by questions concerned with functions (*e.g.*, ability to run 100 meters, walk up stairs, etc.). Even though the disorders and diseases in this study are based on self-assessments, there are also medical diagnoses involved in the assessments. These diagnoses have, in many cases, been made by a physician. By comparing the self-assessed measure with the physician's diagnostic measure, it is possible to check the validity of the individual's responses. However, both the functional and the medical models are questions for further research.

---

[14]We argue that higher educated people have higher wages and incomes than lower educated people. The former people also have better possibilities to obtain information about health policies.

ACKNOWLEDGEMENTS

This work was financially supported by the National Corporation of Swedish Pharmacies. Comments from Per-Anders Edin, Bertil Holmlund, Bengt Jönsson, Mårten Palme and Andreas Terént are highly appreciated.

REFERENCES

Björklund, A., Palme, M., Svensson, I. (1995) Assessing the effects of Swedish tax and benefit reforms on income distribution using different income concepts. Tax reform evaluation. Report no. 13, August 1995. National Institute of Economic Research, Economic Council, Stockholm.

Blaxter, M. (1989) A comparison of measures of inequality in morbidity. in Fox, J., editor, *Health Inequalities in European Countries*. London:Gower, Aldershot

Culyer, A. J. (1993), Health, health expenditure and equity. In van Doorslaer, E, Wagstaff, A, van Rutten, F (eds.), *Equity in the Finance and Delivery of Health Care: An International Perspective*. Oxford: Oxford University Press.

Fritzell, J., Lundberg, O., (red.) (1994) *Vardagens villkor. Levnadsförhållanden i Sverige under tre decennier*. Brombergs förlag. (The conditions of Daily Living).

Institutet för social forskning (1992), *1991 års levnadsnivåundersökning*. Instruktions-och övningsformulär. Institutet för social forskning, Stockholms universitet. (Level of Living Survey 1991. Instruction and Practising).

Jansson, K., (1990) *Inkomst- och förmögenhetsfördelningen 1967 - 1987*. Bilaga 19 till Långtidsutredningen 1990. Finansdepartementet. (The distribution of income- and wealth 1967 - 1987. Appendix 19 to the Medium Term Survey 1990).

Jenkins, S. (1988) Calculating Income Distribution Indices from Micro Data. *National Tax Journal* XLI(1):139-142.

Kakwani, N., Wagstaff, A., van Doorslaer, E. (1996) Socioeconomic inequalities in health: measurement, computation and statistical inference. Forthcoming in *Journal of Econometrics*.

Le Grand, J., Rabin, M. (1986) Trends in British health inequality, 1931-1983. In Culyer, A. J., Jönsson, B., editors, *Public and Private Health Services*. Oxford:Blackwell.

Le Grand, J. (1987) Inequalities in health; some international comparisons. *European Economic Review* 31:182-191.

Le Grand, J. (1989) An International Comparison of Distribution of Ages-at-death. In Fox, J., editor, *Health Inequalities in European Countries*. London:Gower,

Aldershot.

Lundberg, O., (1990) Den ojämlika ohälsan. Om klass- och könsskillnader i sjuklighet. *Institutet för social forskning*, avhandlingsserie 11. (Inequality in Ill Health. On class and sex differences in illness).

Lundberg, O. (1991) Causal explanations for class inequality in health. An empirical analysis. *Social Science and Medicine* 32:385-393.

Lundberg, O., Fritzell, J. (1994) Income distribution, income change and health: on the importance of absolute and relative income for health status in Sweden. In Levin, L. S., McMahon, L., Ziglio, E. editors, *Economic Change, Social Welfare and Health in Europe*. WHO Regional Publications, European Series, No.54, Chapter 3, pp. 37-58. World Health Organization. Regional Office for Europe. Copenhagen.

Sundberg, G. (1996) *Health, Work-Hours, and Wages in Sweden*. Uppsala University, Departments of Economics.

Svensk Författningssamling (1982) SFS 1982:763. *Hälso-och sjukvårdslag*. (The Swedish Health Care Act).

Townsend, P., Davidson, N. (1982) *Inequalities in Health: The Black Report*. Harmondsworth, Penguin Books.

Vågerö, D., Illsley, R. (1995) Explaining health inequalities: beyond Black and Barker. *European Sociological Review* 11:219-241.

van Doorslaer, E, Wagstaff, A. (1992) Equity in the delivery of health care: some international comparisons. *Journal of Health Economics* 11:389 - 411.

van Doorslaer, E., Wagstaff, A., Bleichrodt, H., *et al.* (1997) Income-Related Inequalities in Health: Some International Comparisons. *Journal of Health Economics 16:93-112.*

van Doorslaer, E., Wagstaff, A. and Rutten, F., editors (1993) *Equity in the Finance and Delivery of Health Care: An International Perspective*. Oxford: Oxford University Press.

Wagstaff, A., van Doorslaer, E. (1994) Measuring inequalities in health in the presence of multiple-category morbidity indicators. *Health Economics* 3:281-291.

Wagstaff, A., Paci, P., van Doorslaer, E. (1991a) On the measurement of inequalities in health. *Social Science and Medicine* 33:545-557.

Wagstaff, A., van Doorslaer, E., Paci, P. (1991b) On the measurement of horizontal inequity in the delivery of health care. *Journal of Health Economics* 10:169 - 205.

Wilkinson, R. (1986) Introduction. In Wilkinson, R., editor, *Class and Health*. London:Tavistock.

5

Micro-level Analysis of Distributional Changes in Health Care Financing in Finland

JAN KLAVUS and UNTO HÄKKINEN

STAKES

National Research and Development Centre for Welfare and Health

Helsinki, Finland

ABSTRACT

In the early 1990s the Finnish economy suffered a severe recession, at the same time as certain health care reforms were taking place. This study examined the effects of these changes on the distribution of health care financing. The analysis was based partly on actual income data and partly on simulated data from the base year. The paper applies a new method for estimating confidence intervals for Gini coefficients and progressivity indices. Results indicate that the financing share of poorer households increased during the recession, which was caused purely by

Health, Health Care and Health Economics: Perspectives on Distribution
Edited by Morris L. Barer, Thomas E. Getzen, and Greg L. Stoddart
Copyright 1998 John Wiley & Sons, Ltd.

structural changes. Because of the financial plight of the public sector, the financing share of progressive income taxes decreased, while regressive indirect taxes and out-of-pocket payments contributed more. It seems, however, that aside from the increased financing burden on poorer households, Finland's health care system has withstood the tremendous changes of the early 1990s fairly well.

INTRODUCTION

Nowadays, health care reform is a common policy issue in many countries. The main aim of reforms has been to improve efficiency while preserving equity in the health care system. Policy-makers are usually aware of the potential equity consequences of the reforms, but the empirical evidence to support such concerns is often missing. The reason for this is that collecting population level data covering the entire health care system is both very time consuming and expensive. One possibility is to use existing, updated microdata to evaluate the equity implications of various policy alternatives. Such microsimulation models are widely used in income distribution analysis to provide policy-makers with insight into changes before actual data become available. Although there is also growing interest in this type of analysis in health care research, such studies are still very few in number. In the Netherlands, simulation has been used to estimate the distributional consequences of health insurance reforms (van Doorslaer *et al.*, 1991; Janssen *et al.*, 1993), while in the USA Rivlin and Wiener (1988) and Cohen *et al.*(1993) have simulated the fiscal and distributional impacts of Medicaid reforms.

This paper examines the distributional changes in health care financing in Finland following the deep economic recession and significant health care reforms carried out in the early 1990s. The outcome was measured in terms of progressivity. As baseline material we used the progressivity indices of the various health care financing sources in 1990, which were compared to the corresponding indices in 1994. The analysis builds partly on actual income data from existing income statistics and partly on simulations based on micro-level data from the base year. We employed methods that allowed us to estimate confidence intervals for the base year (1990) indices.

BACKGROUND TO THE ANALYSIS

Health care in Finland is mainly based on public financing and service provision. In 1990 about 85% of total health care expenditure was financed through the public sector: 75% from taxes and tax expenditures, and 10% from sickness insurance payments. The remaining 15% was financed by direct payments from households, including user charges for public services and non-subsidized medicines, and copayments for private sector medical and dental treatment.

Following a period of rapid growth in the late 1980s, the economic situation in Finland worsened abruptly. Between 1990 and 1993 real GDP decreased by 12%, unemployment rose to 18% and central government debt exceeded 50% of GDP. A gradual improvement began in 1994, but in spite of three years of steady growth the GDP still remains below the level of the late 1980s. During the first two years of the economic recession the health care expenditure share of GDP increased from 8.0% to 9.3%, mainly due to a contraction in the GDP (Fig. 1). From 1991 to 1994 health care expenditure per capita decreased by 15%, resulting in a fall in the GDP share to 8.3% in 1994.

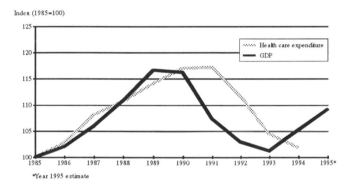

Figure 1 Health care expenditure and GDP per capita in Finland 1985-1995 (at constant prices)

The weakness of public sector finances has also affected the funding of health services. Publicly financed health care decreased its share over four years from about 85% to 75% (Table 1), largely due to a cut-back in the central state contribution.

Table 1 Financing of health care in Finland 1990-1994 (% of total expenditure)

	1990	1991	1992	1993	1994
State:	37.2	36.9	35.1	30.7	29.2
- income tax	14.1	11.2	7.6	5.3	5.6
- indirect tax	22.1	18.1	15.0	11.0	11.4
- net borrowing	1.0	7.6	12.5	14.4	12.2
Municipalities	35.8	35.7	33.3	34.1	33.0
Sickness insurance	10.8	11.3	11.1	12.2	13.0
Total public	**83.8**	**83.9**	**79.5**	**77.0**	**75.2**
Households	**12.6**	**12.6**	**16.6**	**19.1**	**20.8**
Other private	**3.6**	**3.5**	**3.9**	**3.9**	**4.0**
Total	**100.0**	**100.0**	**100.0**	**100.0**	**100.0**

Source: Health care expenditure and financing in Finland 1960-94,
Social Insurance Institution 1996, and own calculations

The structure of the state's revenue base has also changed. In 1993 and 1994 government borrowing became the largest single revenue source, replacing revenue from state income taxes and commodity taxes. This shift towards debt financing means that part of the financial burden of current health care services will be borne by future taxpayers.

Over the four years, the user's share of health care financing rose from 13% to 21%. This increase stemmed partly from the abolition of a tax deduction for medical expenses and partly from increased user fees and copayments for health care services. Health care prices increased in 1990-1994 by 20 percentage points more than consumer prices on average (Table 2). The rise in copayment shares was most striking in outpatient care, hospital inpatient care and prescription medicines (Table 3).

Considerable changes have also emerged in the structure of health care expenditure (Table 4). The most distinct trend is a relative decrease in hospital inpatient care and an increase in specialist and primary outpatient care. This has mainly been caused by a reduction in the number of hospital beds in psychiatric care, but applies also to inpatient care in general.

Table 2 Health care consumer price and utilisation index 1990 and 1994 (1990=100)

	Health Care Price index[a] 1994 (1990=100)	**Change in health care utilisation[b] 1994 (1990=100)**
Hospital in-patient care (specialist care including psychiatric care)	756.3	86
Hospital outpatient care (specialist care)	166.7	115
Health centre visits	227.5	88
Private physician visits	128.5	79
Private examination & treatment	116.0	69
Medicines, of which	136.8	115
-prescription	150.6	95
-over the counter	123.8	136
Eyeglasses	111.0	101
Health care on average	131.2	96
All consumer prices on average	110.9	

Sources: a Consumer price index, Statistica Finland 1996

b Statistical yearbook of the Social Insurance Institution, Social Insurance Institution 1996, and own estimations from various data sources on health care utilisation

In contrast to the opposite trend in the 1980s, expenditure on medicines increased during the recession. In 1994 medicines and pharmaceutical products accounted for 13% of the total health care budget.

These developments reflect changes in the structure of utilisation rather than in the structure of costs (see Table 2). Over the period 1990 - 1994 the average length of stay in hospitals shortened by 15%. Average numbers of visits to health centres and private sector physicians decreased, while visits to hospital outpatient centres became more frequent. In spite of the rise in prices and copayments, the use of medicines increased even during the worst years of the recession.

The State Subsidy System for health and social services was reformed in 1993, during the depths of the economic recession. The aim of the reform was to reduce central government control and allow the local municipalities more freedom in the provision of health and social services. As part of the reform, municipalities were assigned the right to decide whether or not to charge for the use of public services and also the level of any such charges (up to a limit set by the government).

Table 3 Cost-sharing as a proportion (%) of expenditure in health services 1990-1994

	1990	1991	1992	1993	1994
Hospital inpatient care	6.9	6.6	7.6	9.2	10.3
Outpatient care (excl. dental care)	12.1	12.2	12.7	16.2	18.1
of which:					
Health centres	1.4	1.7	1.9	6.9	12.2
Occupational and					
students health care	1.1	1.1	1.3	4.1	4.6
Hospital outpatient care	5.3	4.8	6.3	8.7	10.0
Private services	63.6	65.8	67.3	66.9	65.9
of which:					
Private doctors	61.4	63.9	64.5	64.4	64.0
Private treatments	65.4	67.5	69.8	69.3	67.8
Dental care (incl. prostheses)	53.2	52.0	52.8	55.1	55.6
Medicines	50.6	50.3	52.8	53.9	52.6
of which:					
Prescribed medicines	37.2	36.3	39.8	39.7	39.6
Total	15.6	15.7	16.6	19.1	20.8
Including tax expenditure[a]	12.6	12.6	---	---	---

[a]The tax deduction for medical expenses was removed in 1992
Source: Health care expenditure and financing in Finland 1960-94,
Social Insurance Institution 1996, and own calculations

Because of the major contribution of tax revenues in the Finnish health care financing system, the most obvious distributional effects arise from changes in the burden of taxation. In the early 1990s, two major tax reforms were carried out in Finland. The first, a large-scale reform aimed at reducing the burden of direct taxation, was executed in 1989 - 1991. This involved lowering marginal tax rates in all income groups. In order to simplify and clarify the system of tax allowances, steps were taken to gradually substitute tax deductions by direct income transfers. The reform was to be implemented without altering the distribution of income between income groups.

The second main reform took place in 1994, when the old system of turn-over commodity taxation was replaced by a value-added tax. This reform extended the tax-base by imposing previously exempt elements, such as services, under commodity taxation.

Table 4 Health care expenditure in Finland 1990-1994

	Volume index (1990 = 100)				Share of total expenditure	
	1991	1992	1993	1994	1990 %	1994 %
Inpatient care of which:	99.9	94.7	86.6	82.4	44.7	41.5
Specialist care	97.1	89.7	83.4	76.2	26.6	22.8
Health centres	100.7	96.4	82.4	82.4	13.1	12.1
Other hospital inpatient care	112.8	116.5	114.7	115.7	5.0	6.6
Outpatient care (excl. dental care) of which:	102.8	98.2	93.7	92.9	28.1	29.5
Health centres	102.4	98.1	95.3	94.6	13.3	14.1
Occupational and students health care	97.5	91.4	84.0	89.1	3.0	3.1
Private outpatient care	101.1	89.0	84.8	77.1	4.3	3.9
Outpatient departments of specialist hospitals	107.1	106.6	99.7	100.3	7.5	8.4
Dental care (incl. protheses)	92.4	89.8	87.1	86.3	5.8	5.9
Medicines and pharmaceuticals	110.3	116.4	121.3	127.8	9.4	12.8
Other running expenditure	100.0	99.5	91.4	93.1	7.4	7.8
Total running expenditure	101.7	98.3	92.8	91.8	95.4	97.5
Public investment	91.3	75.3	62.6	55.9	4.6	2.5
Total health care expenditure	101.3	97.3	91.4	89.6	100.0	100.0

Source: Health care expenditure and financing in Finland 1960-94, Social Insurance Institution 1996, and own calculations

In 1991 the proportional sickness insurance payment scale was replaced by a progressive two-tier payment scale. Under the old system all wage and salary earners contributed on average 1.7% of their earnings (adjusted to their local tax) to the National Sickness Insurance fund (NSI), whereas in 1991 the contribution rate was 1.7% for incomes below FIM 80 000 and 2.7% for exceeding income. In 1994 the income division remained unaltered, but the rates were increased to 1.9% and 3.8%, respectively (for pensioners 4.9% and 6.8%).

DATA, VARIABLES AND METHODS

For analysing the distributional consequences of the changes and reforms, three different data sets were used (see Appendix 1). Changes in income, direct taxes, and sickness insurance contributions were examined using data from the 1990 Finnish Household Survey (FHS) and 1994 Income Distribution Statistics (IDS). Changes in indirect taxes and out-of-pocket payments were examined with respect to the FHS data, while to estimate inpatient charges we used data (linked to the FHS 1990 households) from the Finnish Hospital Discharge Registers (FHDR) for 1989, 1990 and 1991.

The FHS is a multipurpose sample survey used to analyse the structure of household consumption and the use of social services. The target population consists of resident households, with those in institutions excluded. In 1990 the sample size was about 11,700 households and complete data were received from 8,258 households.

The IDS is an annual household interview survey describing the level, formation, and distribution of income among the economically active population. It applies a panel technique, where half of the sample consists of households in the previous year's sample. In 1994 the total sample size was 11,876 households and the number of accepted interviews was 8,964 households. Most of the income data come from administrative files such as registers on income taxation, national pensions, sickness insurance, child benefits and housing supports. To test the sensitivity of these results to the choice of survey data (FHS 1990/IDS 1990) progressivity indices were estimated from both data sources.

In the absence of earmarked taxes and social insurance contributions the proportion of each revenue source going to finance health care is not directly observable. This proportion was estimated by weighting all taxes and sickness insurance payments according to the revenue collecting sector's share of total health care expenditure. For example, the share of taxes used to finance health care is equivalent to the government's share of total health care expenditures. Likewise, the proportions of sickness insurance contributions and out-of-pocket payments are equivalent to the expenditure shares of the Social Insurance Institution (SII) and direct payments by households, respectively. Only running expenditures on health care were included; expenditures on environmental health care, and investment were disregarded.

Debt financing amounts to a transfer of income from future to current taxpayers. Since the true distributional outcome of the transfer is unknown, it is reasonable to assume that it is distributed according to state taxation under the present tax system. (An additional, noncash, income transfer is received by those taxpayers who also utilise public health services during the period of consideration). The transfer influences the level of after-payment income and the magnitude of the redistributive effect, but not progressivity, except through changes in the relative shares of the other government revenue sources. Another solution would be to exclude public borrowing altogether. Both of these approaches were used, assuming first that the public borrowing was distributed according to income and indirect taxes in state taxation and, second, that it did not exist.

In estimating sickness insurance payments it was assumed that the employer's share was borne entirely by employees (labor supply was regarded as totally inelastic). Thus, household sickness insurance payments consisted of the payment shares of employers, employees, the state and municipalities. The contributions of the state and the municipalities were assumed to be borne proportional to state and municipality taxes.

The simulation procedure was as follows. Households in the 1990 FHS sample were also assumed to represent the population in 1994. In evaluating the changes in progressivity we took into account the shift in the distribution of income, but assumed that the ranking of households in the income distribution, and thus their relative ranking in the tax/health care payment distribution, had not changed between 1990 and 1994.

The simulated variables were indirect taxes and household out-of-pocket payments. Indirect taxes were estimated from the 1990 FHS data by weighting each household's expenditure by the value-added and excise tax levies on aggregated commodity groups. A total of 47 such commodity groups were used in computations in 1990 and 1994. In addition to incorporating changes in the tax levies on various commodities, we also took account of changes in the level of consumption, as measured by the average expenditure ratios of 10 main commodity groups in 1990 and 1994. The method used for estimating changes in out-of-pocket payments was broadly similar. Data on quantitative changes in the utilisation of health care services between 1990 and 1994 were used and combined with data on changes in the consumer prices of these services (see Table 2).

It was assumed that the changes in expenditure were distributed evenly across all households (the fact that income and price elasticities may differ by income level was not taken into account). In this respect the changes in progressivity reflect relative changes in the expenditure structure on different commodities and health services, as well as changes in their relative prices, but not income group specific changes due to differences in behaviour.

Progressivity was analysed with respect to household gross income. All income, taxes and payments were adjusted by an equivalence scale. We used the OECD-scale, which gives a weight of 1 for the first adult, 0.7 for the second and 0.5 for each child. The individual rather than the household was treated as the relevant income unit. Thus individuals were ranked in ascending order according to their household equivalent income (Danziger and Taussig, 1979).

Progressivity was measured by Kakwani's progressivity index (Kakwani, 1977), which indicates the extent to which the financing system departs from proportionality. It is given by the difference between the concentration curve for health care payments and the Lorenz curve for pre-payment income. A positive value of the index implies that financing is progressive, and a negative value that financing is regressive. Kakwani's index can have values ranging from -2 (when all pre-payment income is concentrated to the richest person and the entire financing burden falls on someone else) to 1 (when pre-payment income is distributed proportionally and the entire financing burden falls on one person).

In order to control for estimation bias arising from systematic nonresponse in the sample, population weighted variables were used. Gini coefficients and progressivity indices were estimated from micro-data by the regression method applied to weighted samples (Kakwani *et al.*, in press, 1997; Klavus, 1996). This approach allowed us to compute standard errors, which were used to construct confidence intervals for the base year indices.

Ranking households by gross income is likely to make successive observations correlate with each other. If the observations are not independently distributed, the standard errors are not entirely accurate. Serial correlation is especially likely to be present among financing sources for which a high value of the dependent variable can be expected to appear together with a high value of the ranked income variable. This applies in particular to the progressive or proportional financing components, such as direct taxes and sickness insurance payments. In this study we used an estimator for standard errors that takes into account serial correlation in the data (for a more detailed technical presentation on the estimation of the indices and standard errors, see Kakwani *et al.*, in press, 1997; and Klavus, 1996).

RESULTS

A remarkable feature of developments in the 1990s is that while real income levels decreased substantially during the recession, the distribution of income remained almost unchanged (Table 5). In this respect the recession seems to have treated all income groups almost equally (this finding lends support to our initial assumption that the ranking of households in the income distribution remained unchanged).

Overall, the progressivity of health care financing decreased over the four years. The most visible changes occurred in the distribution of state income taxes, local taxes and sickness insurance payments. The progressivity indices of these financing sources were outside the confidence intervals of the base year indices. The increase in progressivity of state income taxes is partly explained by the decline in income levels. As a result of a decrease in taxable income, households in all income brackets moved downwards on the tax scale and a larger proportion of households in the lower income brackets fell below the limit of taxable income in state taxation. Another reason for increased progressivity is a forced loan that the government collected from high-income earners in 1993 in the form of an additional, progressive, income tax. This loan was to be returned to taxpayers by the year 1996. At the same time, the levels of certain regressive tax allowances was drastically cut, while others were removed altogether.

The decrease in progressivity of local income taxes is explained by an increase in the average rate of local income taxes. Regardless of the fact that local taxes are proportional to income, regional variation in tax rates increased during the recession. Tax rates rose most in the poorer municipalities, where unemployment and the economic recession were particularly severe and the income level of the population was low.

The increased progressivity of sickness insurance payments is the consequence of adopting a progressive two-tier sickness insurance payment scale. This also increased the level of payments, as indicated by the sharp rise in the revenue share of sickness insurance payments. The distributional consequences of the VAT-reform seem to be rather small. This finding is in line with previous estimations

Table 5 Progressivity and structure of health care financing in Finland 1990 and 1994 (running expenditure)

		State			Municipalities	SII	Households		
	Gross income	Income tax	Indirect taxes	Net public borrowing	Local tax	Sickness insurance	**Total public**	Direct payments	**Total financing**
1990									
Revenue share (%)		14.0	23.0	1.0	37.0	11.0	**86.0**	14.0	**100.0**
Gini coeff.	0.256								
Kakwani's index		0.269	-0.097	0.039	0.077	0.086	**0.061**	-0.198	**0.024**
*se	(0.0051)	(0.0097)	(0.0056)	(0.0030)	(0.0023)	(0.0027)	**(0.0021)**	(0.011)	**(0.0023)**
L95	0.246	0.250	-0.108	0.033	0.072	0.081	**0.057**	-0.219	**0.019**
U95	0.266	0.288	-0.086	0.045	0.082	0.091	**0.065**	-0.177	**0.029**
1994									
Revenue share (%)		6.0	11.0	12.0	34.0	14.0	**77.0**	23.0	**100.0**
Gini coeff.	0.261								
Kakwani's index	0.310	-0.106	0.040	0.064	0.123	**0.066**	-0.198	**0.005**	

*se: standard error accounted for serial correlation
L95 and U95: lower and upper limits of 95% confidence interval

which have considered the distributional outcome of the commodity tax reform (Ritvanen, 1992; Lehtinen and Salomäki, 1993).

In spite of several changes that have occurred in the utilisation and fees of health services, the regressivity of households' direct payments seems to have remained unchanged. This can be examined in more detail by analysing separately the effect of increased out-of-pocket payments and the effect of exclusion of the tax deduction of medical expenses. The distinct effect of the rise in out-of-pocket payments was an increase in regressivity from -0.198 in 1990 to -0.230 in 1994. In this sense the burden of increased payments fell on lower income groups. However, when analysed in connection with out-of-pocket payments, the removal of the tax deduction for medical expenses outweighed this effect and maintained the distribution of direct payments nearly unchanged. The tax deduction particularly favored high income households with larger medical bills and higher marginal tax-rates.

In order to investigate the reasons behind the changes in overall progressivity in more detail, we decomposed the change into the effect arising from changes in the level of progressivity and the effect arising from changes in the financing structure (Table 6).

Table 6 Decomposition of Distributional Changes in Health Care Financing 1990-1994

	Effect of changes in progressivity indices[a]	Effect of changes in financing structure[b]
Kakwani's index, total financing (1994)	0.029	0.003
Net progressivity effect, 1990-1994	+0.005	- 0.021

[a] Calculated from 1994 progressivity indices with 1990 revenue shares
[b] Calculated from 1990 progressivity indices with 1994 revenue shares

It seems that the decrease in overall progressivity was caused solely by structural changes. The net effect of changes in the progressivity of the individual financing sources was to increase progressivity slightly, but structural changes in the relative size of the regressive financing sources reversed this effect, making the overall distribution more regressive.

Our results were not sensitive to whether or not public borrowing was taken into account in the calculation of progressivity. Exclusion of public borrowing made overall financing only slightly less progressive (0.005 vs. 0.0004). Likewise, the choice of the base year survey did not have any significant impact on the conclusions of the analysis (Appendix 2). According to earlier results on the same data, the progressivity indices were rather robust to the choice of equivalence scale (Klavus, 1996).

DISCUSSION AND CONCLUSIONS

Health care financing in Finland has become more regressive in the 1990s. It seems that this has mainly been caused by changes in the financing structure. Resorting to debt financing has decreased the share of progressively distributed income taxes and correspondingly increased the share of regressive indirect taxes and out-of-pocket payments. However, the decrease in progressivity was not very substantial, and overall the health care system remained progressive in 1994. In international comparison of different health care financing systems (Fig. 2), Finland is still grouped among other mainly tax-financed proportional or slightly progressive health care systems (Häkkinen, 1992; van Doorslaer *et al.*, 1992). A striking feature of recent developments is the clear shift in the burden of financing towards the users of services. At the same time, the utilisation of certain services has declined substantially. According to findings on the delivery side, this has not increased income related differences in the utilisation of health care (Häkkinen, *et al.*, 1995). This argument is supported by our earlier observation that income inequality remained almost unchanged throughout the recession. Still, in relative terms, poorer households have suffered worse from the decrease in real income, which may indicate that they have been inclined to more drastic adjustments in their consumption patterns than households with greater consumption potential.

From an equity point of view Finland's health care system seems to have withstood the reforms and changes of the 1990s fairly well. One reason for this success is the wide coverage of the Finnish income maintenance system, which somewhat compensated for income losses due to unemployment and alleviated some of the adverse effects of the recession. Another reason is the redistributive nature of the tax financed health care system, which seems to be capable of apportioning the risks of financial and functional disturbances in an equitable way. The distributional outcome might have been totally different in a health care system that rests more on social insurance and private payments in its financing, and where the delivery of services is linked more closely to the source of the payments.

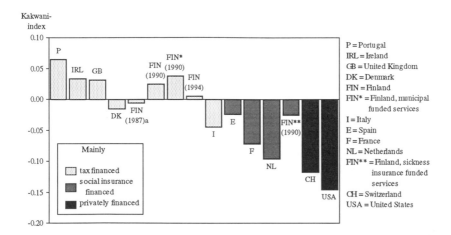

Figure 2 Progressivity of health care financing in 11 OECD-countries
Source: van Doorslaer et al. (1992); Häkkinen (1992)

REFERENCES

Cohen, M.A., Kumar, N., and Wallack, S.S. (1993) Simulating the fiscal and distributional impacts of medicaid eligibility reforms. *Health Care Financing Review* 4:133-150.

Danziger, S. and Taussig, M.K. (1979) The income unit and the anatomy of income distribution. *Review of Income and Wealth* 25:365-375.

Häkkinen, U. (1992) *Health Care Utilization, Health and Socioeconomic Equality in Finland* (in Finnish). Sosiaali- ja terveyshallitus, Tutkimuksia 20, Valtion painatuskeskus.

Häkkinen, U., Rosenqvist, G., and Aro, S. (1995) *Economic Depression and the Use of Physician Services in Finland.* STAKES, Themes 6/95. STAKES, Helsinki.

Kakwani, N.C. (1977) Measurement of tax progressivity: an international comparison. *Economic Journal* 87:71-80.

Kakwani, N.C., Wagstaff, A., and van Doorslaer, E. (1997) Socioeconomic inequality in health: measurement, computation and statistical inference. *Journal of Econometrics* Forthcoming.

Klavus, J. (1996) *Progressivity of Health Care Financing: Estimation and Statistical Inference.* STAKES, Themes 3/97. STAKES, Helsinki.

Janssen, R., van Doorslaer, E., and Wagstaff, A. (1993) Health insurance reform in the Netherlands: assessing the progressivity consequences. ECuity Project Working Paper #1. Erasmus University, Rotterdam

Lehtinen, T., and Salomäki, A. (1993) *The Effect of Changes in the Tax and Transfer Systems on Disposable Income in 1994* (in Finnish). Government Institute for Economic Research, Discussion papers 51, Helsinki.

Ritvanen, K. (1992) The impact of value-added-taxation on consumer prices (in Finnish). In: *Liikevaihtoveropohjan laajentamistyoryhman mietinto.* Helsinki: Komiteamietinto.

Rivlin. A., and Wiener, J. (1988) *Caring for the Disabled Elderly: Who Will Pay?* Washington DC:The Brookings Institution.

van Doorslaer, E., Janssen, R., Wagstaff, A. *et al.* (1991) Equity in the Finance of Health Care: Effectsof the Dutch Health Insurance Reform. In: Lopez-Casanovas, G., editor, *Incentives in Health Systems.* Berlin, Heidelberg: Springer-Verlag, pp. 153-168

van Doorslaer, E., Wagstaff, A., and Rutten, F. (1992) *Equity in the Finance and Delivery of Health Care: an International Perspective.* Oxford: Oxford University Press.

Appendix 1 Description of Data Used in Analysis in 1990 and 1994

	Central government		Municipalities	SII	Households
	Income tax	Indirect taxes	Local tax	Sickness insurance	Direct payments[a]
1990	FHS 1990	FHS 1990	FHS 1990	FHS 1990	FHS 1990
1994	IDS 1994	FHS 1990	IDS 1994	IDS 1994	FHS 1990

[a]Inpatient charges computed from FHDR data
FHS: Finnish Household Survey
IDS: Income Distribution Statistics

Appendix 2 Comparison of Progressivity in FHS 1990 and IDS 1990 Data (Running Expenditure)

	Revenue Share(%)	Kakwani's Index FHS 1990 data	Kakwani's Index IDS 1990 data
State			
Income Tax	14.0	0.269	0.270
Indirect Tax	23.0	-0.097	-0.097[a]
Net Public Borrowing	1.0	0.038	0.038
Municipalities			
Local Tax	37.0	0.077	0.081
Sickness Insurance Institute			
Sickness Insurance	11.0	0.086	0.088
TOTAL PUBLIC	86.0	0.061	0.064
Households			
Direct Payments	14.0	-0.198	-0.198[a]
TOTAL FINANCING	100.0	0.024	0.027

[a] Computed from FHS 1990 data
FHS: Finnish Household Survey
IDS: Income Distribution Statistics

6

Use of Insured Health Care Services in Relation to Household Income in a Canadian Province

CAMERON A. MUSTARD[1,2,4]
MARIAN SHANAHAN[1,2]
SHELLEY DERKSEN[1]
JOHN HORNE[2]
ROBERT G. EVANS[3,4]

[1] Manitoba Centre for Health Policy and Evaluation
[2] Department of Community Health Sciences
Faculty of Medicine, University of Manitoba
[3] Centre for Health Services and Policy Research
University of British Columbia
[4] Population Health Program
Canadian Institute for Advanced Research

Health, Health Care and Health Economics: Perspectives on Distribution
Edited by Morris L. Barer, Thomas E. Getzen, and Greg L. Stoddart
Copyright 1998 John Wiley & Sons, Ltd.

ABSTRACT

Limited information is available on the distribution effects of the financing mechanism of the Canadian health care system, where revenues derived from diverse tax sources are allocated to the provision of health care for those in medical need. One factor accounting for this relative lack of information has been the absence of household-level data which combine comprehensive and longitudinal information on the use of insured health care services with detailed information on household structure and income sources. This presentation describes the utilization of physician and hospital services in relation to household income for a sample of households in the Canadian province of Manitoba in FY86/87. Data are derived from a larger study of net fiscal incidence, examining the incidence of taxation and the use of insured health care services at the household level across the income distribution. In this study, a cross-sectional analysis of a stratified random 5% sample of Manitoba households linking very high quality information on individual health care utilization with detailed socioeconomic information from the 1986 census is presented. On a crude basis, and also adjusting for household structure and age, the analysis estimates the dollar value of household consumption of publicly insured health care services in relation to deciles of household income.

Paradoxically, while hospital utilization was found to increase substantially with descending income decile, results indicate that there was no corresponding gradient in the utilization of ambulatory medical care. The use of ambulatory medical care displayed a shallow U-shaped curve relative to income decile.

The results of this study indicate that the strong income-related differences in hospital utilization, previously described in earlier Canadian studies, persisted after 25 years of universal health insurance. Given that the system is financed by tax revenues which are, on balance, marginally progressive, health care use represents a substantial income redistribution mechanism in this setting.

INTRODUCTION

Limited information is available on the distribution effects of the financing mechanism of the Canadian health care system, where revenues derived from tax sources are allocated to the provision of health care for those in medical need. In part, the relative absence of information on the distribution effects of public health insurance is due to the complexity involved in resolving both macro- and micro-level allocation issues in the incidence of taxation (Barer *et al.*, 1982; Musgrave *et al.*, 1976; Gillespie, 1979). However, a second obstacle has been the absence of household-level data which combine comprehensive and longitudinal information on the use of insured health care services with detailed information on household structure and income sources.

STUDY OBJECTIVE

The objective of this study, based on data describing the use of health care services and household income for a sample of Manitoba households in FY86/87, was to reproduce the approach of the limited number of Canadian analyses that have described the utilization of physician and hospital services in relation to household income (Barer *et al.*, 1982; Boulet *et al.*, 1979; Manga, 1978; Beck, 1973; Beck and Horne, 1976; Siemiatycki *et al.*, 1980; Enterline *et al.*, 1973; Broyles *et al.*, 1983; McIsaac *et al.*, 1993; Manga *et al.*, 1987; Béland, 1995; Kephart *et al.*, 1996; Katz *et al.*, 1996; Health Status of Canadians, 1994). The study used a unique research resource created through the collaboration of Statistics Canada, the Government of Manitoba and the Manitoba Centre for Health Policy and Evaluation, University of Manitoba. In brief outline, the study was a cross-sectional analysis of a stratified random 5% sample of Manitoba households, grouped into deciles on the basis of income. On a crude basis, and also adjusting for household structure and age, the analysis estimated the dollar value of household use of publicly insured health care services. Information on household income and structure was derived from the 1986 census. Health care was enumerated directly from computerized records of individual health care encounters maintained by the Manitoba Health Services Insurance (MHSIP) Plan for the period April 1, 1986 to March 31, 1987.

As this was a descriptive study, no specific hypotheses were tested. Although unmeasured in this study, we assumed that need, indicated by measures of health status, was the primary determinant of the use of health care services. We expected household income would be inversely associated with the consumption of health care services prior to the adjustment for health status, and that accurate measurement of health status would account for income related differences in utilization. It was the expectation of this study that income-related patterns of health care utilization identified in previous Canadian studies would be observed in this setting, namely that the use of physician services would be weakly related to income while the use of hospital care will be strongly and inversely related to income. This divergence in income-related patterns of use of physician and hospital care is one of the central paradoxes of the population's use of health care services in the Canadian health care system.

The study focuses exclusively on the utilization of medical services and hospital care, explicitly excluding other forms of publicly financed health care expenditures, such as hospital capital programs, health care research or the training of health care personnel. Conceptually, these were deemed expenditures to improve access to services, rather than the consumption of services (Evans, 1984). In addition, the study did not attempt to estimate direct and indirect household expenditures on health care services. While estimated to represent approximately 25% of total health expenditures in Canada during the observation period (Table 1), estimating direct expenditures requires household survey data not available to this study.

METHODS

STUDY DESIGN

This study was a cross-sectional analysis of a stratified random sample of Manitoba households estimating the use of publicly insured hospital and medical services by income decile, adjusting for household structure and age. The analysis was comprehensive for all disorders presenting for insured medical and hospital care. In Manitoba in FY 1986/87, the publicly insured health care services described in this study totaled an estimated $961.2 million, representing approximately 50% of the estimated total public and private expenditures on health care (Table 1).

SOURCES OF DATA

The study was based on a database that linked electronic records of the use of insured hospital and medical services with 1986 census records at the individual

**Table 1   Estimated Provincial Government (PG) Health Expenditures
Manitoba 1986/87**

	$ Millions	$ Per Capita	Percent of Total
Total Health Expenditures	2,053.1	1,866.0	100.0
Private Spending	520.0	473.0	25.3
Other Public Spending	167.5	152.0	8.2
PG Health Spending	1,365.6	1,241.0	66.5
Total PG Health Spending	1,365.6	1,241.0	100.0
MHSC Insured Services(a)	1,207.7	1,097.0	88.3
Insured Services Included in Study	961.2	873.0	70.3
Hospital Services	735.1	668.0	
Medical Services (b)	226.1	205.0	
Insured Services Excluded from Study	248.5	226.0	18.2
Pharmacare	37.4	34.0	
Administration	17.5	16.0	
Nursing Home Services	169.1	153.0	
Other Services	24.5	22.0	
(includes transport and ambulance services and other medical services)			

(a)   difference of $158 million between total provincial government spending and MHSC insured services include funds disbursed to Manitoba Cancer Treatment and Research Foundation, Addictions Foundation of Manitoba, provincial diagnostic laboratories, the Mental Health Division of Manitoba Health and programme and policy units of Manitoba Health.

(b)   The study excludes oral and dental surgery, optometric services and chiropractic services ($13.6 million) and is based on an analysis of $207.6 million.

Sources: Preliminary Estimates of Health Expenditures in Canada: Provincial/Territorial Summary Report 1987-91, 1994; National Health Expenditures in Canada 1975-1993, 1994

level, for a stratified random sample of 16,627 Manitoba households that completed the 2B census questionnaire in 1986. Records describing use of services include physician claims for reimbursement of ambulatory and inpatient care, laboratory tests and diagnostic imaging exams in private facilities, and hospital separation abstracts for inpatient and outpatient services in acute care hospitals in the province.

While these utilization data were available for seven consecutive years (1983-1989) in this data set, only information pertaining to a single fiscal year, April, 1986 to March, 1987 was used in these analyses. For each person represented in the sample, records of health care utilization were linked to the complete 1986 census record of information reported on the 2A and 2B census forms, which includes data on sources and amounts of income, attained education, occupation, and labour force participation for all residents of private dwellings over the age of fifteen.

SAMPLE

The sample unit in this study was the census household, which includes residents of private dwellings, non-institutional collective dwellings, and institutions. The methodology and results of the record linkage process are described in detail elsewhere (Mustard *et al.*, 1997; Houle *et al.*, 1996). In summary, all individuals in the 82,728 Manitoba households that completed the 2B questionnaire were eligible for linkage to a file containing person-level demographic information for all known registrants with MHSIP in June, 1986. Deterministic and probabilistic record linkage procedures were performed by Statistics Canada personnel. No actual names or dwelling addresses were used in the linkage. A total of 74% of individual records in the census sample were successfully linked to an identity in the MHSIP insurance registry with 95.5% accuracy. From the pool of linked records, a stratified sample of 16,627 households was drawn (N=47,935 individuals), representing an approximate 5% sample of the Manitoba population.

MEASURES

Health Care Expenditures

In this study, the consumption of insured health care was measured in Canadian dollars. The public administration of insured medical services includes the detailed accounting of payment of fees, and this financial information is included in the computerized records of physician service claims. Estimating the cost of an episode of hospital care, however, has historically been a challenge in the Canadian system, where hospital care is funded globally on an institutional basis, rather than on the basis of direct payment for each service encounter (Black and Frohlich, 1991).

Physician Services: All fee-for-service physician services used by individuals in the sample were enumerated for this study. At the time of this study, approximately 3.0% of total physician services were provided by salaried physicians in provincial mental health institutions, community based clinics, and some hospital emergency and radiology departments. These services were excluded. Care provided to residents of Manitoba in other provinces was enumerated and costed on the basis of actual fees paid. Care provided in out-of-country settings which was reimbursed by the provincial health insurance agency was excluded.

Diagnostic and laboratory services provided by fee-for-service private facilities were included in the enumeration of insured medical services. In the observation period, reimbursement for these services totaled $76.0 million. An additional $34 million of diagnostic services were estimated to have been provided in hospital outpatient services. These hospital-based outpatient services were excluded from these analyses because information on individual patient use was not available (Cheuk *et al.*, 1991).

Hospital Care: Accurate cost information for individual hospital admissions is generally unavailable in Canada, a legacy of the administrative practice of globally funding institutional budgets. Accurate case cost information, which also provides for adjustment for differing degrees of illness severity, is required in studies comparing the efficiency of hospitals (Shanahan *et al.*, 1994). This same requirement pertained to this study, where the cost of hospital care attributable to differing illness and severity profiles may differ across income deciles in ways that are not captured by the use of crude hospital per diems.

In this study we applied an adaptation of the RDRG case costing methodology, which accounts for the severity or complexity of illness. In outline, this method groups hospital admissions into clinically meaningful categories, called refined diagnosis-related groups (RDRGs) on the basis of diagnoses, procedures, and similarity of length of stay and resource use. Each RDRG is assigned a case weight, which reflects the costliness of care relative to the mean hospital admission.

Despite shortcomings, this approach remains the most appropriate method available for accounting for the costs of inpatient hospital care on a case basis. In this application, hospital charge information from the regulated hospital system in the state of Maryland in 1991 and 1992 has been used (Shanahan, *et al.*, 1994). The US hospital charge data are used only to establish the relative cost of care: for example, to quantify the relative cost difference between a gastrointestinal surgical procedure and an open heart procedure. While there is some evidence the Canadian hospital system is more efficient than American hospitals in the use of technology

(Redelmeier and Fuchs, 1993), we know of no work that has demonstrated that the relative distribution of health care resources across RDRG groups differs substantially between the two countries, and it is on this basis that the US hospital charge data were used for the purposes of this study.

Two approaches in applying case weights were implemented to derive estimates of the cost of inpatient care by income decile. The methodology for identifying and allocating costs of inpatient care is described in detail elsewhere (Wall *et al.*, 1994). In the first approach, the case weight assigned to each RDRG was multiplied by the average provincial cost of an inpatient admission. In the second approach, the RDRG case weight was multiplied by the average cost of an admission in the hospital in which the care was provided (Shanahan *et al.*, 1994). This procedure retains information on the relative efficiency of each hospital. In applying both estimation approaches, adjustment was made for the resource use of atypically long stay admissions. No important differences in the use of hospital care by income decile were observed between these two estimation approaches. Accordingly, results are reported only for estimates based on an average provincial inpatient admission cost.

This method is applicable only to the assignment of the cost of inpatient services. No satisfactory methodology currently exists for costing the diverse range of outpatient services provided by Canadian hospitals, which are estimated to represent approximately 21% of total hospital expenditures in Manitoba in this period (Shanahan *et al.*, 1994; Wall *et al.*, 1994). These services range from high cost procedures such as dialysis and diagnostic imaging, to lower cost programs in antenatal care and outpatient mental health care services. Given this shortcoming, an estimated $128 million of outpatient resource use were excluded from analysis in this study.

Other excluded expenditures in the hospital sector were approximately $69 million of services provided in facilities not defined as acute care hospitals and $99.9 million in other costs associated with education and research programs, interest and depreciation charges, and non-patient costs (Shanahan *et al.*, 1994). After these exclusions, a total of $382.9 million inpatient acute care hospital costs (63% of eligible sector costs) are included in this study.

Previous work focused on validating the sample estimates of population health care utilization had established that the sample under-estimated hospital separations in FY86/87 by approximately 4%, and underestimated total days of care by 22% (Technical Note 6, 1995). Two factors were responsible for this substantial underestimation of hospital days: 1) an under-representation of long-stay separations (greater than 60 days) in the sample and 2) an under-representation of hospital care for the treatment of mental health disorders. Approximately 80% of the under-estimate of total days of care was attributable to the sample under-estimation of long-stay admissions. We developed a series of age-specific weights which were applied to each hospital admission in the sample to adjust for this under-estimation. To derive these weights, total days of hospital care observed in the complete Manitoba population within 14 age and sex strata were divided by the total days of hospital care estimated from the weighted sample. This adjustment corrected for age and gender differences in the sample's under-estimation of total days of care, but did not address any residual bias associated with income (for example if low income individuals with long-stay admissions were more likely to be omitted from the study sample).

Household Income: A measure of total economic family income was derived from census responses provided by each household member over the age of 15. This study described 17,210 economic family units that group kinship-related individuals occupying a common private dwelling. Total family monetary income was calculated to include gross wages and salaries from employment, net income from self-employment, pension income, and government transfers, including family allowances, unemployment insurance, child tax credits, workers compensation payments, and other disability benefits. This definition was equivalent to Gillespie's broad income concept (Vermaeten *et al.*, 1994). The census does not collect income information for residents of institutional facilities. Individuals resident in institutions on census day were retained in the analysis of health care utilization, but were not classified to an income decile.

Families were grouped into income deciles, ranked from the poorest 10% to the wealthiest 10% of families, with approximately 5,000 individual observations per decile. A total of 71 economic families reported negative income to the 1986 census. For these families, the reported negative income was converted to its absolute value. An additional 243 individuals were members of economic families in private dwellings that reported a zero income value to the 1986 census. These families were classified to the lowest income decile. Two approaches to the classification of family income were implemented in this study. The first approach ranked individuals on the basis of total family income. The second approach classified individuals on the basis of a per capita equivalent family income measure. This measure implemented an adjustment for household size, where the first adult was valued as 1.0 person equivalents, the second adult was valued as 0.4 person equivalents and each child is valued as 0.3 person equivalents (Wolfson and Evans,

1989). Decile income thresholds are reported in Table 2.

Table 2 Income Decile Thresholds, Manitoba 1986/87

Income Decile	Total Economic Family Income		Per Capita Equivalent Economic Family Income	
1 (lowest)	0	- 9,000	0	- 5,973
2	9,011	- 14,847	5,982	- 8,990
3	14,851	- 20,069	8,990	- 11,565
4	20,073	- 25,696	11,567	- 14,259
5	25,698	- 30,987	14,262	- 16,966
6	30,998	- 36,434	16,971	- 19,936
7	36,435	- 42,694	19,940	- 23,126
8	42,700	- 50,486	23,136	- 27,625
9	50,494	- 62,814	27,631	- 35,137
10 (highest)	62,819 +		35,147 +	

ANALYSIS

The analytic plan focused on estimating the crude and age-adjusted consumption of insured hospital and medical services within ten equal sized population groups, ranked from poorest to wealthiest on two measures of economic family income (Rasell *et al.*, undated). To incorporate the stratified random sampling design, sample weights were applied to estimate population characteristics. Age-adjusted estimates were calculated by direct standardization using 14 age and sex groups with the Manitoba population as the standard.

RESULTS

The total value of physician services reimbursed by MHSIP in FY1986-87 and eligible for inclusion in this study was $207.6 million, which compared well with the estimate of $199.8 million obtained from the study sample. As noted earlier, the total value of hospital care eligible for inclusion in this study was $383 million, approximately 63% of the total hospital sector resource allocation in this period.

Table 3-A Distribution of Sample by Age and Income Decile
Distribution by Total Economic Family Income
Based on Weighted Sample Counts

Income Decile	Age Group						
	0-14 %	15-24 %	25-34 %	35-44 %	45-54 %	55-64 %	65+ %
Not Classified	0.0	1.4	1.2	0.7	1.1	1.4	6.8
1 (lowest)	8.4	12.3	8.8	5.9	7.5	11.3	15.5
2	8.2	9.6	7.9	5.7	5.2	10.1	23.4
3	8.7	8.7	9.7	6.8	6.8	11.2	17.9
4	10.5	9.0	10.7	8.6	7.9	11.0	10.3
5	11.7	8.8	11.5	10.3	8.6	8.8	6.8
6	12.2	8.0	11.8	11.4	9.0	8.6	5.4
7	11.9	8.7	11.3	12.6	9.8	8.5	3.8
8	11.4	8.8	10.8	13.1	11.2	8.5	3.7
9	9.7	10.8	10.0	12.6	13.7	9.4	3.0
10 (highest)	7.2	13.8	6.2	12.3	19.1	11.1	3.4
TOTAL	100.0	100.0	100.0	100.0	100.0	100.0	100.0
N	230,300	169,890	177,026	141,743	98,985	98,962	131,392

Tables 3A and B report the age distribution of the sample over income deciles under the two alternate approaches to the classification of income. In the classification based on total economic family income, persons over the age of 65 are disproportionately represented in the lower income deciles and the income decile distribution of persons aged 35-44 and 45-54 was skewed towards the higher income groups. When classified on the basis of economic family income adjusted for household size, the distribution of persons over the age of 65 was not substantially altered, with the exception that very few elderly are represented in the lowest income decile. The other substantial change in age group distribution under this alternate income measure was an increased proportion of children classified in the lower income deciles relative to the distribution formed by total economic family income.

Table 3-B Distribution of Sample by Age and Income Decile
Distribution by Per Capita Equivalent Economic Family Income
Based on Weighted Sample Counts

	Age Group						
Income Decile	**0-14**	**15-24**	**25-34**	**35-44**	**45-54**	**55-65**	**65+**
	%	%	%	%	%	%	%
Not Classified	1.1	1.4	1.2	0.7	1.1	1.4	6.8
1 (lowest)	13.7	13.6	9.9	7.5	7.8	9.6	2.3
2	11.1	9.6	7.5	6.6	5.7	7.9	19.2
3	10.1	8.5	7.9	6.8	5.6	8.0	21.5
4	12.0	9.4	9.4	9.2	6.5	8.4	12.2
5	12.2	9.0	10.3	10.1	7.3	8.8	8.6
6	11.1	9.6	10.3	11.0	9.3	8.4	7.6
7	10.6	9.1	10.4	13.0	9.7	9.6	5.5
8	8.9	10.3	11.0	11.6	12.3	10.3	5.2
9	6.2	10.3	11.5	11.9	14.7	12.3	5.6
10 (highest)	3.9	9.2	10.4	11.6	19.9	15.3	5.6
TOTAL	100.0	100.0	100.0	100.0	100.0	100.0	100.0
N	230,000	69,890	177,026	141,743	98,985	98,862	131,392

The use of physician services by income decile is reported in Table 4. Utilization of medical care across income decile classified on the basis of economic family income showed a shallow U-shaped curve, with use highest in the lower and the higher income deciles. After age and sex adjustment, utilization over deciles was essentially equivalent, with the exception of the lowest decile, where the ratio of use relative to the mean was 1.17. When classified by economic family income adjusted for household size, the age and sex adjusted profile of use of medical services also did not show any significant gradient in use in relation to income.

In contrast to the general absence of an association between income and physician service utilization, the use of hospital care was strongly related to income decile (Table 5). On the basis of crude economic family income, hospital utilization generally showed an inverse relationship to income. Hospital use weighted by relative resource intensity in the poorest 10% of the population was 3.1 times greater than resource use in the wealthiest 10% of the population. This inverse gradient persists when adjusted for age and sex, although the utilization ratio between the lowest and highest income decile is diminished in magnitude.

TABLE 4 Utilization of Physician Services, By Income Decile

Economic Family Income

Income Decile	Crude $000	Ratio to Mean	Age/Sex Adjusted $000	Ratio to Mean
1 Lowest	24,276.0	1.25	22,995.5	1.17
2	23,086.4	1.18	19,409.4	0.98
3	21,679.1	1.11	19,582.4	0.99
4	19,657.8	1.01	19,871.7	1.01
5	18,168.2	0.93	19,426.1	0.98
6	17,126.3	0.88	18,685.3	0.95
7	16,595.6	0.85	18,349.0	0.93
8	17,221.8	0.88	19,018.2	0.97
9	17,735.8	0.91	19,234.6	0.98
10 Highest	18,993.0	0.97	20,242.9	1.03
Not Classified	5,289.0		2,978.6	
Total	199,838.7		199,838.7	

Economic Family Income, Per Capita Person Equivalent

Income Decile	Crude $000	Ratio to Mean	Age/Sex Adjusted $000	Ratio to Mean
1 Lowest	18,049.5	0.93	19,882.8	1.01
2	21,453.0	1.10	19,802.0	1.00
3	23,016.1	1.18	20,620.7	1.05
4	20,067.4	1.03	20,199.3	1.03
5	18,278.0	0.94	19,255.0	0.98
6	18,296.9	0.94	19,267.4	0.98
7	16,815.8	0.86	18,255.0	0.93
8	18,730.8	0.96	19,939.6	1.01
9	19,563.6	1.00	19,887.2	1.01
10 Highest	20,268.8	1.04	19,845.9	1.01
Not Classified	5,298.7		2,982.8	
Total	199,838.6		199,838.6	

TABLE 5 Utilization of Acute Hospital Care, By Income Decile
(Estimates Based on Provincial Average Cost Per Weighted Case

Economic Family Income

	Crude $000	Ratio to Mean	Age/Sex Adjusted $000	Ratio to Mean
1 Lowest	59,401.7	1.73	55,377.0	1.50
2	59,140.6	1.73	42,027.5	1.14
3	50,805.9	1.48	42,021.4	1.14
4	38,962.0	1.11	42,136.1	1.14
5	26,951.5	0.79	31,951.4	0.86
6	24,604.0	0.72	33,156.7	0.90
7	19,807.5	0.57	28,641.4	0.77
8	21,791.9	0.64	32,979.2	0.89
9	23,235.5	0.68	34,380.6	0.93
10 Highest	18,903.7	0.55	26,766.0	0.72
Not Classified	40,293.4		13,461.4	
Total	382,898.8		382,898.8	

Economic Family Income, Per Capita Person Equivalent

	Crude $000	Ratio to Mean	Age/Sex Adjusted $000	Ratio to Mean
1 Lowest	31,646.6	0.92	44,226.3	1.19
2	66,270.4	1.93	55,305.3	1.49
3	61,049.3	1.78	48,371.3	1.31
4	30,285.9	0.88	32,173.8	0.87
5	34,692.1	1.01	41,706.3	1.13
6	27,168.6	0.79	33,519.3	0.91
7	18,888.1	0.55	24,218.2	0.65
8	23,729.9	0.69	30,648.8	0.83
9	25,039.9	0.73	32,152.6	0.87
10 Highest	23,834.4	0.69	27,046.4	0.73
Not Classified	40,293.4		13,530.6	
Total	382,898.8		382,898.8	

When individuals were classified to an income decile on the basis of per capita adjusted economic family income, the inverse utilization gradient persisted and was of similar magnitude to that observed for unadjusted economic family income. It is important to note, however, that the lowest income decile's use of hospital care was not consistent with the observed income gradient. Possible explanations for this discontinuity are offered in the discussion.

DISCUSSION

In this setting, hospital utilization was found to be substantially higher among lower income deciles. Paradoxically, however, there was no corresponding gradient in the utilization of medical care. The use of medical care displayed a shallow U-shaped curve relative to crude income decile, which was largely eliminated following age adjustment.

In describing the use of insured hospital and medical services across income groups, this study adds to the small number of Canadian studies that have examined this question. Some of these studies contrasted the use of health services before and after the introduction of medicare (Siematycki, 1980; Enterline, 1973). Three subsequent studies conducted in the first decade of public health insurance programs examined the utilization of health care services relative to household income in Ontario (Barer *et al.*, 1982; Manga, 1978), and Saskatchewan (Beck, 1973; Beck and Horne, 1976), as well as in a representative national sample (Boulet and Henderon, 1979). More recently, a number of surveys designed to measure aspects of population health have provided opportunities to describe the pattern of health care utilization in relation to income (Broyles *et al.*, 1983; McIsaac *et al.*, 1993; Manga *et al.*, 1987; Béland, 1995; Kephart *et al.*, 1996; Katz *et al.*, 1996; Health Status of Canadians, 1994; Birch *et al.*, 1993; Santé-Quebec, 1988).

In aggregate, these studies generally have found consistent patterns in the utilization of hospital services in relation to income under universal health insurance. Lower income households typically consume a greater volume of hospital services than median and high income households. This pattern is generally attributed to evidence of a higher prevalence of morbidity among low income households (Birch *et al.*, 1993; Santé-Quebec, 1988; Manga, 1987). Some of this work has not adequately accounted for the age and family structure correlates of household income, which may potentially inflate estimates of income-related differences in utilization. Elderly households, for example, typically have income below the mean of all households, and are consistently high users of health care.

At the same time, these studies have produced inconsistent findings concerning the use of physician services under universally-insured health care programs. Table 6 summarizes descriptions of the utilization of medical services from five important Canadian studies over the past 25 years. There are some contradictory findings in these results. Utilization *per capita* was found to be positively related to family income in Saskatchewan (Beck, 1973) and Ontario (Manga, 1978), while negatively related to family income in Montreal (Siemiatycki *et al.*, 1980). More recent studies from Quebec (Béland, 1995) and Nova Scotia (Kephart *et al.*, 1996) have reported an inverse relationship between income and physician service utilization. In the Quebec study, the differences reported in this table are eliminated following age adjustment, which is consistent with the results reported in this paper. Regression-based age-adjustment did not remove the inverse gradient in the Nova Scotia study. Differences in time period, sampling, and adjustments for age and family size distributions within households are obstacles to comparison across these studies. In addition, while all five studies used a measure of household income to stratify households on a socioeconomic gradient, there was wide variation in the approach to the categorization of income groups. For example, the Saskatchewan study articulated fine divisions at the high end of the income distribution, while this emphasis was inverted in the Ontario study, which chose to describe smaller partitions at the low end of the income distribution. A separate and perhaps more substantial inconsistency is brought forward by these data on income-related patterns in the use of physician services. In general, the use of hospital care is much more strongly associated with household income resources than is the use of physician services.

There are many hypotheses that can be offered to explain this paradox. Members of lower-income households consistently have been shown to use less ambulatory preventive physician care (Goel, 1993; Mustard and Roos, 1994), and some studies have documented a greater use of higher-cost specialist physician care among higher socioeconomic groups (McIsaac *et al.*, 1993; Mustard *et al.*, 1996). These divergent patterns of income-related differences in the use of physician services could accumulate to produce an undifferentiated profile of physician service use across income groups which obscures the need-related utilization assumed to be represented by the use of acute care hospital services.

There are three limitations to this study which warrant caution in the interpretation of the reported findings. First, it is noted that the study sample underestimates long-stay hospital admissions. Although an age adjustment was

**Table 6 Comparison of Studies Describing
the Utilization of Medical Services under Universal Insurance**

Saskatchewan 1967 (Beck, 1976)	$000 Family Income				
	<2.5	**2.5-4.9**	**5-9.9**	**10-14.9**	**15+**
N	6,166	7,497	8,370	2,111	840
%	24.5	29.9	33.3	8.4	3.3
$ per capita	60.77	71.70	96.44	103.59	117.99
Ratio Relative to Highest Income	0.51	0.60	0.81	0.87	1.00

Montreal 1970/71(a) (Siemiatycki, 1980)	$000 Family Income				
	<3	**3-4.9**	**5-8.9**	**9-14.9**	**15+**
N	1,590	2,400	6,921	3,889	1,372
%	8.6	12.9	37.3	21.0	7.4
Mean Annual Physician Visits	7.8	6.0	4.7	4.9	4.8
Ratio Relative to Highest Income	1.60	1.25	0.97	1.02	1.00

Ontario 1974/75 (Manga, 1978)	$000 Family Income				
	<3.9	**4-7.9**	**8-13.9**	**14-19.9**	**20+**
N	157	188	629	704	447
%	7.5	9.0	30.2	33.8	21.4
$ per capita (b)	77.78	56.58	75.58	81.14	86.06
Ratio Relative to Highest Income	0.90	0.66	0.87	0.94	1.00

Quebec 1987 (Béland, 1995)	$ 000 Household Income					
	<12	**12-19.9**	**20-29.9**	**30-39.9**	**40-49.9**	**50+**
N	681	861	1,156	1,115	835	1,161
%	11.7	14.8	19.9	19.2	14.4	20.0
$ per capita (c)	269	237	220	211	195	206
Ratio Relative to Highest Income	1.30	1.15	1.07	1.02	0.95	1.00

(Continued)

Table 6 (continued)

Nova Scotia 1991-94 (Kephart, 1996)			Income Adequacy		
	Lower	Lower Middle	Middle	Upper Middle	Missing
N	144	308	674	599	280
%	7.2	15.3	33.6	29.9	13.9
$ per capita (c)	553.1	530.5	435.0	374.3	565.2
Ratio Relative to Highest Income	1.47	1.42	1.16	1.00	1.51

(a) Income not reported for 2,360 respondents (12.7% of sample), observations excluded from table

(b) Medical services data reported in original study have been age-adjusted across income groups in this presentation

(c) Utilization estimates not adjusted for age

implemented for this under-estimation, a potential bias of unknown direction related to income may be present. Second, the utilization of hospital and physician services by the lowest income decile classified by the measure of *per capita* equivalent economic family income is more consistent with a median income group than a low income group. This pattern raises concerns about the accuracy of income information for some proportion of persons in the lowest income decile. Finally, the study was not able to incorporate a measure of health status in the analysis of health care utilization.

This description of the incidence of benefits under the insurance mechanism of the Canadian health care system is relevant for a number of reasons. First, the majority of previous studies of benefit incidence in Canada date from the first decade of universally insured services. In the following two decades, health expenditures climbed from 7.1% of GNP in 1975 to a current share of 10.1% in 1993 (National Health Expenditures in Canada, 1994), from an estimated 5% of GNP in 1960 (Boulet and Henderson, 1979). As the health share of GNP has increased, the distribution of benefits across income groups may have changed. Second, the current public policy debate concerning the scale and structure of the publicly financed health care sector will potentially benefit from explicit information on income-related patterns of the consumption of health care. For example, the proposition that user fees may be an appropriate mechanism for the partial financing of health care services persists without a clear understanding of the existing income distribution in the consumption of health services. Finally, the work described in this paper is a component of a larger study focused on estimating the net incidence of benefits under a tax-financed universal health insurance program which proposes to integrate analyses of the incidence of taxation and the incidence of health care benefits. This work has not previously been performed in this country.

In summary, strong income-related differences in hospital utilization, previously described in earlier Canadian studies, persist after 25 years of universal health insurance in this setting. Given that the system is financed by tax revenues which are, on balance, marginally progressive, health care benefits represent a substantial income redistribution mechanism in this setting.

ACKNOWLEDGMENTS

An earlier version of this paper was presented to the inaugural meeting of the International Health Economics Association, Vancouver, British Columbia, May 1996.

Funding for this research was provided in part by grants 6607-1730-302 and 6607-1697-302 from the National Health Research and Development Program, Health Canada.

REFERENCES

Barer, M.L., Manga, P., Shillington, E.R., and Siegel, G.C. (1982) *Income class and hospital use in Ontario. Occasional Paper 14*. Toronto: Ontario Economic Council.

Beck, R.G. (1973) Economic class and access to physician services under public medical care insurance. *Int. J. Health. Ser.* 3:341.

Beck, R.G. and Horne, J.M. (1976) Economic class and risk avoidance: experience under public medical care insurance. *Journal of Risk and Insurance* 43:73-86.

Béland, F. (1995) Expenditure on ambulatory medical care over the long term in the Quebec Medicare System. *Canadian Journal on Aging* 14:391-413.

Birch, S., Eyles, J., and Newbold, K.B. (1993) Equitable access to health care: methodological extensions to the analysis of physician utilization in Canada. *Health Economics* 2:87-101.

Black, C. and Frohlich, N. (1991) *Hospital Funding Within the Health Care System: Moving Towards Effectiveness. Report 91.05.* Winnipeg, Manitoba:Manitoba Centre for Health Policy and Evaluation.

Boulet, J-A. and Henderson, D.M. (1979) *Distributional and Redistributional Aspects of Government Health Insurance Programs in Canada.* Economic Council of Canada Discussion Paper #146. Ottawa: ECC.

Broyles, R.W., Manga, P., Binder, D., *et al.* (1983) The use of physician services under a national health insurance scheme. *Medical Care* 21:1037-54.

Cheuk, T., Hammond, G., Horne, J.M., *et al.* (1991) Trends in costs and utilization of medical diagnostic services in Manitoba's private fee-for service sector 1982-87. Unpublished mss.

Enterline, P.E., Salter, V., McDonald, A.D., and McDonald, L.C. (1973) The distribution of medical services before and after 'free' medical care - the Quebec experience. *N. Engl. J. Med.* 289:1174-1178.

Evans, R.G. (1984) *Strained Mercy: The Economics of Canadian Health Care.* Toronto:Butterworths.

Gillespie, W.I. (1979) Taxes, expenditures and the redistribution of income in Canada, 1951-1977. in: *The Conference on Canadian Incomes.* Ottawa, Economic Council of Canada pp 25-50.

Goel, V. (1993) Factors associated with cervical cancer screening: results from the Ontario Health Survey. ICES Working Paper IWP 007, Toronto, May 1993.

Health Status of Canadians: Report of the 1991 General Social Survey. (1994) General Social Survey Analysis Series 11-612E, No 8. 1994, Ottawa:Statistics Canada.

Houle, C., Berthelot, J. M., David P., *et al.* (1996) Project on matching Census 1986 database and Manitoba health care files: private households component. Statistics Canada, Analytic Studies Branch Research Paper Series, No. 91, March 1996.

Katz, S.J., Hofer, T.P., and Manning, W.G. (1996) Physician use in Ontario and the United States: the impact of socioeconomic status and health status. *Am. J. Public Health* 86:520-524.

Kephart, G., Thomas, V.S., and MacLean, D.R. (1996) Socioeconomic differences in the utilization of physician services. Unpublished report, 1996. Population Health Research Unit, Department of Community Health and Epidemiology, Dalhousie University.

Manga, P. (1978) *the Income Distribution Effect of Medical Insurance in Ontario. Occasional Paper 6.* Toronto:Ontario Economic Council.

Manga, P. (1987) Equality of Access and Inequalities in Health Status: Policy Implications of a Paradox. In Coburn, D., D'Arcy, C., Torrance, G., and New. P., editors, *Health and Canadian Society: Sociological Perspectives.* Toronto: Fitzhenry and Whiteside, pp. 637-648.

Manga, P., Broyles, R., Angus, D. (1987) The determinants of hospital utilization under a universal public insurance programme in Canada. *Medical Care* 25:658-70.

McIsaac, W.J., Goel, V., and Naylor, C.D. (1993) The utilization of physician services in Ontario by adults: results from the Ontario Health Survey. ICES Working Paper 20, Toronto, October 1993.

Musgrave, R.A., and Musgrave, P.B. (1976) *Public Finance in Theory and Practice.* New York:McGraw-Hill.

Mustard, C.A., Derksen, S., Berthelot, J.M., *et al.* (1997) Age-specific education and income gradients in morbidity and mortality in a Canadian province. *Social Science and Medicine* 45:383-397.

Mustard, C.A. and Roos, N.P. (1994) The relationship of prenatal care and pregnancy complication to birth weight outcome. *Am. J. Public Health* 84:1450-1457.

Mustard, C.A., Derksen, S., and Tataryn, D. (1996) Persistence of intensive use of mental health care. *Canadian Journal of Psychiatry* 41:93-101.

National Health Expenditures in Canada 1975-1993. (1994) Health Policy and Information Directorate, Policy and Consultation Branch, Health Canada, June 1994.

Preliminary Estimates of Health Expenditures in Canada: Provincial/Territorial Summary Report 1987-91 (1994). Health Information Division, Policy and Consultation Branch, Health Canada, February 1994.

Rasell, E., Bernstein, J., and Tang, K. (Undated) The impact of health care financing on family budgets. Briefing Paper. Economic Policy Institute.

Redelmeier, D.A. and Fuchs, V.R. (1993) Hospital expenditures in the United States and Canada. *N. Engl. J. Med.* 328:772.

Santé-Québec. Et la santé ça va? Rappport de l'Enquête Santé Québec 1987 (1988). Tome I, ministère de la Santé et des Services sociaux, Québec.

Siemiatycki, J., Richardson, L., and Pless, I.B. (1980) Equality in medical care under national health insurance in Montreal. *N. Engl. J. Med.* 303:10.

Shanahan, M., Loyd, M., Roos, N.P., and Brownell, M. (1994) Hospital Case Mix Costing. Manitoba Centre for Health Policy and Evaluation, Winnipeg, Manitoba

Technical Note 6 (1995). Precision of the sample estimate of population utilization of hospital care. Statistics Canada/MCHPE Linkage Project. Unpublished. Manitoba Centre for Health Policy and Evaluation, February 1995.

Vermaeten, F., Gillespie, W,I., and Vermaeten, A. (1994) Tax Incidence in Canada. *Canadian Tax Journal* 42:348-416.

Wall, R., DeCoster, C., and Roos, N. (1994) Estimating per diem costs for Manitoba hospitals: a first step. Manitoba Centre for Health Policy and Evaluation, unpublished, February 1994.

Wolfson, M.C. and Evans, J.M. (1989) Statistics Canada's low income cut-offs: methodological concerns and possibilities. Research Paper Series. Analytic Studies Branch, Statistics Canada, Ottawa.

7

Equity in the Finance and Delivery of Health Care: an Introduction to the ECuity Project

EDDY VAN DOORSLAER[1] and ADAM WAGSTAFF[2]

[1]Department of Health Policy and Management
Erasmus University
[2]School of Social Sciences
University of Sussex

ABSTRACT

This paper presents an introduction to the methods used in and the results obtained from the *ECuity Project*. We show how the overall redistributive effect of health care can be decomposed into three components: progressivity, horizontal equity and reranking. The decomposition is illustrated for selected countries representing the three typical financing systems, *i.e.*, mainly funded through taxes, social insurance, or private payments. We investigate the extent of socioeconomic

Health, Health Care and Health Economics: Perspectives on Distribution
Edited by Morris L. Barer, Thomas E. Getzen, and Greg L. Stoddart
Copyright 1998 John Wiley & Sons, Ltd.

inequalities in self-reported health by using a latent variable approach to measuring health and using concentration indices to measure inequality. Horizontal equity in the delivery of health care is analysed by looking at the association between health care utilisation and rank in the income distribution after indirectly standardising for need. Again, we illustrate the methods with results for some typical countries with either universal public insurance coverage, mixed public/private coverage and mainly private coverage.

INTRODUCTION

This paper presents an overview of the methods used in, and some of the results obtained from, the ECuity Project. The project, which is funded by the European Union's BIOMED I Programme, is a so-called *concerted action* (CA), involving country teams from 13 European countries and the US working together (in concert if not perfect harmony!) on a comparative study of equity in different health care systems. The project builds and extends on a previous comparative study (Van Doorslaer, Wagstaff and Rutten, 1993) and examines equity in both the finance of health care and its delivery. The "building" involves refinement of the methods that were developed and used in the earlier CA to measure and test for inequity in health care financing and delivery. The "extension" involves enlarging the cross-section of countries, the use of more recent datasets and, in some instances, the undertaking of comparisons at different points in time to allow for a longitudinal perspective.

Because this paper aims to provide a general overview of original methods and results which have been written-up elsewhere, it has, inevitably, a somewhat broad-brush perspective. References to the original sources are given to enable readers to obtain further details if they so wish. Moreover, as some of the work presented in this overview was still ongoing at the time of writing, not all of the results presented are definitive and, in some instances, only preliminary and illustrative results were available. This "health warning" applies in particular to the results presented in the sections on "Vertical and horizontal equity in the finance of health care" and "Equity in the delivery of health care."

Apart from the Introduction and Conclusion, the paper is organised around three sections, one concerned with equity in the finance of health care, and two discussing alternative interpretations of equity in health care delivery. The third section examines income-related inequalities in health and explores the extent to which a country's health care system affects the level of health inequality in the country. In the fourth section, the extent to which health care is allocated according to need, and, in particular, the extent to which persons in equal need are treated the same, irrespective of their income are explored. In each section, the project's methods are briefly outlined and empirical results are presented for a subset of participating countries to illustrate these methods.

VERTICAL AND HORIZONTAL EQUITY IN THE FINANCE OF HEALTH CARE

PRINCIPLES

Public finance texts generally distinguish between two competing equity principles: the benefit principle and the ability-to-pay principle. A review of policy documents (Wagstaff and van Doorslaer, 1993) reveals that the benefit principle - requiring payments to be related to benefits received - commands little support in the mainly publicly-financed European health care systems and that instead the guiding principle seems to be solidarity and the notion that payments for publicly funded health care ought to be related to ability to pay (ATP). According to the vertical version of the ATP principle (unequal treatment of unequals), better-off households should make "appropriately" larger payments for their health care than worse-off households, whereas the horizontal version of the principle requires that households with a similar ability to pay should make similar payments for health care.

Obviously, both versions of the ATP principle seem more likely to be violated to the extent that an important share of health care is paid for by *private* payments, as is the case in Switzerland, the Netherlands, and the US. Typically, private payments for health insurance premiums or direct charges are usually not related to ATP, but there are also important differences in the extent to which this is the case for various *public* finance sources, notably in direct versus indirect taxes, local versus central taxation, or social insurance contributions. Therefore the *financing mix*, consisting of the relative shares of taxes, social insurance premiums, private insurance premiums and direct payments, will to a large extent determine the extent of a system's compliance with the ATP principle. But establishing the financing mix is insufficient to predict a system's redistributive effect. It is also important to look beyond the shares of each source and to examine the actual payment rules in order to find out to what degree a financing scheme is horizontally and vertically equitable.

Vertical equity can be seen as the extent to which, *on average*, payments increase (or not) as income increases, whereas horizontal inequity can be seen as the variation in payment *at each income level.* The redistributive effect of a tax or payment scheme is a function of both. In what follows we will (i) explain how vertical and horizontal equity can be measured separately by examining total redistributive effect, (ii) demonstrate how this can be done empirically for health care financing, and (iii) relate the findings to some of the main characteristics of the financing schemes.

MEASUREMENT OF VERTICAL AND HORIZONTAL EQUITY

In contrast to our earlier work, in the ECuity Project we have attempted to investigate not only the issue of vertical equity but also the extent of horizontal inequity. This extension was made possible by applying a method for decomposing the redistributive effect of a tax developed by Aronson, Johnson and Lambert (1994), hereafter AJL. Their work is important because it shows how the vertical and horizontal effects can be measured and compared in terms of the income redistributive effect they induce. Elsewhere (Wagstaff and van Doorslaer, 1997), we have shown how their decomposition method can be applied to the analysis of health care finance. Here we will only give an intuitive explanation.

The total redistributive effect (RE) of any tax can be defined as the change in income inequality induced by paying the tax, and measured, for instance, by the difference between the pre-tax and post-tax Gini coefficient. AJL show that, in general, *RE* can be decomposed into a vertical, a horizontal and a reranking component as follows:

[1]
$$RE = \left(\frac{g}{1-g}\right)K_T - \sum \alpha_x G_{F(x)} - \left[G_{X-T} - C_{X-T}\right]$$
$$= V - H - R.$$

Here V is the redistributive effect that would occur if all households with the same income were treated equally by the tax rules. Where there is some degree of unequal treatment of equals, it can be interpreted as the vertical component of the overall redistributive effect of the tax. V can be computed as the product of K_T, which is Kakwani's (1977) progressivity index computed on the assumption that all equal-income households are treated the same, and $g/(1-g)$, where g is the average tax rate.[1] V is positive (negative) when K_T is positive (negative) because a progressive tax reduces income inequality whereas a regressive tax increases inequality. A proportional tax (with a zero progressivity index) leaves income inequality unchanged. Clearly, the vertical redistributive effect V of any payment will depend on *both* its degree of progressivity (K_T) *and* its relative importance (the average tax rate g).

Because in practice most taxes will not treat all equals identically, V represents an upper bound on RE which can be reduced for two reasons. First, it can be reduced by what AJL label *pure or classical horizontal inequity*, denoted in eqn (1) by H. This is defined as the inequality in post-tax incomes generated in groups of pre-tax equals. Empirically, it can be computed by taking a weighted sum of the post-tax income Gini coefficients $G_{F(x)}$ of households with pre-tax income x. These Gini coefficients are zero only if there is no differential tax treatment of equals. In empirical work, of course, there is a problem of defining what we mean by "equals", since very few households in any dataset have exactly the same income. To get round this, one simply assumes that households within a certain *income range* (say, $500) can be considered "equals". There is a second factor in eqn (1) causing V to diverge from RE, namely R. This measures the extent of *reranking* in the move from the pre-tax distribution to the post-tax distribution, and is measured by comparing the post-tax Gini coefficient with the post-tax concentration coefficient. If there is no reranking, R is zero.

Because H and R are always non-negative, differential treatment always reduces the vertical effect. For our purposes, the difference between H and R is not

---

[1] Kakwani's index is defined as twice the area between the Lorenz curve for pre-tax income and the tax concentration curve, the latter being the curve plotting the cumulative proportion of the population (ranked by pre-tax income) against the cumulative proportion of tax payment. It is equal to the difference between the tax concentration index and the Gini coefficient for pre-tax income, the former being defined in the same manner as the Gini coefficient, but is computed using the tax concentration curve rather than the Lorenz curve for pre-tax income. A more detailed description of Kakwani's progressivity index, its computation, and its application in health care financing can be found in Wagstaff, van Doorslaer, and Paci (1989) and Wagstaff, van Doorslaer, *et al.* (1992).

very important. Empirically, AJL show that H increases and R decreases when the income range used to define "equals" is expanded, but the total differential treatment $(H+R)$ remains fairly constant. Expressing V as a percentage of RE facilitates a comparison of the relative importance of vertical effects versus horizontal inequity and reranking.[2]

CROSS-COUNTRY COMPARISONS

Application of the decomposition method requires detailed micro-data on health care payments and involves making various incidence assumptions in order to be able attribute all payments to individual households. In Wagstaff and van Doorslaer (1997) we have shown how this method can be applied to examine the consequences of financing system changes using micro-simulation. Here we will illustrate the methods using results from Wagstaff, van Doorslaer *et al.* (1997) and van Doorslaer, Wagstaff, *et al.* (1997) for selected prototypical countries. First, we briefly describe the main distinguishing features of the financing systems of the six selected countries. Second, we will show what the progressivity and the vertical redistributive effect would be in these countries in the absence of any differential treatment among groups of equals. Third, we will show how the total redistributive effect is affected by differential treatment.

Health Care Financing Typology

All industrialised countries finance health care using a mix of four possible sources: taxes, social insurance contributions, private insurance premiums and direct payments. Figure 1 summarises the mixes adopted in the six selected countries for the latest year between 1987 and 1992 for which microdata were available. The three clusters that emerged in Wagstaff, van Doorslaer, *et al.* (1992) on the basis of the dominant finance source are represented in this subsample: two countries (the US and Switzerland) finance the majority of their health care from private sources (premiums and direct payments), two countries (France and Germany) mainly rely on social insurance financing while two other countries

---

[2] From Eqn (1) we have $V/RE = 1 + (H + R)/RE$. This is equal to 1 or (100%) if H and R are zero, *i.e.*, if the only factor giving rise to redistribution is the deviation from proportionality of the tax system.

(Finland and the United Kingdom) have primarily tax-based financing systems.[3] These financing mixes will have a large impact on the redistributive effects to be expected in each country, with the public sources typically being more likely to be related to ability to pay than the private payments. It is, however, also important to look beyond the mix.

Two points are especially important to bear in mind. One is that the extent of public or private coverage is often income-related. This is obvious in countries where eligibility criteria for public and private coverage are income-related. This is the case, for instance, in Germany, where persons above a certain income threshold (DM 61200 in 1992) are allowed to opt out of public coverage.[4] Most of the tax-financed and social insurance-based systems provide fairly comprehensive and universal coverage to the entire population. Of the two mainly privately-financed systems in this sample, one, the US, does have two special public schemes (Medicaid and Medicare) which provide public assistance to certain low income groups and the elderly, but still has a substantial proportion of the population without any coverage. The other mainly privately-financed system, Switzerland, does not have such special public schemes but uses subsidies to ensure fairly universal coverage. The second point is that the mix of taxes used to finance health care varies from one country to the next In Germany, Switzerland, the UK and the US, the taxes going to finance health care are general tax revenues, and hence the mix of health care "taxes" mirrors the mix of general tax revenues. In Germany and the UK, the split is fairly even between direct and indirect taxes, whilst in Switzerland and the US, direct taxes play a more important role in raising revenues than indirect taxes. In the Nordic countries, such as Finland, however, the taxes financing health care are not general revenues, but rather a mix of general revenues and local income taxes levied specifically to raise revenue for health care.[5] Both of these points will have to be borne in mind when interpreting the

---

[3] The US financing mix in Figure 1 has not been adjusted for tax deductibility of insurance premiums. Premiums net of tax relief are more regressive, but if one can assume that revenues foregone are compensated by higher taxes, then the overall regressivity of health care financing is not affected very much (Wagstaff, van Doorslaer, *et al.*, 1997).

[4] Other countries with limited public cover for higher income groups include Ireland and the Netherlands. For a more extensive account of these countries' health financing details, see Wagstaff, van Doorslaer, *et al.* (1997).

[5] Some other local government programmes are also financed by these local income taxes, but typically health care absorbs the lion's share of these revenues.

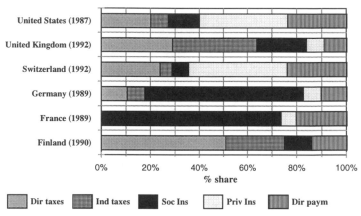

Figure 1 Health care financing mix in 6 ccountries
Source: Wagstaff, van Doorslaer, *et al.* (1997)

progressivity results.

Progressivity

Figure 2 presents the Kakwani indices K_T by source obtained from the cumulative distributions of payments by income when both gross income and payments have been adjusted for household composition using the same equivalence scale for the six selected countries.[6] They have been calculated from grouped observations on the assumption that all households in the same income interval (the equivalent of £260 per year in 1990 prices) are treated the same. The indices for total and subtotal (general taxes, public and private) payments have been calculated as weighted averages of the components using the macro shares as weights.[7]

---

[6] For further details on household expenditure datasets, incidence assumptions and methods of computation used, see Wagstaff, van Doorslaer, *et al.* (1997).

[7] By macro shares we refer to the relative revenue shares of each of the payment sources according to national accounts data. These shares are not in all cases identical to the micro shares that can be obtained from the household expenditure survey data.

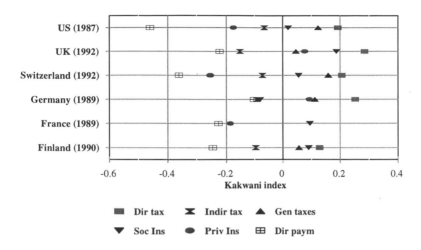

Figure 2 Progressivity of health care finance by source in six countries
Source: Wagstaff, van Doorslaer, *et al.* (1997)

As is clear from Fig. 2, the direct taxes used to finance health care tend to be progressive, whilst indirect taxes tend to be regressive. It is evident that the direct taxes used to finance health care in Finland (principally local income tax) are less progressive than the direct taxes used to finance health care in the other countries (general direct taxation). We can see that financing from general taxation is progressive in all countries, but less so in Finland (due to the near-proportional local income tax) and in the UK (due to the relative importance there of indirect taxes, which are regressive). In fact, general taxation appears to be most progressive in Switzerland, the US and Germany, the three countries that do not rely on tax financing for the majority of their health care funding.

Social insurance has widely differing progressivity implications in the two social insurance countries: it is progressive in France but regressive in Germany. In both countries, the contribution rate is a fixed proportion of earnings but the rules determining rate and eligibility vary greatly.[8] The regressiveness in Germany is mainly a consequence of the opting-out option offered to high-income earners and the self-employed, and of the existence of a contribution ceiling for those in the sickness funds. Social insurance progressivity in France stems mainly from the near exemption of pensioners and unemployed (they pay only 1% of their pension or unemployment benefit) and from the fact that there is no contribution ceiling. For similar reasons, social insurance premiums are also progressive in all other countries that make relatively little use of that source for health care financing.

The degree of progressivity of *private insurance* depends very much on what type of coverage it provides (cf. Wagstaff, van Doorslaer *et al.*, 1992). In the two countries where it is the main source of coverage for the majority of the population (Switzerland and the US), it is very regressive. Private insurance appears as more regressive in Switzerland than in the US because substantial portions of the lower income groups in the US are either uninsured, underinsured or have partial or full coverage from one of the public schemes (Rasell and Tang, 1994) and therefore pay no or lower premiums. But private insurance is also very regressive in France where it is bought by the great majority of the population as coverage for public sector copayments for almost all types of care and extra billing by physicians. Private insurance is only progressive in Germany, where it provides coverage to high income-earners opting out of public coverage, and in the UK, where it is mainly bought by higher income groups to provide additional private coverage on top of NHS coverage ("double coverage").

Finally, in all countries *direct payments* show up as regressive, but very regressive in the two mainly privately financed systems, the US and Switzerland. The overall progressivity of total health care financing in these 6 countries, and of its public and private subtotals, is shown in Fig. 3. Not surprisingly, the countries with the largest share of private payments, Switzerland and the US, have the most regressive financing. The pro- or regressivity of the publicly-financed systems depends on the rules governing the public payments and on the relative shares of more regressive sources such as indirect taxes and private payments. The German case is special. As a result of its opting-out option for the higher income groups, its private funding is less regressive, and its public funding more regressive, than that of other countries.

---

[8] In Germany, the average contribution rate in 1989 was 12.9% (Hoffmeyer, 1994) whereas the contribution rate in 1990 was 19.6% in the French Régime Générale which covers 80% of the population.

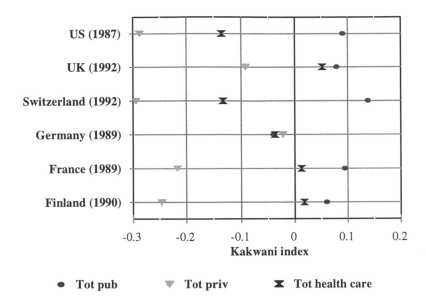

Figure 3 Total progressivity by country
Source: Wagstaff, van Doorslaer, *et al.* **(1997)**

Redistributive Effect, Horizontal Equity and Reranking

As we explained earlier progressivity alone does not provide the entire picture as to how the pre-payment Gini coefficient is changed after payment. As we can see from eqn (1), the vertical redistributive effect, V, is positive (negative) if K_T is positive (negative), but can be reduced if one takes into account the fact that households in the same income interval may not pay the same amount and may change ranking after payment, or, in other words, if H and R are not zero.

It is therefore useful to complement the progressivity analysis by a full decomposition of the redistributive effect into its three components. For those finance components for which data permitted,[9] the results are summarised in two figures presenting the absolute values of *V* and *V* expressed as a percentage of *RE* Recall the former is equal to $[g/(1-g)] K_T$ and the latter is equal to 100% if there is no differential treatment, *i.e.*, if *H* and *R* are zero. When, as a percentage of *RE*, *V* is higher than 100%, it indicates by what percentage the positive redistributive effect would be larger in the absence of any differential treatment. When it is lower than 100%, it indicates by what percentage the (negative) redistributive effect would be reduced.

The values of *V* for the four sources for each of the six countries are shown in Fig. 4. The signs are, of course, the same as those of the corresponding values of K_T. The values, however, are different and indeed the story is rather different.

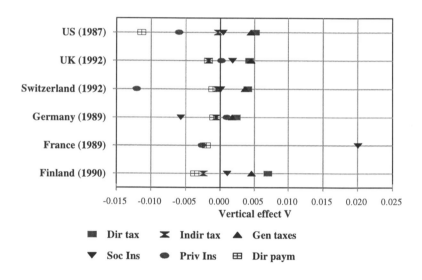

Figure 4 Vertical Redistributive Effect by Source in Six Countries
Source: van Doorslaer, Wagstaff, *et al.* (1997b)

---

[9] For France, Switzerland, and the UK, private payments at the household level could not be estimated reliably because these were recorded in the expenditure surveys for a period of only a few weeks (cf. van Doorslaer, Wagstaff, *et al.*, 1997).

With respect to direct taxes, the UK has the largest value of K_T, whilst the Finnish direct taxes going to fund health care are the least progressive. When it comes to the redistributive effect of direct taxes, however, it is Finland that has the highest value of V, reflecting the relative importance of direct taxes there (*i.e.*, the relatively high value of g). Interestingly, the degree of vertical income redistribution associated with the general taxes used to finance health care is roughly the same in the UK and the US. The high value of V for social insurance in France is striking, reflecting a relatively high value of K_T and a very high value of g.

Figure 5 shows V as a percentage of *RE*. For the most part, these figures are close to 100%, indicating that in terms of redistributive effect, unequal

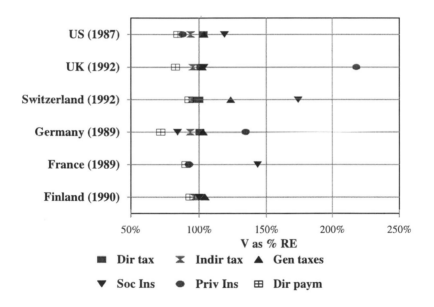

Figure 5 Horizontal Redistributive Effect by Source in Six countries
Source: van Doorslaer, Wagstaff, *et al.* 1997b)

treatment of unequals is far more important than unequal treatment of equals. In general, and not surprisingly, most of the discrepancy between V and RE occurs in the voluntary private payments for which there is little or no relationship between payment and ability to pay: for example, in the UK, private insurance is most popular amongst the better-off but in any given income interval, there is a good deal of variation in coverage (many well-off households having no private coverage at all). But also social insurance payments show a high degree of differential treatment -- higher, indeed, than taxes (except in Finland). This is mainly as a consequence of varying contribution rates and exemptionns on the basis of criteria other than income. Overall, the (positive) redistributive effect would have been 40% larger in Finland and about 20% lower in Germany and the US if there had been no differential treatment.

INCOME-RELATED HEALTH INEQUALITY

PRINCIPLES

It can be argued that all concerns about the distribution of, or access to, health care stem ultimately from a more fundamental concern about the distribution of health itself; therefore any analysis of equity in health care should focus on the extent to which existing delivery systems bring health distributions closer to an equal distribution (cf. Culyer and Wagstaff, 1993). The absence of any health inequality may well be an unattainable goal, but many would subscribe to the view that health care systems are more equitable to the extent that they help to reduce health inequalities that are systematically related to characteristics such as socioeconomic status, place of residence, race, etc. However, any attempt to operationalise this criterion encounters the problems of how to measure health, how to measure inequalities in its distribution and how to establish the marginal impact on this distribution of the various determinants of health inequality. The problem is compounded by the well-known fact that variations in health seem to be largely determined by factors outside of the health care system, some known, some not known, which have to be adequately controlled for when trying to single out the impact of a particular system's characteristics.[10]

Here we simply restrict ourselves to a summary of the project's empirical findings in an examination of the degree of income-related inequalities in (self-reported) health with a view to: (i) assessing whether there is any systematic variation across countries, and (ii) if so, whether there seems to be any relationship with country characteristics, including some features of its health care systems.

MEASURING HEALTH INEQUALITY

It is well-known that in many countries morbidity and mortality have been found to be inversely related with indicators of socioeconomic status. A variety of inequality indices have been employed in the literature on inequalities in health to quantify this phenomenon.[11] We have used the concentration index proposed by Wagstaff, van Doorslaer, and Paci (1989) which is based on the concept of an illness (or health) concentration curve $L(s)$ that plots the cumulative proportion of the population ranked by socio-economic status (*e.g.*, income) against the cumulative proportion of ill-health (see Fig. 6). If this concentration curve coincides with the diagonal, all socio-economic groups report the same relative share of ill-health and there is no inequality. If, by contrast, the concentration curve lies above (below) the diagonal, inequalities in ill-health exist and favour the more (less) advantaged socioeconomic groups.

If one such curve $L(s)$ (say, for one country or for one year) is everywhere closer to the diagonal than another curve $L'(s)$ (for another country or another period), it can be said that $L(s)$ *dominates* $L'(s)$ and unambiguously represents less inequality. When the concentration curves cross, or if one wants to quantify the degree of inequality, one can use an *ill-health concentration index*, C, defined as twice the area between $L(s)$ and the diagonal. It takes the value of zero when $L(s)$ coincides with the diagonal and is negative (positive) when $L(s)$ lies above (below) the diagonal. The upper and lower bounds of C are +1 and -1 respectively.

Clearly, it is not realistic to assume that all income-related health inequality is avoidable. Deviations between $L(s)$ and the diagonal can partly be due to an

---

[10] For a recent account of the wide spectrum of determinants of population health, see *e.g.*, Evans, Barer, and Marmor (1994).

[11] For a review and illustrations of the various measures and their properties, see Wagstaff, Paci, and van Doorslaer (1991).

association between income and demographic factors. One method to control for these *unavoidable* inequalities related to age and sex is to employ the method of direct standardisation to obtain age-sex standardised rates of ill-health by socio-economic status. If age-sex standardisation reduces inequality, the standardised concentration curve $L^+(s)$ derived from this procedure will be *closer* to the diagonal than the unstandardised curve and the resulting standardised index C^+ is smaller (in absolute value) than the unstandardised index.

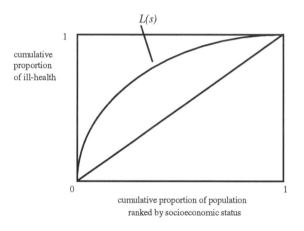

Figure 6 Illness Concentration Curve

If $L^+(s)$ is assumed to be piecewise linear, C^+ can be calculated using the formula proposed by Kakwani, Wagstaff and van Doorslaer (1997), hereafter KWV:

[2]

$$C^+ = \frac{2}{\mu^+} \sum_{t=1}^{T} f_t \mu_t^+ R_t - 1$$

where $\mu^+ = \sum_{t=1}^{T} f_t \mu_t^+$ is the mean standardised rate of ill-health of the sample, f_t is the proportion of the sample in socio-economic group (SEG) t, and R_t is the relative rank of the tth SEG. The latter is defined as:

[3]
$$R_t = \sum_{\gamma=1}^{t-1} f_\gamma + \tfrac{1}{2} f_t$$

and thus indicates the cumulative proportion of the population up to the midpoint of each group interval. Alternative ways of calculating $C+$ and its estimated standard errors from both grouped and individual-level data can be found in KWV. They show how income-related inequality in health can then simply be computed by running a regression from the (ill-) health indicator (of the individual or the group) on the relative rank in the income distribution.

CROSS-COUNTRY COMPARISONS

In van Doorslaer, Wagstaff, *et al.* (1997a) we have presented empirical results of an analysis of income-related inequalities in self-perceived health for nine countries. Ill-health was measured in all countries by the multiple-category responses on a question to rate one's general health status, typically ranging from excellent to poor. Although both the exact wording of the question and the number and type of response categories varied from country to country, it was assumed that the discrete distributions were generated by a continuous, underlying but nobservable, latent health distribution. Using a standard lognormal distribution as the underlying distribution, it is possible to obtain latent ill-health scores for each answer category, to attribute a latent health score for each individual in the sample and to compute average scores of ill-health for socio-economic groups (cf. Wagstaff and van Doorslaer, 1994). The main advantage of this approach is that it avoids a practice in the literature on health inequalities that was (and still is) often used to dichotomise the self-assessed health measure by choosing a cut-off level below which individuals are considered to be not healthy.

Here we will illustrate the methods by presenting 1987 results for just three countries representing "typical" clusters: Finland, the Netherlands and the US.[12] Although the number of answer categories was five in the Finnish and Dutch survey and four in the US survey, the latent variable approach enables the construction of comparable (age-sex standardised) distributions of latent ill-health scores across deciles of equivalent disposable household income. These relative distributions are shown graphically in Fig. 7. Because the scale of the latent ill-

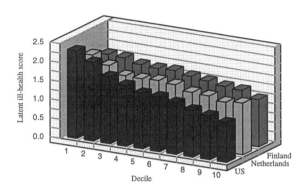

Figure 7 Latent Ill-Health by Income Decile
Source: van Doorslaer, Wagstaff, *et al.* (1997a)

health variable is standardised, all countries have the same mean ill-health but the inverse relationship between average ill-health and income decile is much clearer in the US than in the other two countries, suggesting higher income-related health inequality favouring the better-off in that country. It is more difficult to rank Finland and the Netherlands just by comparison of the relative gradient in the bar charts.[13]

---

[12] The surveys used were the Health and Social Security Survey 1987 (n=11,956) for Finland, the combined 1986, 87, and 89 Health Interview Survey (n=15,457) for the Netherlands, and the 1987 National Medical Expenditure Survey (n=22,226) for the US.
[13] Some authors have suggested running regressions through these observations and deriving indices from the regression slopes to measure health inequality. For a discussion of the disadvantages of these and other indices, see Wagstaff, Paci, and van Doorslaer (1991).

We have based our cross-country comparisons on the ill-health concentration curves and indices. The illness concentration curves for the three countries are shown in Fig. 8. In order to facilitate health dominance-checking, all concentration curves are presented as deviations from the diagonal. It can be seen that all curves lie above the diagonal, indicating inequality favouring the higher income groups in all three countries, but the US curve is clearly *dominated* (*i.e.*, lies *above*) the two other curves. Finland and the Netherlands cannot be ranked *vis-à-vis* one another because the curves cross each other in the eighth decile. The corresponding concentration index values (and 95% confidence intervals) are -0.136 (-0.182; -0.090) for the US, -0.066 (-0.096; -0.036) for the Netherlands and -0.057 (-0.082; -0.032) for Finland. This suggests slightly lower inequality in Finland than in the Netherlands but the difference was not found to be statistically

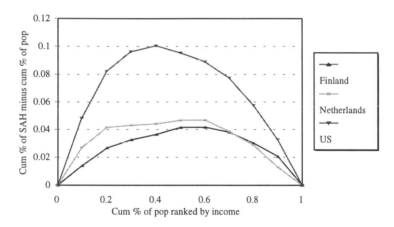

Figure 8 Ill-health concentration curves
Source: van Doorslaer, Wagstaff, *et al.* (1997a)

significant by a *t*-test based on the standard errors. The difference in index value between the US and the other two countries was significant at the 5% level.

The question which arises is: are there any characteristics of these countries' health care systems that might help to explain these differentials in income-related health inequalities? This three-country sample does not really allow any such analysis. One could speculate about the non-universal health insurance coverage in the US versus universal coverage in the other two countries, but in van Doorslaer, Wagstaff, *et al.* (1997a) we went on to explore the statistical association between health inequality indices and two measures of health spending and the level and distribution of income for all nine countries in the study.[14] Neither total health care expenditure per capita, nor the percentage of total expenditure spent publicly appeared to have any statistical association with health inequality, suggesting that neither higher spending, nor higher public sector shares are associated with lower health inequality. Of the two other variables, the GDP *per capita* and the Gini coefficient of income inequality, only the latter proved to bear a consistent and significant positive relationship with health inequality. It appears, therefore, that income-related inequality in health is more related to the distribution of income in a society than to its aggregate income level or its levels of health spending.

EQUITY IN THE DELIVERY OF HEALTH CARE

PRINCIPLES

Not everyone accepts that an equitable distribution of health care is one that reduces health inequality. An alternative interpretation of equity in this area, and one that seems to command a great deal of support amongst health policy makers in Europe, is that health care ought to be allocated on the basis of need[15] Our empirical work on this issue has focused on the measurement and testing of the *horizontal* version of this principle, namely that persons in equal need of care ought to be treated the same, irrespective of their income.

---

[14] These variables were chosen because they had been used before in a cross-country comparison of (non-income-related) health inequality by LeGrand (1987).

[15] Others have argued that it is not the distribution of treatment that matters but rather the distribution of *access* to treatment, and that this ought to be the same for everyone, irrespective of the distributions of health care and health that result from equalising access. There are issues concerning the reasonableness of such a position and how one can distinguish (especially empirically) "treatment" from "access." For a more extensive discussion of equity interpretations, see Wagstaff and van Doorslaer (1993) and Culyer and Wagstaff (1993). On "access" versus "utilisation," see Mooney, *et al.* (1992 a, b) and Culyer, *et al.* (1992 a, b).

MEASURING AND TESTING FOR INEQUITY

In Wagstaff and van Doorslaer (1996), we proposed a new approach to measuring inequity in the delivery of health care, that has several advantages over that used in earlier work.[16] First, it can be used on grouped data but also on individual-level data. Second, it is computationally straightforward. Finally, it is very convenient from the point of view of analysing the effects of reforms by, for instance, simulation methods.

Basically, the method proceeds as follows. It compares the concentration curve of the actual observed medical care utilisation $L_M(p)$ to the concentration curve of the medical care utilisation that can be *expected on the basis of need*, $L_N(p)$. Need-expected utilisation is defined as the indirectly standardised value of medical care utilisation for the individual or group and can be obtained from running a regression of medical care utilisation on a set of need indicator variables. If the $L_N(p)$ lies *above* (below) the $L_M(p)$, as shown in Fig. 9, the lower income

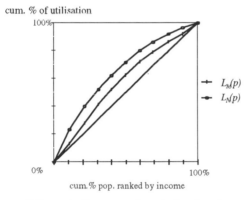

cum. % of utilisation

$L_M(p)$

$L_N(p)$

cum. % pop. ranked by income

Figure 9 Concentration curves for actual and need-expected medical care

groups receive less care than would be expected on the basis of their need and there is horizontal inequity *favouring the better-off* (worse-off).

---

[16] The earlier work, which was reported in van Doorslaer, Wagstaff, *et al.* (1992), employed the index proposed by Wagstaff, van Doorslaer, and Paci (1991).

Horizontal inequity is measured as twice the area between the need and medical care concentration curves, or equivalently as:

[4]

$$HI_{WV} = C_M - C_N$$

where C_M is the concentration index for medical care and C_N is the concentration index for need (*i.e.,* indirectly standardised -- or expected -- medical care consumption). A positive (negative) value of HI_{WV} indicates horizontal inequity favouring the better-off (worse-off), whilst a zero value indicates that the factor of proportionality (between medical care and need) is the same irrespective of income. It is worth pointing out that it is possible that HI_{WV} can be equal to zero even when the two concentration curves $L_M(p)$ and $L_N(p)$ do *not* coincide. This could be the case, for instance, when inequity favouring the poor at the bottom end of the income distribution compensates inequity favouring the rich at the high end of the distribution. In other words, coinciding concentration curves is a sufficient but not a necessary condition for the index value to be zero.

CROSS-COUNTRY COMPARISONS

Wagstaff and van Doorslaer (1996) show how estimates for C_M, C_N and HI_{WV} and their standard errors can be obtained by means of a simple, convenient regression approach as well as through a more accurate but more involved method. Here we illustrate these methods using selected results taken from van Doorslaer, Wagstaff, *et al.* (1997c). Again, we have chosen three countries which can be considered fairly typical of three types of health care systems with a differing public/private mix. Finland is interesting because it has universal public coverage of the entire population but allows the purchasing of private care outside the public system. The Netherlands has universal coverage but the type of coverage differs for higher and lower income groups. Roughly the bottom six deciles are covered publicly through sickness funds while roughly the upper four deciles have to insure privately for routine health care. Potential equity-compromising differences include: (*i*) GPs are paid on a capitation basis for public and fee-for-service for private patients; (*ii*) private patients have direct access to specialists while public patients require a referral by the GP; (*iii*) while medical care is completely free at the point of service to publicly insured, many privately insured voluntarily choose either limited coverage or no coverage for GP services, or have high deductibles; and (*iv*) specialist fees are much higher for private than for public patients. Finally, the US has mainly private insurance coverage for the majority of the population, but also substantial portions -- mainly amongst the lower income groups -- with either public coverage (Medicare and Medicaid) or no coverage at all. In addition, even for those with coverage, there may be substantial direct out-of-pocket payments due to limited coverage or high deductibles.

The empirical analysis focuses on imputed expenditures for three types of care (GP visits, outpatient visits and inpatient days) and the aggregate of these three.[17] The OLS regression specification used to calculate expected expenditures, includes (*i*) a vector of dummy variables for ten age-sex categories, (*ii*) a vector of dummies derived from the responses to the self-assessed health (SAH) question, (*iii*) a vector derived from the responses on the country-specific list of chronic conditions. The wording and response categories of the health indicators and the recording method and period of medical care utilisation are not identical across countries.[18] In the US survey, for instance, primary care (GP) visits could not be distinguished from specialist visits and are therefore both included in the outpatient care visits.

The estimates for HI_{WV} and its standard error for the various medical care types are presented in Table 1. The indices suggest that there is no significant inequity in GP care (except in Finland), that there is substantial and significant pro-rich inequity in the utilisation of outpatient care and that there is a small but statistically insignificant degree of pro-poor inequity in the utilisation of inpatient facilities. In overall imputed expenditure, there seems to be no discernible degree of inequity. Perhaps the most striking finding is that these patterns are very similar across these three countries, despite their widely varying public/private insurance mix arrangements. In Van Doorslaer, Wagstaff, *et al.* (1997c), it is shown that these patterns also hold for a number of other European countries, though not for all. If any inequity in the distribution of health care across income groups can be found at all, it appears to be in favour of the better-off and for the use of specialist

---

[17] Average costs are imputed to value each of these three types of medical care utilisation and to calculate an aggregate figure.

[18] The surveys used are the same as those used in the section on Income-Related Health Inequality (see footnote 12). For further details about the data and variable definitions, see van Doorslaer, Wagstaff, *et al.* (1997). For an alternative analysis of the Dutch results using a two-part model (a probit equation for the probability of positive use, and a negative binomial model for the positive quantity, conditional on use), see Wagstaff and van Doorslaer (1997).

outpatient care only.

Table 1 HI_{WV} indices of horizontal inequity[&]

Type of Care	Finland (1987)	Netherlands (1992)	US (1987)
GP visits	0.022 (2.39)	-0.002 (0.15)	n.a.[&&]
Outpatient	0.077 (5.42)	0.0861 (4.11)	0.044 (7.21)
Inpatient days	-0.010 (-0.28)	-0.060 (-1.48)	-0.008 (-0.40)
Aggregate imputed	0.008 (0.31)	-0.029 (-0.97)	0.009 (0.59)
Actual total	n.a.	n.a.	0.024 (1.55)

[&]   Standardised for need using age, sex, SAH vector and vector of chronic conditions. *t*-values
      in parentheses.
[&&] Outpatient visits in US include primary care physician visits
Source: van Doorslaer, Wagstaff, *et al.* (1997c)

An answer to the question what may be the cause of these findings requires further investigation. In the Netherlands, where the pro-rich outpatient utilisation pattern seems strongest, it may be a consequence of the fact that higher-income privately insured are more inclined to use specialist care than lower-income publicly insured because of their direct access, lower coverage for GP care, and their being more attractive patients to specialists because of higher fees. In Finland, it can be shown to be related to the higher utilisation of private specialist visits by higher income individuals to "jump the public queue." Finally, in the US it may simply be the more comprehensive insurance coverage of the better-off that influences their higher rates of outpatient care utilisation than expected on the basis of our crude need indicators. However, the fact that the finding is fairly widespread irrespective of health care system characteristics begs the question whether these utilisation patterns are not generated by non-economic factors, rather than economic factors such as insurance coverage and physician remuneration. It may simply reflect a tendency on behalf of the better-off and better-educated to be more inclined, at a given level of need, to go and see a specialist physician. One possibility for future research is to test what happens to the HI_{WV} indices after indirectly standardising, via the regression procedure, not only for need but also for the system characteristics which are hypothesised to generate these findings. When van der Burg and van Doorslaer (1997), for instance, included a dummy for private/public insurance status in the Dutch standardisation procedure, the HI_{WV} indices remained virtually unchanged, thereby lending support to the view that other factors than insurance status play an important role in explaining the pro-rich inequity finding for outpatient care utilisation in the Netherlands.

CONCLUSION

This paper presents a brief summary of the main methods used in the ECuity Project in its study of equity in the finance and delivery of health care. The methodology was illustrated with selected results obtained for various European countries and the US.

The analysis of health care finance confirmed earlier findings that tax financed systems tend to be progressive and mainly privately financed systems regressive, while social-insurance systems can go either way depending on the rules governing eligibility and contribution rates. However, it was also shown that in order to evaluate the total income redistributive effect of a financing system, it is important to look beyond these vertical effects. Horizontal inequity and reranking associated with differential treatment of "equals" tend to reduce the positive vertical redistribution or increase the negative vertical effect. This horizontal effect is substantial for all private payments which are becoming increasingly important in most health care systems. Overall, however, income redistributive effects resulting from health care finance are fairly small (*e.g.,* compared to the personal income tax effects). Only in the US the pre-payment income inequality is substantially increased through health care financing.

These findings are worth bearing in mind at a time when many developed countries are rethinking their health care financing methods and considering alternative options (Wagstaff and van Doorslaer, 1995; Hoffmeyer and McCarthy, 1994). Future work on the equity consequences aimed at unraveling the relative contributions of vertical and horizontal effects of health care financing arrangements would benefit from simulation modeling exercises which can keep more factors constant in the comparisons.

Illness concentration curves and indices were shown to be useful in the measurement and testing for cross-country differences in socioeconomic inequalities in morbidity. Significant inequalities favouring the better-off were found in all countries studied and high health inequality appears to be associated with high income inequality. Future work in this area should concentrate on the potential determinants of these cross-country differences in order to distinguish association from causation.

Finally, our method of measuring and testing for horizontal inequity in health care delivery showed little evidence of "unequal treatment for equal need" in GP, inpatient and total health care utilisation. The only type of care for which higher income groups appear to be using consistently and significantly more than would be expected on the basis of need indicators is outpatient care. Whether this finding is due to delivery system characteristics such as differences in insurance coverage or in physician remuneration is unclear. It may also simply reflect a higher propensity of the better-off to use more specialist care because of perceived higher quality. Again, future work should focus on the exploration of potential economic and other determinants of these systematic differences in utilisation patterns.

The cross-sectional datasets used in the ECuity Project so far - though rich and useful in many respects - have serious limitations in two important respects: (*i*) in spite of our efforts at ensuring comparability of variables and procedures, the basic datasets used are all country-specific in design and collected for domestic purposes, and (*ii*) they are all cross-sectional surveys without a longitudinal dimension. For future work to have any serious chance of being successful with respect to the objective of uncovering causal factors in cross-country variation in inequity and inequality, international surveys with a common design and a longitudinal dimension seem indispensable.

ACKNOWLEDGEMENTS

This paper derives from the project "Equity in the finance and delivery of health care in Europe" (the ECuity project), which is funded by the European Union's Biomed Programme (contract BMH1-CT92-608). The paper is based on material presented at the inaugural conference of the International Health Economics Association, Vancouver, 20-23 May, 1996. The authors are grateful to conference participants for comments and to the ECuity Project participants for their concerted efforts and for many helpful discussions at the various project workshops.

REFERENCES

Aaronson, J.R., Johnson, P., and Lambert, P.J. (1994) Redistributive effect and inequal tax treatment. *Economic Journal* 104:262-270.

Burstall, M. and Wallerstein, K. (1994) The health care system in France. In: Hoffmeyer, U.K. and McCarthy, T.R., editors, *Financing Health Care*. Dordrecht: Kluwer Academic Publishers, p. 345-418.

Culyer, A.J., van Doorslaer, E., and Wagstaff, A (1992): Comment: Utilisation as a measure of equity, by Mooney, Hall, Donaldson, and Gerard. *Journal of Health Economics* 11(1): 93-98.

Culyer, A.J., van Doorslaer, E., and Wagstaff, A. (1992) Access, utilisation and equity: a further comment. *Journal of Health Economics* 11(2):207-210.

Culyer, A.J. and Wagstaff, A. (1993) Equity and inequality in health and health care. *Journal of Health Economics* 12:431-457.

Evans, R.G., Barer, M.L., and Marmor, T.R., editors (1994) *Why Are Some People Healthy and Others Not? The Determinants of Health of Populations*. New York: Aldine de Gruyter.

Hoffmeyer, U.K. (1994) The health care system in Germany. In: Hoffmeyer, U.K. and McCarthy, T.R., editors, *Financing Health Care*. Dordrecht: Kluwer Academic Publishers, pp. 419-512.

Hoffmeyer, U.K. and McCarthy, T.R., editors (1994) *Financing Health Care*, Volumes I and II, Dordrecht: Kluwer Academic Publishers.

Kakwani, N.C. (1977) Measurement of tax progressivity: an international comparison. *Economic Journal* 87:71-80.

Kakwani, N., Wagstaff, A., and van Doorslaer, E. (1997) Socioeconomic inequalities in health: measurement, computation, and statistical inference. *Journal of Econometrics* 77:87-103.

Lambert, P.J. and Aronson, J.R. (1993) Inequality decomposition analysis and the Gini coefficient revisited. *Economic Journal* 103:1221-1227.

LeGrand, J. (1987) Inequality in health: some international comparisons. *European Economic Review* 31:182-191.

Mooney, G., Hall, J., Donaldson, C., and Gerard, K. (1991) Utilisation as a measure of equity: weighing heat? *Journal of Health Economics* 10(4):475-480.

Mooney, G., Hall, J., Donaldson, C., and Gerard, K. (1992) Reweighing heat; response to Culyer, van Doorslaer and Wagstaff. *Journal of Health Economics* 111(2): 199.

Rasell, E. and Tang, K. (1994) *Paying for Health Care: Affordability and Equity In Proposals for Health Care Reform*, Working Paper No. 111, Washington, D.C.: Economic Policy Institute.

Van der Burg, H. and van Doorslaer, E. (1997) *Equity in the Distribution of Health Care Finance and Delivery in the Netherlands,* Department of Health Policy and Management, Rotterdam: Erasmus University.

van Doorslaer, E., Wagstaff, A., *et al.* (1992) Equity in the delivery of health care: some cross-country comparisons. *Journal of Health Economics* 11(4):389-411.

van Doorslaer, E., Wagstaff, A., and Rutten, F., editors (1993) *Equity in the Finance and Delivery of Health Care: An International Perspective.* Oxford: Oxford University Press.

van Doorslaer, E., Wagstaff, A., *et al.* (16 authors) (1997a) Income-related inequalities in health: some international comparisons. *Journal of Health Economics* (Forthcoming).

van Doorslaer, E., Wagstaff, A., *et al.* (1997b) *Equity in Health Care financing: Redistributive Effect and Horizontal Inequality.* ECuity Project Working Paper #8. Rotterdam: Erasmus University.

van Doorslaer, E., Wagstaff, A., *et al.* (1997c) *Equity in Health Care Delivery: Some Further International Comparisons,* ECuity Project Working Paper #10. Rotterdam: Erasmus University.

Wagstaff, A. and van Doorslaer, E. (1993) Equity in the finance and delivery of health care: concepts and definitions. In: van Doorslaer, E., Wagstaff, A., and Rutten, F., editors, *Equity in the Finance and Delivery of Health Care: An International Perspective.* Oxford: Oxford University Press, pp. 7-19.

Wagstaff, A. and van Doorslaer, E. (1993) Equity in the delivery of health care: methods and findings. In: van Doorslaer, E., Wagstaff, A., and Rutten, F., editors, *Equity in the Finance and Delivery of Health Care: An International Perspective.* Oxford: Oxford University Press, pp. 49-97.

Wagstaff, A. and van Doorslaer, E. (1994) Measuring inequalities in health in the presence of multiple-category morbidity indicators. *Health Economics* 3:281-291.

Wagstaff, A. and van Doorslaer, E. (1995) *Equity and Health Care Reform: Reforms to Date and Their Likely Consequences.* ECuity Project Working Paper #9. Rotterdam: Erasmus University.

Wagstaff, A. and van Doorslaer, E. (1996) *Measuring and Testing for Inequality in the Delivery of Health Care,* ECuity Project Working Paper #12. Rotterdam: Erasmus University.

Wagstaff A. and van Doorslaer, E. (1997) Progressivity, horizontal equity and reranking in health care finance: a decomposition analysis for the Netherlands. *Journal of Health Economics* (Forthcoming).

Wagstaff, A., van Doorslaer, E., and Paci, P. (1989) Equity in the finance and delivery of health care: some tentative cross-country comparisons. *Oxford Review of Economic Policy* 5:89-112.

Wagstaff, A., van Doorslaer, E., and Paci, P. (1991) On the measurement of horizontal inequity in the delivery of health care. *Journal of Health Economics* 10:169-205.

Wagstaff, A., Paci, P., and van Doorslaer, E. (1991) On the measurement of inequalities in health. *Social Science and Medicine* 33:545-557.

Wagstaff, A., van Doorslaer, E., *et al.* (1992) Equity in the finance of health care: some cross-country comparisons. *Journal of Health Economics* 11(4):361-387.

Wagstaff, A., van Doorslaer, E., *et al.* (1997) *Equity in Health Care Financing: an Update and Trends in Progressivity.* ECuity Project Working Paper #11. Rotterdam: Erasmus University.

8

Vouchers and Choice: the Impact of MSAs on Medicare Beneficiaries

JACK RODGERS and KAREN E. SMITH

Price Waterhouse LLP
Health Policy Economics Group
Washington, DC

ABSTRACT

This paper assesses the effect of expanding Medicare beneficiaries' health plan choices to include medical savings accounts (MSA). The analysis is based on a two-part econometric model using the 1992 Medicare Current Beneficiary Survey that predicts the characteristics of the Medicare beneficiaries who would choose to enroll in MSAs, and the cost of MSA enrollment to Medicare. Our model shows that MSA plans would experience favorable selection. Under the spending

---

Health, Health Care and Health Economics: Perspectives on Distribution
Edited by Morris L. Barer, Thomas E. Getzen, and Greg L. Stoddart
Copyright 1998 John Wiley & Sons, Ltd.

cap provisions of the Balanced Budget Act, healthy enrollees are likely to receive higher payments on their behalf, while less healthy ones are likely to receive lower payments, after accounting for the current AAPCC rates. For example, if 11% of Medicare beneficiaries enroll in MSAs, fee-for-service payments would need to be cut by 4%.

INTRODUCTION

The Medicare program currently offers its beneficiaries only a choice between the fee-for-service (FFS) health plan and a limited number of pre-paid health plans (typically HMO coverage). However, the Balanced Budget Act (BBA) of 1995 (which was passed by the Congress in November 1995 but vetoed by President Clinton) would have greatly expanded the plan choices for Medicare enrollees.

Looking at the effects of expanding Medicare health plan choice on Medicare beneficiaries is important because Medicare reform appears inevitable in the long run for a number of reasons. First, the rapid growth of Medicare spending has contributed significantly to the federal deficit, and it continues to "crowd out" spending on other domestic programs. Second, the Republicans are ideologically committed to the privatization of Medicare and it is believed by some that the private sector can run health plans more efficiently than the government. Finally, the private health care sector has changed substantially during the past decade. Advocates of change argue that Medicare must "catch up" with the private sector and incorporate some of the newest health delivery system changes that are beginning to occur.

The BBA would have transformed Medicare from an entitlement program that covers a defined set of benefits to an entitlement program with a defined contribution. Medicare beneficiaries who enroll in one of the expanded choice plans would have a set amount of their premiums paid by Medicare. For those people left in fee-for-service, there would be a pre-set, average *per capita* Medicare payment during the fiscal year for all covered services provided to beneficiaries.

The purpose of this paper is to assess the effect of expanding Medicare beneficiaries' health plan choices to include medical savings accounts (MSA). The paper describes the development of a model to predict Medicare enrollment in MSAs. We then use the model to evaluate the characteristics of the Medicare beneficiaries who would choose to enroll in MSAs and who would choose to remain in the FFS health plan. We estimate the cost of favorable selection on the level of Medicare outlays for both MSA enrollees and beneficiaries who would remain in the FFS health plan.

MODELING HEALTH PLAN CHOICE

People make choices about what type of health plan to enroll in based on many factors, including individual out-of-pocket health spending, the amount of financial risk associated with the health plan, preference for style of care, location and access to care, and preference for specific physicians. When modeling an individual's health plan choice, his or her current choice gives some indication of the individual's preference. Given a new list of health plan choices, individuals are faced with the task of evaluating whether any of the new plans would make him or her "better off," and thus willing to change to the new plan.

To evaluate whether an individual would be better off under a traditional fee-for-service plan (FFS) or a medical savings account (MSA), we compare their expected out-of-pocket health spending for each health plan type. Unfortunately, it is not sufficient to simply assign the individual to the health plan that would yield the lowest out-of-pocket spending, because the value of other individual preferences needs to be accounted for as well.

The general strategy we adopted to model individual health plan choice given an opportunity to enroll in a MSA, is to calculate the individual's expected out-of-pocket health spending under both a FFS and a MSA plan. We then apply a "risk aversion" factor, to capture the value of the other individual preferences. Unfortunately, we know very little about the precise value of these preferences. Rather than select a specific value, we apply several values designed to exemplify a plausible range. We assume that the true value is within the range. The range of values ranges from low risk aversion, to medium risk aversion, and finally to high risk aversion. Finally, individuals would choose the health plan that would give them the lowest out-of-pocket health spending adjusted for risk aversion.

Under the BBA, the cost to Medicare of offering MSAs to its beneficiaries depends on three factors: 1) the number of beneficiaries who choose to enroll in MSAs, 2) the amount Medicare pays for MSA enrollees, and 3) the average cost of the beneficiaries remaining in the FFS sector. The cost to Medicare for each MSA enrollee would be 95% of a pre-determined payment. This payment is based on the average *per capita* cost for FFS enrollees adjusted for the beneficiaries' age, gender, and risk group (institutionalized, non-institutionalized Medicaid, working aged, other). This payment is called the AAPCC. If the Medicare beneficiaries who choose to enroll in MSAs are systematically healthier than the beneficiaries who remain in the FFS sector, then we say MSAs experience favorable selection. If the Medicare beneficiaries who choose to enroll in MSAs are systematically less healthy than the beneficiaries who remain in the FFS sector, then we say MSAs experience adverse selection. If MSAs experience favorable selection, then the average *per capita* cost of the remaining FFS beneficiaries will systematically increase. The BBA, however, caps the *per capita* cost for these FFS beneficiaries. To the extent that favorable selection causes the FFS *per capita* cost to increase, the BBA would reduce the *per capita* cost by an equivalent amount. The cost to Medicare, after expanding health plan choices to include MSAs, will either remain constant in the case of favorable selection into MSAs, or will be lower by the amount the AAPCC payment for MSA enrollees saves Medicare costs in the case of adverse selection into MSAs.

DATA

We model health plan choice using data from the Medicare Current Beneficiary Survey (MCBS). The MCBS is a continuous, multi-purpose survey of a representative sample of the aged and disabled Medicare population. The purpose of the MCBS is to provide current and accurate information on health service use and sources of payments for Medicare beneficiaries. The survey links information from existing Medicare databases, such as Medicare claims files and other administrative data, to enhance the analytical power of the survey.

The MCBS collects information on the use of health care services, Medicare expenditures, and factors that affect health use and ability to pay. It also collects information on demographics, self-reported health status and functioning, access to care, insurance coverage, and financial resources. The longitudinal design of the MCBS allows researchers to monitor changes in the Medicare program and subsequent beneficiary utilization and expenditures.

The MCBS is a sample of selected Medicare enrollees from 107 geographical primary sampling units (or PSUs) in 46 states, the District of Columbia, and

Puerto Rico, consisting of counties chosen to represent the nation.[1] The sample beneficiaries were selected randomly by age groups (0-44, 45-64, 65-69, 70-74, 75-79, 80-84, and 85 and over). The survey is based on quarterly round respondent interviews.

Our analysis is based on Round 4, the latest available MCBS round. This round was conducted between September and December 1992. There were 11,924 respondents in Round 4 of the survey who were entitled to Medicare as of January 1992. We deleted the 70 end-stage-renal-disease (ESRD) respondents and 2 respondents missing the county identifier, leaving 11,852 respondents in the sample. Each record is weighted to reflect U.S. population totals.

METHODOLOGY

The MSA choice model is based on the concept that each Medicare beneficiary chooses whether or not to enroll in a MSA plan based on a comparison of out-of-pocket costs under the FFS plan and under a MSA plan. Our model is based on three related health cost measures: 1) Medicare reimbursement, 2) expected health expenditure, and 3) expected out-of-pocket health spending. These measures are described below.

Medicare Reimbursement. Medicare reimbursement is the amount Medicare pays for covered services. Medicare covered services include:

Part A
- in-patient hospital care, up to 90 days per benefit period plus 60 lifetime reserve days,
- skilled nursing facility care for 100 days,
- intermittent home-health care,
- hospice care;

---

[1] Alaska, Hawaii, Montana, and South Dakota are excluded from the MCBS. The MCBS has 564 counties.

Part B
- physician services (including visits, surgeries, consultations),
- lab and other diagnostic tests,
- out-patient services at hospitals, and
- mental health services.

Expected Health Expenditure. Expected health expenditure is the Medicare reimbursement amount each Medicare beneficiary expects to spend in the next year. To the extent that any specific health episode experienced in the current year may or may not repeat itself, or a chronic condition may become more costly with age, their expected health expenditure may be higher or lower than their current year's Medicare reimbursement.

Expected Out-of-Pocket Health Spending. Expected out-of-pocket health spending is the amount each Medicare beneficiary expects to spend on next year's Medicare charges.

Medicare reimbursement is available on the MCBS for all FFS beneficiaries and, except for inflation, does not need to be modeled. Expected health expenditure is not available from the data. This value is estimated as a function of Medicare reimbursement. We estimate it using a probability model described below. The expected out-of-pocket health spending depends on both the beneficiary's expected health expenditure and health plan type. Once we estimate the beneficiary's expected health expenditure, we then calculate the expected out-of-pocket health spending for both a FFS plan and a MSA plan.

MODEL OF EXPECTED HEALTH EXPENDITURE

We use a two-part regression model to calculate expected health expenditure for each individual Medicare beneficiary. This two-part model first estimates the probability of having spending. For those respondents with spending, it then estimates the amount of spending. The equations for the two-part model are as follows:

(1) $P(S>0)=L(B_1X_1)$
(2) $\log(S)=B_2X_2 + \epsilon$

where P is the probability of having positive spending estimated by the logit function L. S is Medicare spending, X_1 and X_2 are vectors of explanatory variables such as age, gender, health status, history of chronic health conditions, ability to perform activities of daily living, etc.. B_1 and B_2 are vectors of estimated parameters, and ϵ is a vector of error terms. Using the predicted values from the two-part model, expected health spending is the probability of having positive spending predicted by equation (1) multiplied by the spending predicted by equation (2). Since equation (2) is the logarithm of spending, the predicted spending must be retransformed using the inverse logarithm function to get nominal spending. The retransformed spending must be adjusted by a "smearing factor" to correct for the distribution of the retransformed error term.[2] The predicted spending is as follows:

(3) $E(S) = P * \exp(B_2X_2) * \phi$

where E(S) is expected health expenditure, exp is the inverse logarithm function, and ϕ is the smearing adjustment. Part A and Part B expected health expenditures are calculated separately and then added together to calculate total expected health expenditure.

More than four out of five Medicare beneficiaries (81.4%) have no Medicare Part A spending, which covers hospital, home health, hospice, and skilled nursing facility care. Eight percent of Medicare beneficiaries spend less than $5,000 per year. The remaining 11% spend over $5,000 per year, and that spending can be very large (see Table 1). Slightly less than one out of five Medicare beneficiaries (19.6%) have no Medicare Part B spending, which covers physician services. About two out of three Medicare beneficiaries (66.7%) spend less than $2,500 per year. The remaining 14% spend over $2,500 per year, and that spending, while not as large as Part A spending, can still be very large. Both distributions are skewed to the right.

---

[2] The smearing estimate for a logarithmic transformation is

$$\phi = \frac{1}{n} \sum_{i=1}^{n} (\epsilon_i)$$

For more information on the smearing estimate see "*A comparison of Alternative Models for the Demand for Medical Care.*" RAND R-2754-HHS. Duan, Naihua, Willard G. Manning, Jr., Carl N. Morris, Joseph P. Newhouse. January 1982.

A two-part regression model predicts actual spending better than a single linear ordinary least squares regression model when spending is highly skewed to the right (i.e., its right tail is elongated). In other words, a large proportion of the population has no spending and a small proportion has a fairly long distribution of positive spending. The logarithmic transformation of spending as the dependent variable in the second equation corrects for heteroskedasticity associated with skewed data.[3] Both of these properties are characteristic of Medicare spending.

TABLE 1 Distribution of Average Annual Medicare Spending, 1992

Average Annual Medicare Spending (1992 Dollars)	Part A Enrollees (Percent)	Part B Enrollees (Percent)
$0	81.4	19.6
$1 - $2,500	3.2	66.7
$2,501 - $5,000	4.8	9.0
$5,001 - $7,500	2.5	2.6
$7,501 - $10,000	2.0	1.1
$10,000 - $15,000	2.5	0.6
More than $15,000	3.6	0.4

Source: Price Waterhouse L.L.P. tabulations of the 1992 Medicare Current Beneficiary Survey

Notes: The universe is all FFS enrollees.

MODEL OF OUT-OF-POCKET HEALTH SPENDING

What matters to individuals in determining which health plan makes them better off is expected out-of-pocket health spending, and this varies depending on the type of health plan.

Fee-For-Service. In 1996, Medicare beneficiaries enrolled in the fee-for-service sector must pay:

---

[3] An assumption of the classic linear regression model is that variance of the error term is constant for the range of the dependent variable. Heteroskedasticity is when the variance of the error term is dependent on the dependent variable. The least squares estimate of a regression that is heteroskedastic is unbiased but is not efficient.

Part A
- $736 deductible per hospital episode,
- $184 per hospital inpatient day between 61 to 90 days,
- $368 per hospital inpatient day in excess of 90 days, up to a limit of 60 lifetime reserve days,
- $92 per day for skilled nursing facility days between 21 and 100 days;

Part B
- $100 deductible for Part B,
- 20% of all covered charges in excess of the Part B deductible,
- 50% of approved outpatient mental health therapy amount.

Medical Savings Account. The specific parameters for MSAs are not detailed in the BBA. We have had to make assumptions about the limits on out-of-pocket health spending. We modeled MSAs such that Medicare beneficiaries enrolled in MSAs would pay up to $5,000 deductible on all health costs.

Expected out-of-pocket health spending is dependent on expected health expenditure. Individuals have some uncertainty about their own expected out-of-pocket health spending given their expected health expenditure. For individuals with low expected health expenditure, a higher proportion of their out-of-pocket spending would be below the deductible. Conversely, for beneficiaries with high expected health expenditure, a higher proportion of their out-of-pocket spending would be above the deductible.

We constructed a distribution of expected out-of-pocket health spending for both MSA and FFS plans based on a scaled distribution of Medicare reimbursement and applying the appropriate out-of-pocket spending formula to the scaled reimbursement (see Table 2). For given ranges of expected health expenditure, we calculate the average out-of-pocket spending. We then apply the ratio of average out-of-pocket spending to average expected health expenditure to calculate the individual's estimated out-of-pocket spending. For example, the average out-of-pocket spending for a FFS beneficiary with expected health expenditure of $250 is $62, or 25% of their expected expenditure. The average out-of-pocket for the same beneficiary enrolled in a MSA is $245, or 98% of their expected expenditure. As expected health expenditure increases, average out-of-pocket spending increases, but the ratio of out-of-pocket spending to expected health expenditure decreases. The average out-of-pocket spending for a FFS beneficiary with expected health expenditure of $10,000 is $1,150, or 12% of their expected expenditure. The average out-of-pocket for the same beneficiary enrolled in a MSA is $2,124, or 21% of their expected expenditure.

TABLE 2   Average Out-of-Pocket Spending and Out-of-Pocket Rate
by Expected Health Expenditure and Insurance Type (1996 Dollars)

Expected Health Expenditure (Dollars)	MSA Plan		FFS Plan	
	Average Out-of-Pocket Spending (Dollars)	Out-of-Pocket Rate	Average Out-of-Pocket Spending (Dollars)	Out-of-Pocket Rate
$0 - $375	245	0.979	62	0.249
$375 - $750	450	0.899	99	0.198
$750 - $1,250	744	0.844	161	0.161
$1,250 - $1,750	945	0.630	219	0.146
$1,750 - $2,250	1,099	0.550	275	0.138
$2,250 - $2.750	1,225	0.490	331	0.132
$2.750 - $3,250	1,333	0.444	386	0.129
$3,250 - $3,750	1,425	0.407	441	0.126
$3,750 - $4,500	1,507	0.377	496	0.124
$4,500 - $5,500	1,648	0.330	605	0.121
$5,500 - $6,500	1,767	0.294	715	0.119
$6,500 - $7,500	1,871	0.267	824	0.118
$7,500 - $8,500	1,964	0.245	933	0.117
$8,500 - $9,500	2,048	0.228	1,042	0.116
More than $9,500	2,124	0.212	1,150	0.115

Source: Price Waterhouse LLP tabulations of the 1992 Medicare Current Beneficiary Survey

MSA DECISION MODEL

We estimate MSA enrollment by comparing each individual's out-of-pocket health spending in the FFS sector with a risk adjusted out-of-pocket health spending in a MSA. Each beneficiary would choose the plan that gives him or her the lowest out-of-pocket health spending. Since we do not know the true value of the risk adjustment factor, we model out-of-pocket spending with four risk aversion factors: no risk aversion, low risk aversion, medium risk aversion, and high risk aversion. These factors are designed to represent a plausible range of MSA participation. The model is specified as follows:

(4) $O_f = s * E(S)$
(5) $O_m = (\alpha * r * E(S)) - M$
where

O_f is out-of-pocket under fee-for-service (FFS),

s   is the out-of-pocket rate under a FFS plan (this is a function of $E(S)$ from Table 2),

$E(S)$ is expected health expenditures from equation (3),

O_m is the adjusted out-of-pocket under a MSA,

α is a vector of risk aversion factors,

r   is the out-of-pocket rate under a MSA (this is a function of $E(S)$ from Table 2),

M   is the cash payment for the beneficiary to enroll in a MSA.

Each Medicare beneficiary would choose to enroll in a MSA if their adjusted out-of-pocket spending under a MSA plan would be less than their out-of-pocket spending under a FFS plan, or $O_m < O_f$. Otherwise the beneficiary would choose to remain in the FFS plan.

For this simulation, M is assumed to be $1,000 and α is 1.0 for no risk aversion, 1.2 for low risk aversion, 1.3 for medium risk aversion, and 1.4 for high risk aversion.

COST TO MEDICARE

The total cost to Medicare before MSA enrollment is the total expected health expenditure. The total cost to Medicare after MSA enrollment is the total expected health expenditure for the beneficiaries remaining in the FFS health plan plus the sum of the AAPCC amount for the beneficiaries who choose MSAs. Under the BBA, the average *per capita* cost for FFS beneficiaries would be held constant. If, after MSA enrollment, the average *per capita* cost for FFS beneficiaries increases, we reduce the *per capita* payment by a factor that holds the average *per capita* cost constant. The cost model is as follows:

(6) $C_0 = \sum_{i=1}^{n} E(S)$

(7) $C_1 = (1 - h) * C_f + C_m$

$$(8) \quad C_f = \sum_{i=1}^{ffs} E(S)$$

$$(9) \quad C_m = \sum_{i=1}^{msa} A$$

$$(10) \quad h = \frac{(C_f + C_m - C_0)}{C_f}$$

where

C_0	is the cost to Medicare before MSA enrollment,
$E(S)$	is the expected health expenditure from equation (3),
n	is the number of Medicare beneficiaries,
C_1	is the cost to Medicare after MSA enrollment,
h	is the FFS average *per capita* cost adjustment factor,
C_f	is the cost to Medicare for FFS beneficiaries before applying the average cost cap,
C_m	is the cost to Medicare for MSA beneficiaries,
ffs	is the number of beneficiaries who remain in the FFS plan,
msa	is the number of beneficiaries who enroll in MSA plans,
A	is the AAPCC payment (this payment is 95% of the risk adjusted average *per capita* cost for FFS beneficiaries in the beneficiary's county).

RESULTS

EXPECTED HEALTH EXPENDITURE

The purpose of the two-part regression model is to calculate expected health expenditure controlling for factors expected to affect spending. We include dummy variables for mortality, age group, institutional status, Medicaid status, gender, self-reported health status, presence of chronic conditions, health insurance from a current employer, and income. The regression equations also include the number of limitations in activities of daily living (ADLs), and the number of instrumental activities of daily living (IADLs). The ADLs include difficulty bathing, difficulty dressing, difficulty using the toilet, difficulty eating, and difficulty getting out of chairs. The IADLs include difficulty using the telephone, difficulty making meals, difficulty managing money, difficulty shopping, and difficulty doing light housework. The cost regression also includes the unadjusted county AAPCC payment to control for county-specific cost variation.

Table 3 lists the parameter estimates for the probability of having positive spending from equation (1). We estimated a separate equation for Medicare Part A and Medicare Part B spending. The dependent variable is a dummy variable for whether the FFS beneficiary has positive Medicare spending. The dummy variable equals one if spending is positive and zero if spending is zero. We use all FFS beneficiaries in the logistic regressions. The omitted group is 65- to 69-year-old, non-institutionalized, non-Medicaid, non-white women in good health with annual family income below $25,000.

All of the independent variables in Table 3 are statistically significant based on a chi-square test, and the regression predicts whether the FFS beneficiary had Medicare spending correctly (true for positive spending and false for no spending) 82% of the time for Part A spending, and 81% of the time for Part B spending.

Table 4 lists the parameter estimates for the logarithm of spending from equation (3). We estimated a separate equation for Medicare Part A and Medicare Part B spending. The dependent variables are the logarithm of Medicare Part A costs and the logarithm of Medicare Part B costs. We use only FFS beneficiaries with positive costs in the cost regressions. The omitted group is 65- to 69-year-old, non-institutionalized, non-Medicaid, non-white women in good health with annual family income below $25,000.

Many of the explanatory variables are highly multi collinear. For example, institutionalized Medicare enrollees are likely to have a large number of ADLs. Medicare enrollees in advanced age are likely to have more chronic health conditions. Medicare enrollees with chronic conditions are likely to report being in poor health. Some of the signs of the parameter estimates are counterintuitive. Given the multicollinearity, a parameter estimate for each independent variable cannot be evaluated alone.

Even with the multicollinearity, many of the parameter estimates are consistent with prior expectations. For example, the probability of having positive Medicare spending increases monotonically with age (see Table 3). The probability of

**TABLE 3 Logistic Regression Results for Predicting the Probability
of Having Positive Medicare Spending**

	Parameter Estimates	
Independent Variable	**Part A**	**Part B**
Intercept [a]	-2.40	0.71
Dead as of December 31, 1992	2.13	0.57
Disabled (Age Under 65)	-0.23	-0.46
Age 70 - 74	0.16	0.15
Age 75 - 79	0.25	0.33
Age 80 - 84	0.42	0.36
Age 85 and Over	0.46	0.35
Institutionalized	-0.34	1.36
Medicaid	0.22	0.55
Male	-0.03	-0.61
Health Insurance from Current Employer	-0.59	-1.10
Excellent Health	-0.59	-0.52
Very Good Health	-0.36	-0.26
Fair Health	0.16	0.09
Poor Health	0.34	0.16
Number of IADLs	0.26	0.06
Cancer	0.52	0.67
Diabetes	0.34	0.63
Stroke	0.47	0.30
Asthma or Emphysema	0.31	0.39
Hypertension	0.13	0.43
Hardening of the Arteries	0.11	0.26
Myocardial Infarction	0.57	-0.05
Angina Pectoris	0.15	0.21
Other Heart Condition	0.72	0.58
Annual Income More than $25,000	-0.12	0.36
White	0.18	0.51
Probability of Having Positive Spending	0.19	0.80
Regression Predicts Actual Spending (Percent)	82	81
Observations	11,293	11,293

Source: Price Waterhouse LLP tabulations of the 1992 Medicare Current Beneficiary Survey.

Notes: The regression includes Medicare costs for all FFS enrollees.

a.   The omitted group is 65- to 69-year-old, non-Medicaid, non-institutionalized, low-income, non-white women in good health with annual income below $25,000.

TABLE 4 Regression Results for Predicting the Logarithm of Medicare Spending

Independent Variable	Parameter Estimates	
	Part A	Part B
Intercept[a]	5.327	2.361
	(0.000)	(0.000)
Dead as of December 31, 1992	0.787	0.964
	(0.000)	(0.000)
Disabled (Age Under 65)	-0.051	0.016
	(0.576)	(0.791)
Age 70 - 74	-0.047	0.139
	(0.506)	(0.001)
Age 75 - 79	-0.063	0.123
	(0.389)	(0.008)
Age 80 - 84	-0.150	0.205
	(0.054)	(0.000)
Age 85 and Over	-0.122	0.106
	(0.148)	(0.087)
Institutionalized	0.104	0.058
	(0.249)	(0.438)
Medicaid	-0.081	0.078
	(0.217)	(0.122)
Male	0.118	0.017
	(0.016)	(0.604)
Health Insurance from Current Employer	-0.280	-0.700
	(0.057)	(0.000)
Excellent Health	0.013	-0.351
	(0.893)	(0.000)
Very Good Health	-0.207	-0.208
	(0.004)	(0.000)
Fair Health	0.014	0.165
	(0.816)	(0.000)
Poor Health	0.250	0.314
	(0.001)	(0.000)
Number of ADLs	0.026	0.034
	(0.258)	(0.071)
Number of IADLs	0.041	0.025
	(0.046)	(0.142)
Difficulty Walking	-0.067	0.119
	(0.253)	(0.005)
Cancer	0.074	0.523
	(0.240)	(0.000)

(Continued)

Table 4 (Continued)

Independent Variable	Parameter Estimates	
	Part A	Part B
Diabetes	-0.024	0.150
	(0.639)	(0.000)
Stroke	-0.040	0.198
	(0.627)	(0.008)
Asthma or Emphysema	0.047	0.215
	(0.422)	(0.000)
Hypertension	-0.052	0.007
	(0.268)	(0.830)
Hardening of the Arteries	-0.083	0.151
	(0.142)	(0.000)
Myocardial Infarction	0.356	0.202
	(0.000)	(0.004)
Angina Pectoris	-0.044	0.067
	(0.545)	(0.282)
Other Heart Condition	0.135	0.431
	(0.013)	(0.000)
Broken Hip	0.602	0.240
	(0.000)	(0.022)
Paralysis	0.258	0.221
	(0.024)	(0.027)
Amputation	0.445	0.324
	(0.004)	(0.019)
AAPCC[b]	0.004	0.008
	(0.000)	(0.000)
Annual Income More than $25,000	-0.003	0.031
	(0.968)	(0.464)
White	-0.055	0.121
	(0.445)	(0.016)
Dependent Variable Mean[c]	6.21	3.82
R-Square	0.12	0.15
Observations	2,234	9,097

Source: Price Waterhouse LLP tabulations of the 1992 Medicare Current Beneficiary Survey.

Notes: The regression includes only FFS enrollees with positive Medicare Spending. The numbers in parentheses are p-values for 2-tailed tests of the hypothesis that the coefficient is zero for the population. Thus, values below 0.05 indicate that the effect of the variable on the logarithm of cost is significantly different from zero at the 0.05 level.

a.   The omitted group is 65- to 69-year-old, non-Medicaid, non-institutionalized, non-white women in good health with annual income below $25,000.

b.   AAPCC is the unadjusted county AAPCC (Part A for column 1 and Part B for column 2).

c.   Logarithm of monthly of Medicare FFS cost (Part A for column 1 and Part B for column 2).

having positive Medicare spending increases monotonically as health status decreases. The parameter estimates are positive for mortality and presence of chronic conditions. The logarithm of Medicare spending increases as health status decreases (see Table 4). The parameter estimate for current employer health insurance is negative. This measures the better health status of Medicare enrollees who continue to work. The parameter estimates for the age dummy variables in the Part A regression decrease as age increases, which implies that Part A spending goes down for advanced age. This finding is consistent with recent research on life-time Medicare spending, which found that doctors tend not to perform very costly procedures on the elderly in poor health.

MSA DECISION MODEL RESULTS

Our model shows that expected health expenditure is highly correlated with age, health status, risk status (institutionalized, non-institutionalized Medicaid, non-institutionalized non-Medicaid, working aged), and income. Younger, healthier, and wealthier Medicare beneficiaries tend to have lower expected health expenditures. The average expected health expenditure for 65- to 69-year-old Medicare beneficiaries is $4,494 per year compared to $9,939 per year for beneficiaries age 85 and older (see Table 5). The average expected health expenditure for the healthiest Medicare beneficiaries is $2,721 per year compared to $14,984 per year for the sickest beneficiaries. The average expected health expenditure for the working aged is $2,108 per year compared to $13,308 per year for institutionalized beneficiaries. The average expected health expenditure for beneficiaries with family income above $50,000 per year (1996 dollars) is $4,497 compared to $6,322 per year for beneficiaries with family income below $10,000 per year.

Characteristics of MSA Enrollees. In the simplest model, we assume no risk aversion. In this model, individuals would choose to enroll in a MSA if their expected out-of-pocket spending under a MSA is lower than their expected out-of-pocket spending under a FFS plan. Assuming no risk aversion ($\alpha=1$), sixty-eight percent of all beneficiaries would be better off under a MSA plan (see Table 5). In other words, their expected out-of-pocket spending under a MSA plan after $1,000 annual cash contribution to join the MSA plan would be lower than their out-of-pocket spending under the traditional FFS Medicare plan. Beneficiaries with lower expected out-of-pocket spending are better off than beneficiaries with

TABLE 5 **Percent of Medicare Beneficiaries Who Enroll in Medical Savings Accounts by Demographic Characteristics and Risk Aversion Level**

	Average Expected Health Expenditure (1996 Dollars)	Medicare Beneficiaries Who Enroll in Medicare Savings Accounts (Percent)			
		No Risk Aversion	Low Risk Aversion	Medium Risk Aversion	High Risk Aversion
All	6,000	67.5	11.4	5.1	3.2
Age					
64 and under	5,243	70.5	16.5	10.3	7.1
65-69	4,494	77.4	20.8	10.3	5.9
70-74	5,471	69.4	10.0	3.4	2.4
75-79	6,389	64.3	5.8	1.4	1.0
80-84	7,939	55.4	2.2	0.4	0.2
85 and over	9,939	48.8	1.8	0.3	0.3
Gender					
Male	5,860	69.3	14.0	5.9	4.4
Female	6,103	66.2	9.6	3.8	2.4
AAPCC Risk Category					
Institutionalized	13,308	34.7	0.5	0	0
Medicaid	7,660	56.5	3.5	1.2	0.6
No Risk	5,508	69.7	10.2	3.3	1.4
Working Aged	2,108	92.8	71.6	62.1	53.1
Self-Reported Health Status					
Excellent Health	2,721	91.1	33.9	15.5	9.2
Very Good Health	3,141	85.5	17.4	6.4	4.2
Good Health	5,738	63.5	3.2	2.0	1.4
Fair Health	8,513	48.3	2.6	1.7	1.2
Poor Health	14,984	29.6	0.7	0.4	0.3
Family Income					
Less than $10,000	6,322	64.7	8.8	3.7	2.2
$10,000-$20,000	5,899	67.4	11.8	5.2	3.2
$20,000-$30,000	5,781	69.9	12.7	5.1	2.9
$30,000-$40,000	4,883	74.3	14.2	7.0	4.6
$40,000-$50,000	4,497	76.5	21.6	11.4	8.6
More than $50,000	4,497	76.5	21.6	11.4	8.6

Source: Price Waterhouse LLP tabulations of the MSA Selection Model

higher expected out-of-pocket spending. On average, these beneficiaries tend to be younger, healthier, and wealthier Medicare beneficiaries. Seventy-seven percent of 65- to 69-year-old Medicare beneficiaries are better off under a MSA plan compared to only 49% of beneficiaries age 85 and older. Ninety-one percent of the healthiest Medicare beneficiaries are better off under a MSA plan compared to only 30% of the sickest beneficiaries. Ninety-three percent of the working aged are better off under a MSA plan compared to only 35% of the institutionalized beneficiaries. Seventy-seven percent of Medicare beneficiaries with family income above $50,000 per year (1996 dollars) are better off under a MSA plan compared to only 65% of beneficiaries with family income below $10,000 per year.

Risk aversion substantially reduces the number of Medicare beneficiaries who would choose to enroll in a MSA. The risk aversion assumption corrects for the fact that the individual must be compensated for bearing a higher potential out-of-pocket spending. Even though their expected out-of-pocket spending under a MSA may be lower than their expected out-of-pocket spending in the FFS plan, there is some chance that their actual spending will be higher. Assuming low risk aversion (α=1.2), 11% of all Medicare beneficiaries would be better off under a MSA plan (see Table 5). Twenty-one percent of 65- to 69-year-old Medicare beneficiaries are better off under a MSA plan compared to only 2% of the beneficiaries age 85 and older. Thirty-four percent of the healthiest Medicare beneficiaries are better off under a MSA plan compared to only 1% of the sickest beneficiaries. Seventy-two percent of the working aged are better off under a MSA plan compared to only 1% of the institutionalized beneficiaries. Twenty-two percent of Medicare beneficiaries with family income above $50,000 per year (1996 dollars) are better off under a MSA plan compared to only 9% of beneficiaries with family income below $10,000 per year.

Increasing the risk aversion level, or the cost of bearing the risk, substantially reduces the number of Medicare beneficiaries willing to join a MSA plan. Assuming high risk aversion (α=1.4), only 3% of all Medicare beneficiaries would be better off under a MSA plan (see Table 5). Six percent of 65- to 69-year-old Medicare beneficiaries are better off under a MSA plan compared to less than 1% of beneficiaries aged 85 and older. Nine percent of the healthiest Medicare beneficiaries are better off under a MSA plan compared to less than 1% of the sickest beneficiaries. Fifty-three percent of the working aged are better off under a MSA plan, while no institutionalized beneficiaries are. Nine percent of Medicare beneficiaries with family income above $50,000 per year (1996 dollars) are better off under a MSA plan compared to only 2% of beneficiaries with family income below $10,000 per year.

The difference in the FFS and MSA out-of-pocket spending formulas causes a dramatic difference in the characteristics of the Medicare beneficiaries choosing each plan type, regardless of the assumed level of risk aversion. In all cases, only the least costly Medicare beneficiaries would choose MSAs and these beneficiaries are systematically younger and healthier than those remaining in the FFS sector.

ESTIMATED COST TO MEDICARE

Our model shows that MSA plans would experience favorable selection. In other words, the cost to Medicare for the beneficiaries who would enroll in MSAs is systematically lower than the amount Medicare would spend for the enrollee had the enrollee remained in the FFS sector. Because MSA enrollees are systematically less costly than the FFS counterparts, the average *per capita* cost for the FFS beneficiaries would increase. Under the spending cap provision of the BBA, the average *per capita* cost for FFS beneficiaries would get reduced by the proportion the average *per capita* cost would increase.

If MSAs were not offered to Medicare beneficiaries in 1996, total Medicare reimbursement would be $199 billion (see Table 6). Once Medicare beneficiaries enroll in MSAs, Medicare would then pay out both payments for MSA enrollees and FFS beneficiaries. The cost to Medicare after MSA enrollment would depend on both the number of beneficiaries who enroll in MSAs and their relative cost. Our risk aversion assumption affects both factors.

Assuming no risk aversion, the cost to Medicare for FFS beneficiaries would be $117 billion, and the cost for MSA enrollees would be $116 billion. Before applying the BBA cap, total cost to Medicare with MSAs would be $233 billion. Sixty-eight percent of Medicare beneficiaries would enroll in MSAs, but unadjusted FFS cost would decline by 41%. In order to keep total Medicare costs constant, as required in the BBA, Medicare would have to reduce FFS costs by 28.5%. After applying the BBA cap, total Medicare cost would once again be $199 billion.

Assuming low risk aversion, the cost to Medicare for FFS beneficiaries would be $194 billion, and the cost for MSA enrollees would be $13 billion. Before applying the BBA cap, total cost to Medicare with MSAs would be $207 billion. Eleven percent of Medicare beneficiaries would enroll in MSAs, but unadjusted FFS cost would decline by only 3%. To keep total Medicare costs constant, as required in the BBA, Medicare would have to reduce FFS costs by 4.2%. After applying the BBA cap, total Medicare cost would once again be $199 billion.

**TABLE 6 Cost to Medicare of Expanding Choice to MSAs
by Risk Aversion Level (1996 Dollars)**

	No Risk	Low Risk	Medium Risk	High Risk
	Billions of Dollars			
Cost to Medicare				
Before MSA Enrollment (C_0)	199	199	199	199
For FFS Beneficiaries after MSA Enrollment (C_f)	117	194	197	198
For MSA Enrollees after MSA Enrollment (C_m)	116	13	5	3
With MSA Enrollment Before BBA ($C_f + C_m$)	233	207	202	201
With MSA Enrollment After BBA (C_1)	199	199	199	199
	Percent			
MSA Enrollment	67.5	11.4	5.1	3.2
Reduction in FFS *Per Capita* Cost (h)	28.5	4.2	1.6	1.0

Source: Price Waterhouse LLP tabulations of the MSA Selection Model.

Assuming high risk aversion, the cost to Medicare for FFS beneficiaries would be $198 billion and the cost for MSA enrollees would be $3 billion. Before applying the BBA cap, total cost to Medicare with MSA would be $201 billion. Three percent of Medicare beneficiaries would enroll in MSAs, but unadjusted FFS cost would decline by only 0.1%. In order to keep total Medicare costs constant, as required in the BBA, Medicare would have to reduce FFS costs by 1.0%. After applying the BBA cap, total Medicare cost would once again be $199 billion.

The higher the rate of risk aversion, the lower the number of Medicare beneficiaries would be who would choose to enroll in a MSA. As risk aversion increases, only the healthiest beneficiaries would choose MSAs. While the rate of favorable selection increases, the proportion of the population that would choose MSAs decreases. As MSA enrollment decreases, a smaller BBA reduction would be required to keep Medicare costs constant.

CONCLUSIONS

The major downside of expanding Medicare choice to include MSAs is that healthy enrollees are likely to receive higher payments on their behalf, while less healthy ones are likely to receive lower payments. The magnitude of the problem with respect to less healthy enrollees depends on how many additional enrollees leave the traditional program and join a MSA plan. If substantial numbers of beneficiaries enrolled in MSAs, there would be large costs to the elderly in terms of reduced Medicare payments for FFS care. The reduced FFS payments will result in either higher copayments and deductibles for the FFS beneficiaries, or lower reimbursements to health care providers. Both outcomes have their opponents.

Is there some way to design an expansion of choice that is low-risk? The easiest way to protect Medicare enrollees who remain in the traditional program is to limit the types of choices that are available. MSAs could be introduced in selected areas on a demonstration basis. The overall impact of favorable selection in a limited geographic area would be small when compared to the entire Medicare program. If evaluations showed that favorable selection would be minimal, or if the demonstration found a method of adjusting for health status that was powerful enough to offset selection, then MSAs could be implemented for the entire Medicare population.

Finally, the expansion of choice could be phased-in and monitored to make sure that selection was under control or at least not significant enough to cause major problems. The phase-in could be accomplished easily in a number of ways, such as the following:

- **Limiting disenrollment from MSA plans.** For example, once a Medicare beneficiary enrolles in a MSA, they could become ineligible to return to the FFS plan. This would prevent a beneficiary from enrolling in a MSA while they are healthy and less costly, only to switch to the FFS plan when their health fails.
- **Limiting the types of enrollees who are allowed to join new plans.** For example, MSAs could be open only to enrollees who enter the program after a certain date.
- **Reducing the reimbursement rate.** For example, reimbursement for MSAs could be set at 80% of the AAPCC in the short-run when younger, healthier people are expected to enroll, then gradually increase to 95% as the population in the capitated plans matures and becomes less healthy.

9

Is Community Financing Necessary and Feasible for Rural China?

YUANLI LIU,[1] SHANLIAN HU,[2] WEI FU,[3]
and WILLIAM C. HSIAO[1]
[1] Department of Health Policy and Management
Harvard University School of Public Health
Cambridge, Massachusetts
[2]Training Center For Health Administrators
Shanghai Medical University
Shanghai, P.R. China
[3]National Health Economics Institute
Ministry of Health
Beijing, P.R. China

ABSTRACT

The collapse of Cooperative Medical System (CMS) in China after the agricultural reforms of the early 1980s caused serious concerns and doubts about the viability of community financing of basic health care for the low-income population. This

---

Health, Health Care and Health Economics: Perspectives on Distribution
Edited by Morris L. Barer, Thomas E. Getzen, and Greg L. Stoddart
Copyright 1998 John Wiley & Sons, Ltd.

paper examines the rise and fall of China's community financing schemes and ascertains the need for and feasibility of community financing. Ninety-percent of the Chinese rural population now pays out-of-pocket for their health services. Both the problems with the fee-for-service system and the observed advantages of the existing community financing schemes indicate the necessity for revitalizing community financing as a major rural health care reform strategy. The feasibility of the community financing approach depends on adequate financial and social resources. Our study found that there are multiple potential funding sources for health care in rural areas, including households, village welfare funds, local enterprises, and the government. We designed several illustrative benefit packages and estimated their costs. It seems a basic benefit package with high co-insurance would be affordable if funds can be mobilized from multiple sources. More importantly, community financing would require governmental promotion and support.

INTRODUCTION

China was the first large nation in the world to develop a nationwide community financing scheme, called the "Rural Cooperative Medical System" (CMS), to fund and organize prevention, primary care, and secondary health services for its rural population. China's relatively successful experience in extending health care coverage to most of its rural population at a fairly low cost through mobilizing local resources had once stimulated interest throughout the developing world in the potential role of community financing of health care (Abel-Smith and Dua, 1987). After the agricultural reform in the early 1980s, however, this community financing of rural health care has given way to predominantly private payment schemes. Nearly 90% of the rural households now pay out-of-pocket for health services. Many village doctors have either left for full time farming or become private practitioners. Township health centers and county hospitals are also largely financed by fee-for-service.

China faces several major problems in providing basic health care for its rural population: reduced access, the financial burden of high medical costs for the low income population, and inefficiency. Therefore, questions and doubts arise: Doesn't the Chinese experience show that community financing is not a viable approach? Is there a better way to finance basic health care for the rural population, especially for the rural poor? Addressing these questions, this paper first provides a description of the rise and fall of CMS and discusses the problems associated with the collapse of CMS. Then major issues on the financial, social and political feasibility of community financing in rural China are discussed. Finally, we summarize the major lessons that can be learned from the Chinese experience.

THE RISE AND FALL OF CHINA'S COMMUNITY FINANCING SCHEMES

HEALTH CARE DELIVERY IN RURAL CHINA

As many as 800 million Chinese live in rural areas, and most of the households engage in farming. The average disposable income per person was 922 yuan[1] in 1993, ranging from under 200 yuan per capita for the poorest households to 1390 yuan for those in the highest income quartile (Statistical Yearbook of China, 1994).

Health care **delivery** in rural China is through village health stations (each serving on average 500-1000 villagers), township health centers (serving about 15,000 to 20,000 people), and county hospitals (serving a catchment area of 200,000 to 300,000 people). Village stations are staffed by part-time village doctors whose training consists of three to six months basic medical education after junior middle school; they provide basic preventive care (*e.g.*, immunization and prenatal consultation) and curative services (treating common illnesses and injuries). Most township health centers are owned and operated by the local government. An average facility has 7-10 beds and 10 staff members, led by a physician with a three-year medical school education after senior middle school. County hospitals, serving as rural medical referral centers, are owned and operated by the county government and staffed by physicians with 4 to 5 years of medical school training. The average county hospital has 135 beds and 186 staff members, of whom 8% have Bachelor of Medicine degrees.

---

[1] US$1 was equivalent to 7 yuan in 1993.

DEVELOPMENT OF CMS, 1960-1983

Before the 1980's agricultural reform, health services for China's rural population were organized and financed through the Cooperative Medical System (CMS), which was an integrated part of the overall system of collective agriculture production and social services.

CMS organized rural health care into a three-tier structure. The first tier was comprised of "barefoot doctors" who provided both preventive and primary-care services, including prescription drugs. The barefoot doctors, like the peasants who worked on farming, received a certain number of work points for each working day in a health post. For more serious illnesses, barefoot doctors referred patients to the second tier: township health centers. The medical workers at the health centers received a modest salary funded by subsidies from the government and revenues generated by the services they provided. Finally, the most seriously ill patients were referred to the third tier: county hospitals. In rare cases, the patient may be referred to an urban tertiary hospital. Village health stations, township health centers and county hospitals were integrated by a vertical administrative system supervised by the county bureau of health. County hospitals and township health centers provided regular technical assistance and supervision to the lower-level organizations. Under CMS, the financing of health care relied on a pre-payment plan. Most of the villages funded CMS from three sources: (1) Premium assessments. Depending on the benefit structure of the plan and the local community's economic status, 0.5% to 2% of a peasant family's annual income (4-8 yuan) were to be paid as premiums to the Fund; (2) Collective Welfare Fund. According to the State's guidelines, each village contributed a certain portion of its income from collective agricultural production or rural enterprises to a welfare fund; (3) Subsidies from higher level governments. In most cases, this subsidy was used to compensate health workers and to purchase medical equipment.

Gradually developed in the 1950s as a mutual assistance mechanism to establish access to basic drugs and primary health care (Zhang, 1992), the Cooperative Medical System was given political priority and developed rapidly during the "Cultural Revolution" (1960's-1970's). At the peak, 90% of the rural population was covered by CMS schemes (Zhu, 1988).

This model of community financing and organization of health care was believed by many to have contributed in a significant way to China's success in accomplishing its "first health care revolution" by providing preventive and primary care services to the majority of the Chinese population, reducing the infant mortality rate from about 200/1000 life births (1949) to 47/1000 life births (1973-1975), and increasing life expectancy from 35 to about 65 years (Hsiao, 1984; Gu, 1993; Sidel and Sidel, 1984; and Halstead, 1985).

THE COLLAPSE OF CMS IN THE EARLY 1980s

Following the implementation of the agricultural reforms[2] in the early 1980s, the Cooperative Medical System (CMS) collapsed. Figure 1 shows the significant decrease of the number of villages covered by CMS after reform. The demise of China's CMS system can be explained by several factors.

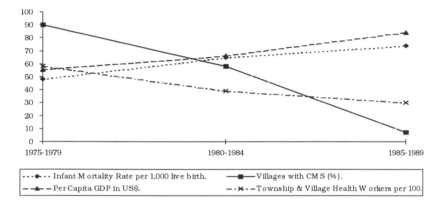

Figure 1

First, when China shifted from a system of agricultural collectives to the individual household responsibility system beginning in the late 1970s, both the communal administrative structure which employed barefoot doctors as health "workers" and the collective welfare fund (the major source of financing for drugs

---

[2] The two principal components of China's rural reforms were the decollectivization of agricultural production and the gradual adjustment of pricing and production of agricultural commodities toward a free market.

and other services) disappeared. The government did not replace CMS with a new organized financing structure, but instead adopted a laissez-faire policy. In response, many communities voluntarily designed their own new funding mechanisms, and many villages fell back on a fee-for-service (FFS) payment system. The poorest farmers, who could not afford to pay for services, could ask for support from the village welfare fund, which was maintained by a special tax of just under 5% of the village's net output from farm production. One fifth of this agricultural tax was designated for welfare assistance and to defray health care costs of those in need.

Second, the ideology on which China's economic system and its social services were based dramatically shifted in the post-Mao era. To speed national economic development the once dominant party dictum of "Serve the People" has been replaced by "Let Some People Get Rich First." Hence, economic efficiency is emphasized and equality is ignored. As a result of disbanding of China's communes, just 40-45% of China's villages were still covered by CMS by 1983. At about that time, an ideological shift prompted some high government officials to declare that the remaining CMS programs should be abolished. Thus, most communities that still had CMS were forced to disband their system by the mid-1980s, much to the dismay of the local people (Zhou *et al.*, 1991).

Last but not least, patronage and corruption as well as poor management contributed to the downfall of CMS. The CMS, even though based in local communities, was controlled and managed by local officials who were not held accountable to the people, some of whom used their power for selfish gains. As a result, people lost confidence in the government-run CMS program and refused to make financial contributions once the system became voluntary in the early 1980s. This experience underscores the importance of effective organization and management of any new community financing scheme, and the need for an adequate financial base.

HEALTH CARE PROBLEMS IN THE POST-CMS ERA

The collapse of CMS seems to be closely related to the deterioration of rural health care conditions in China. For example a recent World Bank study (1997) has indicated that China's earlier progress in improving child health appears, in the aggregate, to have come to a stop, despite rapid economic growth in the past decade. The analysis concludes that under-five mortality declined steadily until the early 1980s and then began a slight upward drift. Experiences from other countries suggest that the under-five mortality rate need not plateau as China's has done. This indicates that China's performance has deteriorated not only in absolute terms but also relative to other countries.

This major change appears to be confirmed by our 30 poverty county study which collected historical data on economic and health status in those underdeveloped areas. As depicted in Figure 1, even though of relatively modest magnitude, China's poverty areas had experienced steady economic growth after economic reform. *Per capita* GDP (in real terms) increased from $56 in the late 1970s to $88 in the late 1980s. However, the median infant mortality rate in the surveyed counties increased from about 50 per 1,000 live births to 72 per 1,000 live births during the same period of time.

Multiple factors may be responsible for this disturbing trend. Among other things (*e.g.*, changes in fertility rate and poverty reduction), China's relative performance in health during the 1970s and 1980s tracks closely with the rise and decline in percentage of the rural population covered by the CMS (Figure 1). Several major problems are associated with the collapse of CMS and thus may explain the mechanisms through which the collapse of CMS had a health impact.

First, access to primary health care has been reduced as a result of increased physical and financial barriers for the rural population.

Many barefoot doctors left the health profession with the introduction of the household production responsibility system. The agricultural reforms improved the income derived from farming, and many barefoot doctors left the health sector for full-time farming, particularly when they could no longer be compensated by the CMS for their health work. Some barefoot doctors, however, converted their health posts into private practices on a fee-for-service bases without adequate supervision. As depicted in Figure 1, the number of township and village health workers per 1000 population decreased by 48% from the late 1970s to late 1980s. Our 30 poverty county study also found that in 1979, 71% of villages had at least one health station, whereas only 55% of villages had a functioning health station in 1993. In light of the isolated geographical location of many poor villages (80% of the poverty region population live in mountainous areas), there might be serious physical barriers to accessing basic health care.

Increased financial barriers are reflected in the increase of health care costs relative to farmers' income. Inflation-adjusted health care costs rose an average of 10-15% each year over the decade 1983-1993, a rate which is two times that of the average growth rate of farmers' disposable income (Ministry of Health, 1984;

Chinese Statistics Bureau, 1994). With most Chinese farmers having to pay out-of-pocket, financial barriers to health care have increased significantly. According to our 30 poverty county study, there is a gap between need and effective demand for services. Twenty eight percent of the interviewed farmers do not seek health care when seriously ill, and 51% of rural patients refuse hospitalization when recommended by physicians. Financial difficulties are cited as the major reason for forgoing professional care. Our descriptive and regression analyses indicate that lower utilization rates are related to the poor health status of the rural population. For example, Figure 2 shows that the percentage of women experiencing better birth outcomes is significantly higher among women who received professional birth assistance than those without professional care. Therefore, increasing effective demand for needed services can generate significant marginal health improvement in China, especially for the rural poor. There is empirical evidence to indicate that controlling for income, people covered by community financing schemes tend to use more health care services than the uninsured (see Table 1).

Figure 2 Birth Outcomes by Assisted and Non-Assisted Deliveries

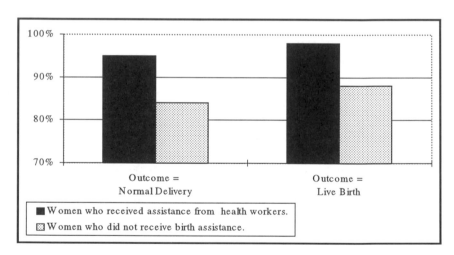

Second, high health expenses are a major cause of poverty in rural areas. In China, health care costs are high relative to farmers' income. Those with modest incomes must spend one-third of a week's average income per person to pay for village doctors and prescriptions and nearly double that for a visit to a township health center. A poor farmer would have to spend 1.2 years of his disposable income to pay for an episode of hospitalization at a county hospital (see Table 2). We found that 18% of the households using health services incurred health expenditures that exceeded their total household income in 1993. Of the 11,044 rural households interviewed, 24.5% borrowed or became indebted to pay for health expenses. Another 5.5% sold or mortgaged properties to pay for health care. Once a household is seriously in debt, its living standards and nutrition may decline, adversely affecting the health status of household members. In our 30 county survey, 47% of the medically indebted households reported having suffered from hunger. This interaction between income and health could start a vicious cycle of illness, poverty, and more illness.

Table 1 Comparing households covered by community financing schemes (CF)
and the uninsured in China's poverty regions

	Households under CF	Uninsured
Use of MCH services		
Pre-natal care (%)	82.8	39.4
Post-natal care (%)	48.6	21.7
Self-delivery (%)	13.5	43.5
Costs & utilization pattern		
Costs/visit (yuan)	1.5	3.0
Medical expenses/year (yuan)	15.5	27.9
Visits at village (%)	66.8	39.7
Hospitalization at Town (%)	75.0	58.0

Third, inefficiency is associated with the current fee-for-service system. There is an incentive to over-prescribe drugs and diagnostic tests with no significant gain in marginal health benefits (sometimes with even harmful effects to the patients), because the incomes of village doctors and health facilities depend on charges for drugs, injections, and new-technology tests, and because prices for drugs and some diagnostic procedures were set higher than average costs. County hospitals, township health centers and village health stations as well as private practitioners are allowed to mark up their prescribed drugs by 15-20%. Moreover, user fees charged for previously free preventive services have had detrimental effects on public health through reduced demand for and supply of preventive services. The

Epidemic Prevention Service workers shifted their attention to services for which fees could easily be charged -- such as cosmetic product inspection and food safety -- which were not necessarily the highest priority and the most cost-effective activities (Jin, 1995).

**Table 2 The financial burden of health care costs for households
with different income levels in China's poverty regions**

Level of facilities	Households with income/capita 200 yuan	Households with income/capita 400 yuan
	Cost of an outpatient visit as % of weekly income	
Village	38%	36%
Township	151%	71%
County	170%	84%
	Cost of an inpatient episode as % of annual income	
Township	28%	22%
County	116%	138%

Community financing schemes reduce the incentive for the providers to over-prescribe and overuse services as in FFS system. Our 30 poverty county study found that the average charge per outpatient visit for the uninsured patients is almost three times that of the patients under CMS (see Table 1), because community financing schemes can exercise their bargaining power in demanding discounted prices or the providers can be paid on a partial-capitation basis. Furthermore, through a referral system, CMS manages patients at lower-level facilities wherever possible. As indicated in Table 1, 66.8% of outpatient visits and 75% of hospitalization by patients with CMS coverage happened at village and township levels, while only 39.7% of ambulatory patients and 58% of hospitalized patients who were not insured use village and township level health facilities. Without CMS, many farmers in more affluent communities went directly to county hospitals for medical services. The shift in demand toward services rendered at higher levels has put additional pressure on the already overtaxed medical facilities at the county levels. Furthermore, the inter-connection and cooperation among different rural health facilities also weakened or disappeared after reforms. Under CMS, county hospitals and township health centers provided regular technical assistance and supervision to the lower level organizations. After the collapse of CMS, however, these health care organizations became independent institutions. Often they compete for patients to increase revenues (Zhu *et al.*, 1988). This disintegration of the three-tier system may also have implications for the quality of services provided by uncoordinated rural health workers.

CAN COMMUNITY FINANCING BE REVITALIZED IN CHINA?

The current self-financing and fee-for-service system in rural China, which is plagued with many problems as discussed above, clearly needs to be reformed. Instead of relying on current user fees, rural health care can be financed by a combination of sources: general revenues, earmarked taxes, social insurance, private insurance, and community financing. In light of their fiscal conditions and expected slow growth of general revenues, it seems unlikely that the Chinese central and provincial governments would provide a large portion of the required funds to finance rural health care needs. Mandatory social insurance funded by a wage tax or premiums is infeasible because it relies on employers to pay and China's farmers are self-employed. Moreover, China lacks the institutional and organizational capacity to manage large social insurance programs.

Private commercial insurance is also problematic for covering the rural population because private insurance is not an equitable or efficient approach to insure basic health benefits. Information asymmetry and adverse selection by individuals, which often lead to premium costs spiraling, severely limit risk pooling. On the other hand, risk selection by insurance companies can leave the disabled, elderly, and less healthy population uninsured. This may explain why to date China's "People's Insurance Companies" have offered rural medical insurance only in some high-income counties.

Community financing is one promising approach to organized financing for China's rural population. Its advantages include improved access and efficiency as well as popular support. However, a question may arise: if community financing is such a good idea, why have only a few rural communities reestablished CMS in the past decade? Multiple factors affect the voluntary development of community-based schemes (Hsiao, 1995; Coleman, 1990; Esman and Upoff, 1984; and Fukuyama, 1995). Unattractive benefit packages or packages that cost more than people's willingness and ability to pay can deter participation. We investigated these questions by designing a reasonable basic benefit package (BBP) and estimating its costs. Then we evaluated whether the people have the capacity and willingness to pay for this BBP.

BASIC BENEFIT PACKAGES AND FINANCIAL FEASIBILITY

Whether community financing is feasible for rural China will first of all depend on its benefit structure: a low benefit package (*e.g.*, only covering cost-effective preventive services) is affordable but may not meet the rural population's need for protection from catastrophic medical expenses. On the other hand, a high benefit package, even though desirable, may not be feasible because people's willingness and ability to pay is limited. Illnesses are uncertain; thus the payoff from participating in community financing schemes is uncertain for the households. We found that about 11% of the rural population consumed 70% of the total medical expenditures. This finding illustrates the need for catastrophic insurance and the potential problems of adverse selection and risk selection under a voluntary insurance program. The core issue in designing an appropriate and feasible basic benefit package is the balance between three considerations: the cost-effectiveness of the services covered, people's desired coverage, and the financial constraints of those paying for the coverage.

Household responses to some surveys indicate that people prefer a wide range of services, from drugs and village doctors to township health centers, and they prefer coverage of hospital inpatient services (catastrophic expenses) with willingness to accept coinsurance (Luo *et al.*, 1995; Gu *et al.*, 1991). For illustrative purposes, we developed several basic benefit packages for the low income rural population based on the data of the 30 poverty county survey. The following principles and assumptions were used in designing the benefit packages: a) first cover the most cost-effective services, but take into account that health care delivery is not organized by disease; b) coinsurance should vary for different services depending on demand elasticity; c) people are risk-adverse and demand coverage for catastrophic expenses. From a societal perspective, the coverage of catastrophic medical expenses also reduces the poverty rate.

The simulation results are shown in Table 3. Depending on the coinsurance level, the estimated per capita cost is between 28 and 31 yuan (about $4 - $5) for providing a basic benefit package which includes specified maternal and child health care services and a stop-loss provision of approximately 500-600 yuan in 1993. The following section discusses the feasibility of financing the BBP for the low-income rural population.

Table 3
Two Prototype Benefit Packages for China's Rural Poor (Benefit Structure & Costs)

Type of Expenses Covered	Level of Coinsurance	
	High	Medium
Village Post		
*Service fees	20%	20%
*Drug expenses	50%	40%
Township Health Center		
*Outpatient service fees	30%	30%
*Outpatient drug expenses	50%	40%
*Inpatient	35%	30%
County Hospital		
*Outpatient service fees	40%	35%
*Outpatient drug expenses	50%	40%
*Inpatient	45%	35%
Catastrophic protection		
stop-loss at	600 yuan	500 yuan
Estimated *per capita* costs	28 yuan	31 yuan

In poverty areas, households already spend a significant amount of their income on health care. According to our survey, annual medical expenditures by such households were 24 yuan per capita in 1993 (see Table 4). However, it would be unrealistic to expect that people are willing to prepay this amount to support an organized financing scheme. Although the majority of individuals surveyed expressed their support for CMS, their willingness to prepay into the system was only about 5 yuan per capita. *Per capita* contributions to existing community financing schemes range from 1.05 yuan to 6.14 yuan. With effective social marketing it might be expected that 10 yuan per capita could be obtained from households.

As there are few rural enterprises in the poor regions, collective welfare funds -- averaging 7 yuan per capita and managed by the township government -- constitute the most important potential source of local community funding. Currently less than 1 yuan per capita from this fund is spent on health. Most township officials interviewed said that if they received matching support from higher levels of government an increasing portion of the funds could be used to finance a community scheme. Doubling the current spending level would amount to 2 yuan per capita from this source. Therefore, potentially 12 yuan could be collected from individuals and local communities, covering less than half the expected costs of a comprehensive package. The rest of the resource gap will have to be filled by public assistance. Otherwise, without government support, community financing schemes in the poverty regions can only finance a very limited package for the low-income households.

Table 4
Current Financing of Health Spending by Source in China's Poverty Regions

Source	Expenditure *per capita* in 1993	%
Household	23.41 yuan	59.32
Government	13.18 yuan	33.40
Insurance for public employees	2.31 yuan	5.85
Collective fund	0.31 yuan	0.80
Other	0.25 yuan	0.63
Total	**39.46 yuan**	**100.0**

There are several possible sources of government assistance. First, some resources can be freed up by improving the efficiency of current health care provision. For example, if 50% of the current level of inefficiency in the township health centers could be reduced by reducing government subsidies (direct government subsidies to the centers are 3001 yuan per worker per annum -- almost two times that of the national rural average), this would result in a resource gain of one yuan per township resident (Liu *et al.*, 1996). Second, our study found that over 70% of the poor counties have received various funds from the central government for poverty alleviation purposes, but very little of those funds is currently channeled to the health sector. We found that most of the local fund managers are willing to consider supporting organized health care financing if a more consolidated and coordinated system could be set up. Third, the government can use earmarked taxes to support health care for the rural poor. One approach would be through a "sin-tax" on cigarette consumption. Smoking has serious public health consequences and is on the rise in China. Based on 1992 consumption data, the government could raise 8 billion yuan in additional revenue with a tax of 0.1 yuan per packet sold (Ding and Zhao, 1995). If a fraction of this tax revenue were to be channeled to support organized health care financing, the benefits for the rural poor would be tremendous. Therefore, the successful development of organized financing schemes will depend not only on mobilizing existing financial resources, but also on government policy to generate additional resources designated for subsidizing the poor.

OTHER NECESSARY CONDITIONS

The preceding discussion makes it clear that a reasonable basic benefit package is financially feasible, because even among low-income groups a significant share of health care costs can be financed by the people themselves, and there are multiple channels through which the government can provide additional financial support. However, financial capital is just one of the necessary conditions for success. Our 30 poverty county study compared communities with CMS to those without and found that the average household income is comparable in those two areas. However, the CMS-communities somehow managed to establish a bigger collective welfare fund despite having a less developed rural industry (a condition believed by many experts to be the key factor for CMS). The village welfare fund per capita is only 1.27 yuan in villages without CMS, whereas the average welfare fund in CMS villages is 6.41 yuan. This finding indicates that the formation of financial capital for community financing is not influenced by economic conditions alone.

Several large household interview surveys have found that a majority of Chinese peasants want cooperative financing established in their communities (Zhou *et al.*, 1991; Hsiao, 1995; and Li, 1988). Moreover, in spite of the government edict in the mid-1980s to abolish the Cooperative Medical System, close to 10% of the rural villages continue to maintain their system. This empirical evidence suggests that there is a significant amount of social support in many villages for establishing community financing schemes. However, voluntary development of CMS is very limited even in affluent areas. For example, only about 6% of the villages have established CMS in Fujian, a high-income province in China (The World Bank, China, 1997). In our 30 poverty county study survey, 70% of villages that reinstated CMS did so at the request of the government. Experience from China and other countries demonstrated that government can play a significant role as initiator and enable for community financing (Hsiao, 1995;

Suwandono, *et al.*, 1995; and Jarrett and Ofosu-Amaah, 1992).

Many policy decisions in China are driven by ideology. Because of the ideological shift after economic reform, any discussion about nationwide rehabilitation of CMS was politically taboo for quite a while. This lack of political legitimacy may have had a negative impact on the development of community financing schemes in China. In 1994, after years of experience with serious financial and physical barriers to basic health care for the rural population without CMS, the Chinese government announced a new policy direction for the financing of health care for the rural population (Yuan and Chen, 1994). The announcement declared that China would rely on community-based organized financing to fund and organize health care for its rural population. Several principles were enunciated to guide this approach: local communities are encouraged to organize their own collective financing for basic health care with funding from multiple sources; the schemes would vary between communities according to their socioeconomic conditions; the organization should adopt scientific management methods and be held accountable to the people.

However, there are ambiguities and inconsistencies remaining in Chinese government policy. First, the government required that schemes be voluntary; no mandatory enrollment is allowed. Faced with potential adverse selection problems, many rural communities, especially those lacking cohesive social structure, neither have the incentive nor the capacity to establish and maintain the scheme. Second, simply acknowledging and legitimizing the benefit and organizational variation among different communities, the government has not spelled out its role in welfare redistribution and how it will help the poor communities which do not have the necessary financial and social capital. Third, health policy and other related economic and social policies are not well coordinated in China. Despite the announced government support of community financing from some top officials, the State Council and the Ministry of Agriculture prohibit local taxes for community financing of health care from exceeding a taxing cap of .8% of the average net income of the farmers (State Council Research Office, 1994). Although well intentioned (to protect farmers from over-taxation), this policy makes it illegitimate for local leaders to ask for extra contributions to finance a basic benefit package. Even though 88% of the 2,235 interviewed township and village officials in our 30 county survey said that it is necessary to establish community financing in the rural areas, many of them indicated that they were reluctant to play a leading role in mobilizing community resources for fear of violating the government tax policy. When asked about the major reasons for lack of community financing initiatives, 52% of the community leaders cited financial difficulties. However, about a third of the interviewed leaders listed non-financial reasons such as lack of organizational capacity and lack of policy support from higher-level government (see Figure 3).

Figure 3 Percentage of 2,236 Surveyed Community Leaders Citing Major Reasons for lack of Rural Community Financing.

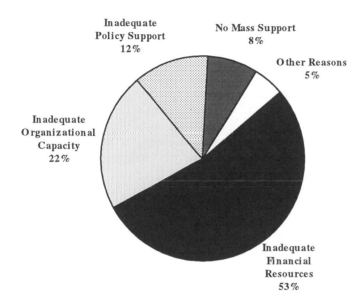

The preceding analysis indicates that several measures have to be taken by the government to activate and organize the community financing schemes. Foremost is a consistent and well coordinated official policy to legitimize the community financing approach as an effective strategy to finance and organize health care. Often official approval for a strategy gives impetus for its acceptance and wider adoption. Second, initial investment is required to build the clinics (where there are none or they are poorly equipped) and to stock them with basic drug supplies. In the event that willingness to participate is insufficient and adverse selection is present, the government may have to make enrollment in community financing schemes mandatory or provide some subsidy as incentive for people to join. Moreover, qualified managerial, financial, and health personnel are needed to operate a community financing scheme successfully. The government can develop these human resources by offering training programs. Finally, the government can set forth appropriate regulations to control fraud and abuse and to monitor the quality and availability of health services.

CONCLUSION

After the collapse of CMS in the early 1980s, China's rural health care system was plagued with many problems. At China's level of development, however, the government does not have adequate public resources to finance all health services. The majority of health care costs may have to be borne by communities or individuals. Therefore, community financing seems to be both a necessary and effective approach to provide an organized way to finance and deliver basic health services.

For community financing to be feasible, there has to be adequate financial and social support in place. The fact that community financing exists in some of China's poorest regions but is not well developed in much more affluent areas may underscore the importance of other social factors, such as community cohesiveness, which might affect financial capital formation for the common good.

China's experience also illustrates that government still has a very important role to play as initiator and enabler. Just as many rural communities were once forced to disband CMS due to misguided political pressures, the majority of villages that either continued or reinstated CMS had not been able to do so without strong support from the local government. Therefore, governmental promotion and support is required to initiate and sustain community financing schemes, especially in areas lacking adequate financial resources as well as technical know-how.

Government involvement, on the other hand, should not crowd out community participation. The ultimate control and management of community financing schemes will have to be at the local community level for the schemes to be effective and sustainable. One of the major reasons for the downfall of CMS was the excessive government control and related corruption. The new community financing schemes need to avoid the problems of the old CMS. Community participation and control can be embodied in different ways, including increasing consumer representation in the local management board and granting different responsibilities to different levels of decentralized administration. However, for risk-pooling purposes, community financing schemes need to be sufficiently large. Hence, there will be a trade-off between accountability by local control and risk sharing by "law of large numbers." A community financing model that balances the two aspects could be jointly run by the village and township, with the village responsible for managing the prepayment part of the scheme (*e.g.*, outpatient visits, drugs, etc.), and the insurance part of the scheme (*e.g.*, inpatient care and coverage of catastrophic expenses) managed at the township level (a more adequate risk-pooling base than the small village).

In conclusion, this paper demonstrates that community financing of a basic benefit package is feasible for rural China if resources from multiple channels can be mobilized and if the government and local communities form a cooperative partnership according to the principles discussed above. Moreover, if community financing can be successfully adopted throughout China by adapting the government-community partnership to fit the socioeconomic conditions of different local communities, China could regain its position as an international leader in improving the health of its vast population at low cost. If China fails to take prompt action, access to basic health care will remain a major problem in the rural areas and the health of the poor rural population could further deteriorate, jeopardizing efforts to eliminate poverty and promote equity.

ACKNOWLEDGMENTS

This paper draws in part on a cooperative study in 30 poverty counties in China by the China Network of Health Economics Institutions and the Harvard School of Public Health funded by UNICEF, IHPP, and the Chinese Ministry of Health. We wish to thank Dean Jamison and Jacques van der Gaag for helpful suggestions and comments. Karen Eggleston and Maria Leo provided excellent editing assistance. The authors are solely responsible for the contents of this paper.

This paper was published in *Health Policy* 38 (1996) 155-171, and is reprinted with the kind permission of Elsevier Science.

REFERENCES

Abel-Smith, B. and Dua, A. (1987) The potential of community financing of the health sector in developing countries. In: *Asian Development Bank, Health Care Financing,*. pp. 42-70.

Coleman, J.S. (1990) Foundations of Social Capital Theory. Cambridge, MA: Harvard university Press.

Ding, H. and Shao, Z. (1995) Economics of smoking, *Chinese Health Economics* 148(4):65-71.

Esman, M.J. and Upoff, N.T. (1984) *Local Organizations: Intermediaries in Rural Development.* New York: Cornell University Press.

Fukuyama, F. (1995) *Trust: The Social Virtues and the Creation of Prosperity.* New York: The Free Press.

Gu, X. *et al.* (1993) Financing health care in rural China: preliminary report of a nationwide study. *Soc. Sci. Med.* 36: 385-391.

Gu, X., *et al.* (1991) Medical services research of the rural population in the PRC. In The Health Policy and Management Expert Council of the Chinese Ministry of Health, editors, *The Rural Medical Care System in China.* Shanghai: Shanghai Science and Technology Publishing House.

Halstead, S.B. *et al.* (1985) *Good Health at Low Cost.* New York: Rockefeller Foundation, New York.

Hsiao, W.C. (1984) Transformation of health care in China. *New England Journal of Medicine* 310: 932-936.

Hsiao, W.C. (1995) Community Health Care. Presented at the International Seminar on Financing and Organization of Health Care for the Poor Rural Population in China, Fragrant Hill Hotel, Beijing, October 8-10, 1995.

Jarrett, S.W. and Ofosu-Amaah, S. (1992) Strengthening health services for MCH in Africa: the first four years of the "Bamako Initiative" *Health Policy and Planning* 4:110 120.

Jin, S. (1995) Case Study on Health Finance of Shanxi, Jiangsu, and Guizhou Province. Presented at the Health Care Seminar in Beijing, China, 2-5 May, 1995.

Li, X. (1988) Cooperative Medical System is a good form of health care financing in poor areas. *Chinese Rural Health Services Administration* 25(3):45-48

Liu, Y. *et al.*, (1996) Efficiency in China's Rural Health Care: A Stochastic Frontier Approach. Presented at the Inaugural Conference of the

International Health Economics Association, Hyatt Hotel, Vancouver, B.C., Canada, May 19-23, 1996.

Luo, W. *et al.* (1995) Study of Health Care Financing and Organization in Poor Rural Areas of China, presented at the IHPP Research, Writing and Dissemination Workshop, Washington D.C., March 1-9, 1995.

Ministry of Health (1994) Research on National Health Services - An Analysis Report of the National Health Services Survey in 1993, Chinese Ministry of Health, Beijing.

National Statistics Bureau (1994) *China Statistics Digest.* Beijing: The Chinese Statistics Publishing House.

National Statistics Bureau (1994) *Statistical Yearbook of China 1994.* Beijing: The Chinese Statistics Publishing.

Sidel, R. and Sidel, V.W. (1984) *The Health of China: Current Conflicts in Medical and Human Services for one Billion People* Beacon: Boston, 1984.

State Council Research Office (1994) *A Study on the Rural Cooperative Medical System.* Beijing: Beijing Medical University Press.

Suwandono, A. *et al.* (1995) The Indonesian Experiences on Rural Health Financing, presented at the International Seminar on Financing and Organization of Health Care for the Poor Rural Population in China, Fragrant Hill Hotel, Beijing, October 8-10, 1995.

The World Bank, China (1997) *Issues and Options in Health Financing.* Washington, DC: The World Bank.

Yuan, M. and Chen, M. (1994) The Chinese rural health care reform. *People's Daily.* July 2, 1994.

Zhang, Z. (1992) Review of the early period of Cooperative Medical System. *Chinese Health Economics* 52(1):88-95.

Zhou, S., *et al.* (1991) The need for reestablishing Cooperative Medical System. *Chinese Rural Health Services Administration* 65:92):78-81.

Zhu, A. *et al.* (1988) Systematic study of rural cooperative medical system. *Chinese Rural Health Services Administration* 2(3):21-30.

10

Inequality of Health Finance, Resources, and Mortality in Russia: Potential Implications for Health and Medical Care Policy

DOV CHERNICHOVSKY[1]
TATIANA KIRSANOVA[2]
ELENA POTAPCHIK[2]
ELENA SOSENSKAYA[2]

[1]Health Policy and Management Unit
Health Policy Program for Economies Under Stress
Ben-Gurion of the Negev University, Israel
[2]New Economic School, Moscow. Russia

Health, Health Care and Health Economics: Perspectives on Distribution
Edited by Morris L. Barer, Thomas E. Getzen, and Greg L. Stoddart
Copyright 1998 John Wiley & Sons, Ltd.

ABSTRACT

Soon after the breakup of the Soviet Union and the re-establishment of Russia as an independent federation in 1991, regional oblast- (state/province-) level authorities became responsible for their own health care administrations and budgets. This was a dramatic deviation from the former Soviet system in which management and financing responsibilities rested with the central authorities in Moscow. As a result of this shift in responsibilities, the regional distribution of *per capita* health expenditure across the Russian Federation started changing, during the study period 1990-1993, to resemble the distribution of the regional product or income *per capita*. This marked the beginning of a process which has been gradually offsetting the Soviet legacy of allocation of medical resources according to standardized mortality rates. At the same time, no correlation was observed during that period between regional variations in mortality levels, which rose, and the regional changes in levels of health financing. Cross-sectional data from the period 1989-90, before the breakup of the Soviet Union, indicate that there was no apparent effect on mortality of health finance and real medical resources in Russia even before the onset of the social and economic transition. In contrast, by the same data, there was a negative effect on mortality of education and "life-styles." These observations from the earlier and stable period can contribute to the explanation of the unobserved correlation between health finance and mortality across the Russia Federation during the period 1991-1993. Namely, within the observed data range, mortality is insensitive to variations in levels of health finance. This finding, taken together with the observations (a) that mortality in Russia is higher than in the West even considering its comparatively low levels of income (not education), and (b) that there is scope to improve life expectancy in Russia through medical intervention, has a major policy implication. It suggests that the levels of health financing and real medical resources might make a difference in Russia, especially if expended to change Russia's medical care approach and technology.

INTRODUCTION

The objective of this paper is to assess the potential impact of recent changes in the administration and distribution of health care financing across the Russian Federation on the health of the Russian people. By implication, the paper draws conclusions about the potential effect on health of the current medical care approach and technology in Russia. These objectives are accomplished through studying regional variations in health financing in Russia and their health and medical correlates.

BACKGROUND

The Russian Federation comprises three levels of administration organized according to the following hierarchy: (a) The Russian Federation; (b) Republics, Krais, Oblasts, National Okrugs, and the cities of Moscow and St. Petersburg; and (c) Local entities. These local entities are divided into (1) rayons and cities, and (2) towns, villages, and rural settlements. A city, depending on its size, may be divided into several rayons or may form a rayon by itself.

Territories below the federal level — republics, krais, oblasts, okrugs, and the two main cities of Moscow and St. Petersburg — are called territories of "oblast-level" which are analogous to states or provinces in Western federations (*e.g.*, Australia, Canada, and the United States of America). The oblasts comprise the Russian Federation. Under the Soviet Union in 1990, the Russian Republic comprised 73 oblast-level administrative territories, including 15 republics, six krais, 50 oblasts, and the two cities. Today, following administrative changes in Russia since 1991 and the 1993 constitution, the federation is comprised of 89 oblast- (state-) level subjects: 21 republics, six krais, 49 oblasts, one autonomous oblast, two cities and 10 autonomous okrugs. All are of equal status.[1]

Until the late 1980s with the unfolding of "Perestroika," financing and management of the Soviet health care system was completely centralized. The Soviet Federal Ministry of Health (SFMOH) regulated management and resource allocation of the entire system through each republic's ministry, including the Russian Federal Ministry of Health (RFMOH) which was then part of the Soviet Union. Other ministries managed their medical systems, accounting for about 10%

---

[1] Russian statistics often aggregate the Russian Federation into 12 economic regions, grouping together geographically and economically close oblasts. This aggregation has no administrative significance but is often used for presentation of data. It is used here as well for summary of data. At the same time, all statistics and calculations reported in this paper are based on individual oblast-level data. About the administrative organization of the health system, see Chernichovsky and Potapchik 1996a.

of total medical resources, independently but similarly (Rowland and Telyukov, 1991; Chernichovsky, Barnum, and Potapchik, 1996; Chernichovsky and Potapchik, 1996).

Centralized management had several key manifestations. Heads of the oblast-level health authorities and of major medical institutions were appointed only after SFMOH confirmation. Although financed through territorial budgets, mandatory resource allocation criteria were established and enforced by the Soviet Federal Ministry of Finance and the SFMOH. Those two ministries approved both current and capital expenditures throughout the system. Periodically, the SFMOH conducted surveys that established development needs dealing with investment in, and upgrading of, medical facilities, notably hospitals (beds) and community polyclinics. Need was based on demographic characteristics as discussed below. The last survey of this kind was conducted in 1988. Subsequently, operating budgets for hospitals and polyclinics were established and decreed according to expenditure coefficients assigned correspondingly to hospital beds and to patient-visit capacity in polyclinics. Some adjustment was made for differences in wages of medical personnel in remote areas (Chernichovsky, Barnum, and Potapchik, 1996).

With the breakup of the Soviet Union and the re-establishment of Russia as an independent federation in 1991, oblast-level territories still had to confirm their health budgets with the Russian federal MOH (RFMOH) and have their budgets approved by the Russian Federal Ministry of Finance. However, these procedures have become increasingly declaratory, especially since 1991-92 when the decentralization process in the Russian health system was overtaken by broader changes in the general administration and budgetary systems, giving almost complete budgetary freedom to oblast-level authorities. According to the pertinent legislation, oblast- and local-level administrations (cities and rayons) manage their own medical services (Supreme Soviet of the Russian Federation, 1991a, 1991b, 1991c; Wallich, 1992; Chernichovsky and Potapchik, 1996). Contrary to the Soviet legacy, those administrations now appoint new heads of territorial health authorities and the heads of appropriate medical facilities without the RFMOH's approval. In addition, they are almost exclusively responsible for health budgets.[2]

The 1993 Russian health insurance legislation stipulated the creation of

---

[2] A notable exception is the State Committee for Sanitary and Epidemiological Surveillance which has remained a federal organ responsible mainly for prevention of the spread of infectious diseases. See Chernichovsky and Potapchik, 1996.

regional and federal health insurance funds financed through a 3.6% tax on the (local) wage bill. Of this tax, 0.2% is allocated to the Federal Fund for regional equalization purposes. However, the legislation did not provide appropriate funds for the equalization role; neither does the Fund have the needed financial mechanisms to perform this role (Supreme Soviet of the Russian Federation, 1993; Chernichovsky, Barnum and Potapchik, 1996; Chernichovsky and Potapchik, 1997).

GROWING INEQUALITY IN HEALTH CARE FINANCING

Although in 1993 national health system revenues recovered, after declines in 1991-92, to the 1990 level (Table 1), the disparities among regions have been growing; some regions have gained in health financing (*e.g.*, Northern, Urals, Far East), while others have fallen behind (*e.g.*, Northern Caucasus, Kaliningradskaya oblast and Volgo-vyatsky).

Table 1 *Per capita* **health expenditure by economic regions.**
Russia. 1990 and 1993 (in 1990 Prices)

Region	1990	1993	Deviation, %
Russia	95.52	95.30	0.88%
Northern region	116.76	127.67	9.35%
North-western region	99.02	89.76	-9.36%
Central region	92.64	96.54	4.21%
Volgo-vyatsky region	84.937	2.36	-14.80%
Central-chernozemny region	84.16	75.01	-10.88%
Povolzhsky region	3.57	88.24	5.59%
Northern Caucases region	77.20	57.70	-25.27%
Urals region	91.06	106.30	16.74%
Western Siberia region	105.76	113.65	7.46%
Eastern-Siberia region	103.01	97.97	-4.89%
Far East region	138.28	152.39	10.20%
Kaliningradskaya obl	86.49	73.14	-15.44%
Weighted Standard Deviation	21.31	35.04	

Notes: (a) 1993 health funds comprise health expenditures through local health budgets plus revenues of Territorial Health Insurance Funds. (b) 1993/90 GDP price index is used. (c) Weighted statistics are based on oblast populations.
Sources: Goskomstat 1994, pp. 9, 12, 441-443; Ministry of Health working tables.

Based on a re-aggregation (for comparative purposes) of Russia's original 72 oblast-level entities, the Lorenz curves (Figure 1) display the rising inequality in health financing, and its regression to the inequalities existing among local economies as estimated by the local *per capita* incomes or products.[3] Through these curves and the underlying inequality indexes or Gini coefficients, health expenditure distributions for 1990 and 1992 are compared with a hypothetical

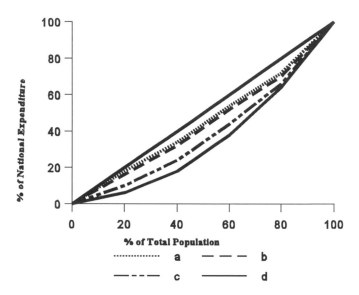

Figure 1 Lorenz Curves -- health expenditure and estimated gross product across the Russian Federation

a - simulated "need-based" local health expenditures, 1992; b - local health expenditures, 1990; c- local health expenditures 1992; d - GDP estimate, 1992

---

[3]The Chechnya and Ingushetia Republics are not included in the calculations because (a) since 1991 Chechnya has not submitted its statistics to the Russian Federal authorities, and (b) there is no clear split between Chechnya and Ingushetia in available statistical sources. In 1993 Russia comprised 89 oblast-level territories as opposed to 73 in 1990 covering the same territories. Consequently for comparative purposes, 1993 data are re-aggregated according to the 1990 administrative units.

"need-based" health expenditure distribution for 1992 (curve "a," Figure 1) and with the estimated *per capita* GDP distribution for 1992 (curve "d").[4] The Gini Coefficient is 0.052 for the 1990 actual distribution (Table 2). This coefficient is close to the coefficient, 0.038, for the "need-based" distribution. In 1992 the coefficient, measuring inequality, rose to 0.102, and is 0.096 in 1993. For 1992, the year for which both Gross Domestic Product (GDP) and health financing data are available, the coefficient for health care expenditure, 0.102, was approaching the coefficient, 0.120, for the GDP distribution. Namely, the distribution of health care expenditure regresses to the distribution of the estimated regional GDP as demonstrated by curve "c" approaching curve "d" in Figure 1.

Table 2 Inequality indexes or Gini Coefficients - domestic product and health. Russia. 1990, 1992, and 1993

Indicator	1990	1992	1993
Net Material Product (NMP)	0.081		
Estimate of Gross Domestic Product (GDP)		0.120	
Local health expend.	0.052	0.102	0.096
"Need-based" health expend		0.038	

Note: To construct the Lorenz Curves and establish the Gini Coefficients, oblasts were ranked by their health expenditure *per capita*.

Sources: see Table 1.

Simultaneously, during the same period there was a rise in mortality rates across the Russian Federation (Table 3). Evidently, the observed deterioration in health status, as measured by crude mortality rates (CMR), is also coupled with a slightly worsening distribution in these rates, showed by the Standard Deviation statistic. Statistically speaking, however, there is no correlation between the aforementioned changes in health finance and the change in crude mortality rates; based on the 72 oblast-level observations (making up today 87 of Russia's 89

---

[4]"Need-based" health expenditures are calculated by re-allocating regional health expenditures according to the British capitation formula, but with Russian SMR, age-and-gender, as well as regional cost coefficients. Regional GDPs were estimated as the sum of gross industrial product, gross agricultural product and volume of paid services.

territories), this (first order) correlation is -0.090.[5]

Table 3 Crude Mortality Rates per 1,000 Population and Rate of Increase by Region.
Russia. 1990 and 1993.

Regions	1990	1993	Increase %
RUSSIA (total)	11.2	14.5	29.46%
Northern	9.1	13.3	46.15%
North-Western	12.7	17.9	40.94%
Central	13.0	16.6	27.69%
Volgo-Vyatsky	11.9	14.6	22.69%
Central-Chernozemny	13.7	16.3	18.98%
Povolzhsky	11.0	13.4	21.82%
Northern Caucases	11.1	13.6	22.52%
Uralsky	10.4	13.8	32.69%
Western Siberia	9.6	13.0	35.42%
Eastern Siberia	9.5	13.0	36.84%
Far Eastern	8.2	11.8	43.90%
Kaliningradsk. obl.	9.8	13.5	37.76%
Weighted Standard Deviation	2.00	2.26	

Source: Goskomstat 1994b, Tab.2.2, pp.40-50.

This lack of correlation between regional changes in mortality patterns and changes in regional allocations to health care may reflect particular realities. Real medical resources, namely personnel and facilities, remained in place in spite of variations in financing; changes in levels of financing manifested themselves in a fall in real salaries of medical personnel, reduced levels of supplies, and a deteriorating state of medical facilities (Chernichovsky *et al.*, 1996). These realities, plus the shortness of the study's observation period, can contribute to the lack of a statistical correlation between variation in health finance and mortality.

At the same time, this lack of correlation may also lead to a cardinal hypothesis about the efficacy of the Soviet and current Russian health care approach and medical technology. It may be that the "tight" organization of life under the Soviet regime, *e.g.*, guaranteed work, income, etc., maintained mortality levels below the

---

[5]Crude mortality rates are used here for comparative purposes, as the age structure within regions is unlikely to have changed during the period.

point where they would otherwise be, given the general standards of living, environment, public health, nutrition and medical services. With the changes in the economy and society, mortality levels may be reaching their "more natural levels," given the other factors, mainly life styles, which may have little to do with variations in spending on medical care (in the observation range).[6]

Moreover, the situation may also suggest the "lack of relevance" of current health care approach in Russia *vis a vis* major causes of mortality in that nation: trauma, malignancies, and other degenerative disorders. The latter two have been traditionally higher in Russia than in the West and have been aggravated, along with trauma, during the transition period. These diseases relate to risk factors associated with life styles: diet, stress, smoking, alcoholism, accidents, and violence. These risk factors have been deteriorating during the transition period. There is evidence that the Russian health care system has been ill equipped to deal with these medically-related public health situations (Chernichovsky *et al.*, 1996).

That is, while particular medical practices and interventions are beneficial to health, aggregate crude mortality levels appear insensitive, on the average, to a fall or even a rise of up to the observed 30% in health financing or medical resources in Russia. Investigation of this particular hypothesis, which has important policy implications, is the subject of the following empirical discussion in which we try to assess, from the period prior to the breakup of the Soviet Union when the situation was stable, the potential correlation between medical resources and mortality in Russia.

HEALTH CARE FINANCING AND HEALTH: BASIC CONCEPTUAL AND STATISTICAL CONSIDERATIONS

With the available cross-sectional data, summarized in Table 4, statistical estimation of the potential long term impact of the growing regional inequalities in health care financing on health as measured by mortality, is based on correlating regional variations in these two and other related variables. This is done within a framework that attempts to capture the pertinent behavioral and policy aspects of

---

[6]It should be emphasized that while infant mortality rates are higher in Russia than in almost all OECD nations, those rates are below levels of developing nations. Russia's life expectancy is severely affected by high mortality rates in ages 15-45 mainly due to trauma and cardiovascular problems (see Chernichovsky *et al.* 1996).

Table 4 Data Used for Regression Estimates

Weighted Parameter	Variable description	Year	Mean	S.Deviation
E	Local health expenditures *per capita*, rbs.	1990	96.02	21.77
H	Standardized Mortality Rate (SMR), percent	1989	100.16	7.90
G	Age and gender structure of the population is not used; accounted in SMR			
SE				
	Population age 15 and over with primary education or incomplete secondary education per 1,000 of the population age 15 and over	1989	195.75	4.91
	Population age 15 and over with secondary or incomplete higher education per 1,000 of the population age 15 and over	1989	481.61	46.03
	Population age 15 and over with higher education per 1,000 population age 15 and over	1989	111.73	47.24
	Percent of urban population	1990	64.59	22.97
EN				
	Air pollution, tons *per capita*	1990	0.23	0.22
	Percent of treated compounds in air pollution, percent	1990	67.81	17.55
	Ratio of up-to-standard treated sewage, percent	1990	16.10	22.79
R	Annual consumption of bread, kg *per capita*	1990	119.39	14.71
	Annual consumption of meat, kg *per capita*	1990	75.25	11.78
	Annual consumption of milk, kg *per capita*	1990	386.77	38.85
	Annual consumption of sugar, kg *per capita*	1990	47.28	4.20
	Annual consumption of eggs, units *per capita*	1990	298.11	39.08
	State sale of alcohol, liters *per capita*	1990	5.47	1.27
B	Hospital beds per 10,000 population	1990	137.67	9.97
Y	Net Material Product (NMP) *per capita*, Rbs.	1990	2982.96	1146.21

the former Soviet and now Russian system. For such correlations, a system of structural equations is estimated employing available cross-sectional regional pre-1991 data pertaining to the averages of 73 entities comprising the Russian Federation at the time. This system is as follows:

a $H^* = h \ (E^*, \ SE, \ EN, \ R)$
b. $E^* = e \ (H^*, \ Y, \ B^*)$
c. $B^* = b \ (H^*, \ Y)^7$

where:

H=Health status of the population measured by standardized mortality rates (SMR),[8]
E=Health expenditure *per capita*,
SE=Socioeconomic status measured by education level
EN=Environmental conditions measured by air and water pollution
R=Health behavior measured through food sales/consumption
B=Hospital beds *per capita*,
Y=Income *per capita*, and
* = Endogenous variable.

The first equation stands for the "health production function." It includes variables which are hypothesized to affect health either directly through genetics, behavior and environment, or indirectly through socioeconomic status indicating availability of resources to the population and how efficiently they are used.[9] This function is assumed to be identical for all regions. This assumption is fairly realistic given the uniformity of the Soviet centrally planned system.[10]

The last two equations delineate the commonly hypothesized short- and long-term aspects of resource allocation to health care in Russia under the former Soviet Union. In the short-term, as depicted by the second equation, budgeting (E) was (and by-and-large still is) based on number of beds (B), with some modification

---

[7] A graphical presentation of this system is provided in Appendix A.

[8] As such, this variable measures also "genetic" effects approximated by age and gender.

[9] The potential effect of socioeconomic status (*e.g.*, education) on behavior (*e.g.*, nutrition) is disregarded.

[10] The cities of Moscow, St. Petersburg and possibly other centers in particular localities serving the nomenclature, may have benefitted from superior technology and services

according to local health (H) and economic circumstances (Y). In turn, as described by the third equation, the number of beds (B) was based, in the long-term, on health status (H) and local economic circumstances (Y).[11]

This basic system of equations, where H, E, and B are simultaneously or co-determined, attempts to capture the relation between medical resources and mortality before the breakup of the Soviet Union when the situation was still stable. This is the situation Russia inherited, and can help explain the longer term relationship between variations in finance and changes in mortality in Russia today.[12]

The Health Production Function

The reported estimates, representing those with the best statistical fit and most explanatory power, at least for the health production function, are linear (Table 5). The measured effect of "health expenditure" on SMR is statistically insignificant. This suggests that, on the average and within the relevant data range, levels of health care expenditure across the Russian Federation (before the breakup of the Soviet Union) did not affect mortality.[13] This situation may also persist now, within the observed range.

The health behavior aspects of the health production function are estimated through consumption and education. Higher levels of bread consumption (per kilo of meat) are associated, although with limited statistical significance, with lower SMR.[14] These estimates support the hypothesized negative effect on health of risk

---

[11] The last two structural equations can be combined into a single reduced form equation which does not separate between long- and short-term allocation decisions mechanisms.

[12] Clearly, unless under severe conditions, as often happens in particular cases during the current transition period, E may not affect contemporary H. For estimation purposes, it is assumed, however, that there was a serial auto-correlation in each variable, $[\text{cov}(x_t, x_{t-1}) > 0$, where t indicates time], and that the data (Table 4) depict a reality that has been established over the years with the appropriate lags between dependent and independent variables.

[13] Some variables have been retained in the equation in spite of their statistical insignificance (*e.g.*, "treated air" for pollution) because they contributed to the fit of the estimated equations.

[14] Because *per capita* levels of consumption or sales of commodities are highly correlated, all commodities are expressed in terms of "per kilo of meat." High correlations still persist nonetheless among levels of consumption. The ratio of kilos of bread (per kilo of meat) is highly correlated with the ratios of fruit (0.48), milk (0.62), and sugar (0.67). These items can be considered the comparatively "good diet." At the same time, the ratio of kilos of eggs to meat is highly correlated with sales of liters of alcohol (0.60). These items and meat can be considered the comparatively "bad diet." Indeed, the first group has a negative effect on mortality. The effects of diet are more

factors such as animal-fat and energy-rich diets.

At the same time, levels of air pollution do not have the negative estimated effect on SMR. This finding may be related to better medical services in more densely urban centers. Still, the "urbanization" variable *per se* has no measurable effect on mortality.

Table 5 Two-stage least squares -
SMR, health expenditure *per capita* and beds as endogenous variables

Dependent variable	Standard Mortality Rate (SMR)		Health Expenditure		Beds	
	Coefficient	t Stat.	Coefficient	t Stat.	Coefficient	t Stat.
	(eq.1)		(eq.2)		(eq.3)	
Endogenous Variables						
Hlt. Exp.	-.1914145	-0.492				
SMR	.0963554	0.149	.7527026	3.384		
Beds	.7754963	1.510				
Exogenous Variables						
N.M.Prod.			.0062928	2.454	-.0003475	-0.317
R. Eggs	1.129818	0.309				
R. Bread	-11.56957	-1.842				
Air Pol.	-12.5536	-1.613				
Prim. Ed	-.2314875	-2.146				
Seco. Ed.	-.0948689	-1.156				
High Ed.	-.2813658	-2.548				
Treat.Air	.0357348	0.307				
% Urban	-.1581657	-0.859				
nca_reg	-8.977406	-1.521				
wes_reg	8.371794	1.738				
eas_reg	11.79001	1.768				
Constant	266.8839	3.272	-36.71578	-0.583	66.5356	2.936
Number of obs.	73		73		73	
F	2.11		3.17		5.78	
Adj R-square	0.1566		0.0829		0.1173	

pronounced in OLS estimates which are not reported here but available on request from the authors.

Education has the expected positive effect on health. Areas with more educated populations experience lower SMR, *ceteris paribus*. Education affects health positively in many ways, usually associated with better health behavior. It is noteworthy that, when the regional variables are removed from the equation, the education coefficients become more significant statistically, suggesting that part of the regional differences in SMR may be associated with regional differences in educational levels.

Even when controlling other variables including education that are hypothesized effects on SMR, some regional variations in SMR persist across regions, as measured by the coefficients on regional "dummy variables." Although with limited statistical significance, the eastern (eas_reg) and western regions (wes_reg) fare worse while the north Caucasus (nca_reg) fares better than the rest of the Federation.

The findings lend support to the argument about the apparently dominant effect of life-styles rather than of medical resources on mortality in Russia.

The Regional Resource Allocation Policy

The estimates reflecting medical resource allocation policy and mechanism (equations 2 and 3, Table 5) as "solidified" over the years by the Soviet regime, confirm the common hypotheses regarding allocation of health care resources in the former Soviet Union. Health care expenditures have been influenced, in the short term (equation 2), by the number of beds and by the state of the local economy, but not by SMR. In addition, while the effect of the "beds" is of limited statistical significance, the impact on health expenditure of the state of the local economy, as measured by the Net Material Product (NMP), is statistically robust. In terms of actual impact, the estimates, at the mean values of the relevant variables, suggest however that, on the average, a 10% higher number of beds (per 10,000 population) was associated with an 11% higher health budget, while a 10% higher NMP *per capita* was followed by a 2% higher health budget. That is, the health budget was particularly sensitive to the number of beds, as decreed by the Soviet authorities.

Simultaneously, in the longer term (equation 3), the number of beds was indeed determined, on the average, mainly by SMR, and not by the local income *per capita*. This lends support to the equalitarian approach of the Soviet authorities who, at least by this statistical account, invested in beds (whether effective or not) by SMR rather than by local income. Combining the results of the last two equations by substituting the third into the second equation, yields:

Health exp. = 15.3 + 1.55 SMR + 0.0057 NMP.

This particular reduced form presentation of the results suggests that, on the average, a 10% higher SMR induced a 22% higher allocation to health through the number of beds, compared with a 1.7% higher allocation for a 10% rise in the local product.

These combined estimates suggest a long term equalitarian allocation policy of health finance and resources by the Soviet authorities. "Beds" and local income levels influenced levels of health care expenditure in the short term. At the same time, "beds" were influenced by SMR, and not by local income. The findings shows a dominant effect of SMR and not local income on number of beds and level of health finance in a region.[15]

To sum up, at the end of the day, the system, while equalitarian, was ineffective and inefficient. Health finance and medical resources have not influenced mortality levels, while all other elements remained constant.

CONCLUSION

The statistical estimates discussed here capture mainly the Soviet legacy during the period before the break-up of the Soviet Union. Contrary to the currently unfolding state of affairs of growing inter-regional inequalities in health financing, the data suggest an equalitarian Soviet resource allocation policy to health. This policy appears to have been responsive to SMR and, by implication, to basic demographic variables, rather than to the state of the local economy. At the same time, within their range of data variation, the (cross sectional) data also suggest an ineffective system: levels of health care expenditures and medical resources did not influence SMR, although the potential to do so was there. This assertion is supported by long term data. Between 1965 and 1992 the number of beds per

---

[15] Capital expenditure norms for facilities, such as beds per population, were last approved in 1987. The most recent survey of medical facilities to determine their condition and general reconstruction needs was carried out in 1989. Thus the system was clearly left without federal norms and equalization mechanisms (Strusov, 1990).

1,000 increased in Russia from 9.8 to 13.1, a rise of 33.7%. Life expectancy at birth hardly changed over the period, and it remained at about 62.0 years for men and 74.0 for women. Crude mortality rates increased from 77 per 10,000 to 12.2 during the same period (Chernichovsky *et al.*, 1996). By comparison, in the United Kingdom, for example, the number of beds fell from 9.9 to 6.3 (1965-1990) during a comparable period, life expectancy for males rose from 67.9 to 72.8 (1961-1989), and for females from 73.8 to 78.2, with a change in crude mortality rates from 11.5 to 11.2 (Health Financing Review, 1992).

Hence, the data appear to suggest that, on the average, with Russian current medical technology and approach, health care financing -- within the 30% range of variation of the data -- may not influence health outcomes. That is, to raise life expectancy Russia needs to adopt new medical approaches, including health promotion, to combat the major causes of preventable morbidity and mortality (Chernichovsky *et al.*, 1996; Tulchinsky and Varavikova, 1996).

As for the future, even with the current Russian medical approaches and technology, it can be expected that the growing regression of health financing will resemble the state of each local economy, will eventually manifest itself beyond reduced supplies, deterioration of physical state of medical facilities, and lower real wages of medical personnel. Eventually, medical personnel, which has generally remained stable since 1991, will start migrating to wealthier areas. While this may lead to some gains in efficiency, in the regions falling behind, real resources may deteriorate to levels not yet captured by data that will inevitably adversely affect the already compromised health status of the population. This will also suppress developing new medical technology and approaches in those regions.

REFERENCES

ABT Associates (1993) Russian Federation and Territories Data Base. Mimeo. Moscow.

Chernichovsky, D., Barnum, H., and Potapchik, E. (1996) Health Sector Reform in Russia; the Perspective of Finance. *Economics of Transition*. 4(1): 113-134.

Chernichovsky, D., Potapchik, E., Barnum, H., and Tulchinsky, T. (1996) Health System Reform in Russia; Meeting Old and New Challenges. Mimeo. Ben-Gurion University of the Negev, Beer-Sheva, Israel.

Chernichovsky, D. and Potapchik, E. (1996) From Centralism to Federalism in the Russian Health Care Syste. Mimeo. New Economic School Moscow.

Chernichovsky, D. and Potapchik, E. (1997) Needed Financial Mechanisms to Achieve Health Sector Reform Under the Russian Health Insurance Legislation. *International Journal of Health Planning and Management* 12(4) In press.

Goskomstat (1993) *The Russian Federation in 1992.* Moscow.

Goskomstat (1994a) *Russian Statistical Yearbook.* Moscow.

Goskomstat (1994b) *Demographic Yearbook of the Russian Federation.* Moscow *Health Financing Review.* (1992) Tables 12,20,21,27,28.

Rowland, D. and Telyukov, A.V. (1991) Soviet Health Care from Two Perspectives. *Health Affairs.* Fall. 10(3):71-76.

Strusov, V.A. (1990) Results of Material and Technical Base of Medical Facilities, 1989. *All-Union Seminar on the Results of Pasportization (Census) of Medical Facilities.* Moscow. (Russian).

Supreme Soviet of the Russian Federation. (1991a) *The Law on the Local Authorities in RSFSR. Moscow.* (Russian).

Supreme Soviet of the Russian Federation. (1991b) *The Law on the Forming of the Budgets of Rayons, Cities, City Rayons, Towns, Rural Settlements and Other Administrative Territorial Units of RSFSR in 1991.* Moscow. (Russian).

Supreme Soviet of the Russian Federation. (1991c) *The Law on the Foundations of Budgets Structure and Budgetary Process in RSFSR.* Moscow. (Russian).

Supreme Soviet of the Russian Federation. (1993) *The Law on the Amendments and Additions to the Law on the Health Insurance of the Citizens in RSFSR.* Moscow. (Russian).

Tulchinsky, T.A. and Varavikova E.A. (1966) Addressing the Epidemiological Transition in the Former Soviet Union: Strategies for Health System and Public Health Reform in Russia. *American Journal of Public Health.* 86: 312-320.

Wallich, C. (1992) *Intergovernmental Relations in the Russian Federation.* World Bank: Washington, D.C.

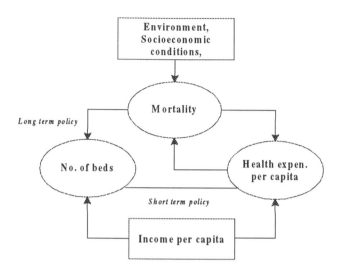

Appendix A Inter-relations between key variables

11

A Needs-Based, Weighted-Capitation Formula in Support of Equity and Primary Health Care: a South African Case Study

JANE DOHERTY and ALEX VAN DEN HEEVER
Centre for Health Policy
Department of Community Health
University of the Witwatersrand
South Africa

ABSTRACT

Government planners in South Africa are currently engaged in a complex debate regarding the proper approach to allocating financial resources to provincial health care services. This debate originates in a needs-based formula used by the Department of Health (DOH) to allocate the national health budget in 1995/96.

This paper critiques both the approach of the DOH and subsequent government proposals for the creation of consolidated, multi-sectoral budgets for 1997/98. The paper motivates for the continued use of a needs-based health care formula, but recommends adjusting it in crucial ways. More importantly, the paper points out

Health, Health Care and Health Economics: Perspectives on Distribution
Edited by Morris L. Barer, Thomas E. Getzen, and Greg L. Stoddart
Copyright 1998 John Wiley & Sons, Ltd.

that, if the government attempts to redress inequities too rapidly, it runs the risk of destabilising services and impeding the redistribution of real resources (such as personnel, facilities, equipment, and pharmaceuticals) to disadvantaged communities.

INTRODUCTION

The new South African government divided its first national health budget (1995/96) among the nine provinces on the basis of a needs-based, weighted capitation formula. Following criticism from several quarters, the formula was revised for the 1996/97 budget. In addition, discussions are afoot regarding the 1997/98 budget which, for the first time under the new system of fiscal federalism, will be distributed to provinces on a consolidated basis, rather than by individual sector (such as health, education, and transport). This will do away with a national health budget and a health care formula, allowing individual provinces to decide on the appropriate allocation to their health services.

The research on which this paper is based grew out of a concern that these government strategies for re-allocating resources have flaws which might inadvertently undermine the very health care goals they are meant to reflect, namely, the reduction of inequity and the strengthening of the district health system.[1] We believe that these concerns have been substantiated by recent developments and that a more carefully formulated and comprehensive approach to budgeting is required to achieve real shifts in resources towards under-developed areas and services.

This paper summarises our proposals for reforming the resource allocation process in South Africa, focusing on issues that may be of relevance to other countries, especially those middle-income countries experiencing considerable social inequity. The objectives of the paper are to:

1. examine methodological options for devising a needs-based formula within a data-poor context;

---

[1] The research was funded by the Health Systems Trust of South Africa. A detailed research report is available from: Centre for Health Policy, c/o SAIMR, P.O. Box 1038, Johannesburg, 2000, South Africa. The reports includes an extensive literature review of the experience of other countries with regard to resource allocation formulae.

2. suggest how such a formula may be applied to best effect;

3. highlight the political and technical constraints facing the development and application of a formula;

4. defend the need for a health formula as an instrument for ensuring an equitable distribution of resources between provinces, even within a federal system where consolidated provincial budgets are anticipated; and

5. highlight the limits of such a formula as an instrument of change.

The paper begins by commenting briefly on the structure of the government's health care formula and then discussing in more detail the problems associated with the timescale over which the formula was to be implemented. The paper then describes one approach to modifying the formula as well as its implementation, and proposes a continuing role for the formula within the new process of provincial budgeting. Finally, the paper concludes by suggesting processes and topics for research which are necessary to achieve more effective budgetary reform and enhance the re-allocation of resources.

DEFINITIONS

Before continuing it is necessary to clarify the terminology we use to describe health care facilities and the care that is delivered within them (see Box 1) (Doherty, 1994; Hospital Strategy Project, 1995 a, b). This terminology is useful for conceptualising the elements of a needs-based formula.

BOX 1
HOSPITAL CATEGORIES AND LEVEL OF CARE DEFINITIONS

Primary health care includes personal promotive, preventive, curative, and rehabilitative ambulatory care available through an outpatient department in a hospital, clinic, or GP's office, as well as non-personal health care.

Acute hospital care is provided in three categories of institutions:

> *Level I* patients require treatment which may be adequately and appropriately provided at a *district hospital* (the first level of referral) by a generalist with access to basic diagnostic and therapeutic facilities.

> *Level II* patients require the use of equipment and facilities found at a *regional or secondary hospital* (which represents the second level of referral), as well as the expertise and care associated with any of the following specialists: physicians (internists), general surgeons, orthopaedic surgeons, anaesthetists, paediatricians, obstetrician-gynaecologists, psychiatrists, general radiologists, and general pathologists. The hospital would be equipped with an intensive care unit. Level I patients can also be treated at a secondary hospital.

> *Level III* patients require the expertise and care associated with the sub-specialties and less common specialities (such as cardiology, endocrinology, oncology, organ transplantation, plastic and trauma surgery, neonatology, sophisticated paediatarics, and specialised imaging), or require access to scarce, expensive and specialised therapeutic and diagnostic equipment found only at a *central or tertiary hospital* (the third level of referral). Patients with uncommon ambulatory conditions who attend the hospital for highly specialised outpatient services are also classified as receiving care at this level. Level I and Level II patients can also be treated at a tertiary hospital.

> A tertiary hospital may also serve *Level IV* patients. These patients require sub-specialist care that is currently very costly or requires significant expertise. This type of care is not routinely available in the sub-specialty, is very new, and is usually found in only one or two hospitals in the country.

A *chronic hospital* is a hospital that provides long-term care for patients, usually after discharge from acute care hospitals. Psychiatric hospitals and tuberculosis hospitals are chronic hospitals. Psychiatric and tuberculosis beds may also occur in acute hospitals.

Academic care is care that is associated with a Medical Faculty. Academic care may be delivered from a hospital with beds at any level of care, or it may be delivered from a primary care facility in an ambulatory setting.

THE FORMULAE OF THE
NATIONAL DEPARTMENT OF HEALTH

THE STRUCTURE OF THE 1995/96 AND 1996/97 FORMULA

The 1995/96 formula was developed over the period of a month by a small group of provincial representatives. Pressure was intense to reach consensus on the structure of the formula quickly, and to demonstrate a commitment to redressing inequities rapidly. In the end, the 1995/96 national health budget was divided into a "top-slice" representing expenditure on activities that are of nation-wide relevance, and a "bottom-slice" representing expenditure on intra-provincial activities.[2]

The bottom-slice was redistributed between provinces according to a calculation that weighted the base-year population of each province by the ratio of the provincial to national average per capita income, multiplied by a factor of 0.25. The weighting was supposed to reflect relative need for public health care due both to health status as well as the ability to afford private health care, but was not based on any systematic research. In 1996/97, the only major change to the formula was in the calculation of the base-year population as the crude population minus beneficiaries of medical schemes. These beneficiaries were assumed to make use of private health care.[3]

The top-slice was made up of allocations for the national Department of Health (DOH), nursing colleges and the supra-provincial activities of academic hospitals. These activities include training and research as well as the provision of highly specialised, referral services (that is, Level III and Level IV care).[4] These supra-provincial activities were funded by a single allocation which became known as the National Increment for Teaching, Education and Research (or NITER). NITER was assumed to be 25% of the budget of provinces which have academic hospitals.

---

[2] In this paper the term "formula" is used to describe the series of calculations which make up the top-slice and the bottom-slice. The formula is used for the allocation of recurrent budgets only.

[3] The formula did assume that beneficiaries do make some use of the public sector, estimated as 0.5 visits per capita per annum.

[4] These activities are regarded as supra-provincial as they contribute to the national pool of personnel and research, and also provide referral services to provinces without academic hospitals (under the current structure of the health system in South Africa, Level III and Level IV care are only provided by academic hospitals).

The top-slice achieved some re-distribution in two ways. First, in 1995/96 a 5% cut of the budget of academic hospitals was allocated to an equalisation fund, to be spent on the recurrent cost of new clinics built under the government's Reconstruction and Development Programme. Second, we estimated that the method for calculating NITER implied large cuts for the provinces of Gauteng and Western Cape which have several academic hospitals, and increases for Eastern Cape and KwaZulu/Natal which have few academic hospitals (see Table 1). This was because the figure of 25% was applied to all the provinces with academic hospitals, regardless of the actual ratio in each province of expenditure on academic hospitals to expenditure on other health services.

**Table 1 Our Estimation of the Costs of Supra-Provincial Activities
as a Percentage of Provincial Expenditure (1995/96)**

Provinces with academic hospitals	Supra-provincial expenditure as a % of total provincial expenditures (1995 Prices)
Eastern Cape	6*
Free State	24
Gauteng	38
KwaZulu/Natal	10
Western Cape	33
Total	**25****

* This province was not allocated any funds for NITER according to the 1995/96 DOH formula
** It is coincidental that this national average is the same as the figure used by the 1995/96 formula

THE TIMESCALE FOR IMPLEMENTATION

The DOH proposed that the equitable allocation of the bottom-slice should be achieved by the year 2000. This means that the gap between the position of the most over-resourced province (Western Cape at 46% above the target allocation at equity) and the most under-resourced province (Northern Province at 85% below target) has to be closed within five years. Furthermore, the DOH believed that provinces should move 30% of the distance towards their target allocations in the first year. This meant that in 1995/96, Northern Province and Northern Cape experienced the largest increases in their total budgets[5] (14% and 10% respectively, in real terms) while Western Cape and Gauteng experienced the largest cuts of 21% and 20% respectively, in real terms (see Table 2).

Table 2 Target Percentages of the 1999/2000 Budget, and the Percentage Change in the Budget in the First Year of Implementation, as Calculated by the 1995/96 Governmental Health Care Formula, By Province

Province	% of population (1993)	target % of 1999/2000 budget*	% change in the budget in the first year of the formula (in real terms)**
Eastern Cape	16.37	14.8	- 7.60
Free State	6.89	7.1	-13.24
Gauteng	16.82	17.6	-20.01
KwaZulu/Natal	21.00	21.9	- 7.50
Mpumalanga	6.97	5.5	4.46
Northern Cape	1.88	1.7	10.06
Northern Province	12.58	14.5	14.04
North West	8.61	7.2	- 5.73
Western Cape	8.89	9.7	-21.58

* These percentages refer to the total budget, including both the bottom-slice and NITER allocations
** An inflation rate of 10% is assumed

THE LIMITATIONS OF THE DOH FORMULAE

We believe that the DOH formulae attempt a redistribution of resources that is both too extensive and too rapid, particularly given the necessarily slow pace of planning for change. The consequences are summarised in Box 2 and point to both the creation of instability in the health services as well as the failure to re-distribute real resources (such as personnel, drugs and supplies, and facilities and equipment) on the ground.

---

[5] The total budget of provinces includes both the bottom-slice and NITER allocations.

BOX 2: UNINTENDED CONSEQUENCES OF THE DOH FORMULAE

In under-resourced areas new funds may not be absorbed into the services for which they are intended because it takes time to create new facilities, employ new personnel, and otherwise develop capacity. As a result, spending could occur on services which are not the highest priority, especially when these services are already up and running or have a high public profile (such as hospitals in urban areas).

There is poor staff morale in provinces targeted for large cuts. Skilled staff leave the services, staff strike or productivity worsens. On the whole, services are de-stabilised and community members are dissatisfied.

Access to referral services for poor provinces could worsen as referral centres cut back on their activities across the board, rather than focusing on cutting low priority activities.

The large poor populations in the provinces receiving large budget cuts may not experience an improvement in services commensurate with other parts of the country.

The poorer provinces experience a surplus at the end of the year, while the richer provinces have deficits.

As a result of the above factors, re-distribution does not occur as planned (and some money may even be wasted on low-priority services) leading to disaffection amongst political constituencies.

Unrealistic budgeting could be encouraged because there is only a weak association between budgets and actual expenditure. As in the past, this could lead to health planners disregarding the budgetary process as a planning tool and indulging in "budget games". This is a problem not only in provinces which experience large cut-backs, but also in poorer provinces which feel they did not receive a fair allocation.

As the assumptions of the formula are contested, rivalry between provinces is promoted instead of co-operative, integrated planning. Revisions to the formula become associated with the interests of individual provinces rather than with the real needs of the country.

With the introduction of the new provincial budgeting system, previously planned changes to the size of provincial health budgets (especially rapid growth) are rejected by provincial administrations because they imply budget reductions for other sectors in the province, rather than reductions in the health budget of other provinces.

Interestingly, evidence is already beginning to emerge that provinces receiving large increases in their allocations have been unable to consume their entire budgets, while provinces which received large budget cuts have in reality maintained their expenditure. It also seems that the equalisation fund has not been spent.

AN ALTERNATIVE FORMULA: METHODOLOGY

OVERVIEW

We have suggested that the DOH formulae might result in inappropriate shifts of funds between provinces which will lead to limited transformation of health services on the ground. We believe this for two reasons. First, the data and methodology used to construct the formula are flawed. Even within the severe data constraints faced by South Africa we believe that it is both necessary and possible to design a more accurate formula based on rational assumptions derived from the available information. Second, the proposed pace of re-allocation is unrealistically rapid, failing to take into account macro-economic factors and organisational constraints. We address these two issues separately in the following paragraphs, focusing on our approach rather than our results. To make our discussion less abstract, however, Table 3 shows how the relative allocations to provinces would differ from that proposed by the 1995/96 DOH formula, using our methodology. Both the relative positions of provinces at equity, and their projected positions in 2000/01 according to three possible scenarios, are presented. We believe that Scenario 3, which assumes zero real growth in the national health budget, is the

Table 3 Comparison of the Relative Position of Provinces Using the DOH Formula, Our Formula and Likely Scenarios for the Pace of Change

Province	Target % of budget in 1999/ 2000 (DOH)	Target % of budget (Doherty and van den Heever)	Projected % distance from target in 2000/01, Scenario 1: 2% real growth p.a.	Projected % distance from target in 2000/01, Scenario 2: 0.5% real growth p.a.	Projected % distance from target in 2000/01, Scenario 2: 0.0% real growth p.a.
Eastern Cape	14.8	15.7	-14.67	-15.32	-14.93
Free State	7.1	7.4	-1.82	- 1.79	- 2.27
Gauteng	17.6	21.4	10.59	12.77	12.68
KwaZulu/Natal	21.9	19.1	-1.08	0.73	1.14
Northern Cape	1.7	1.3	18.31	20.84	20.88
Nothern Province	14.5	12.1	-13.33	-14.83	-14.55
North West	7.2	7.5	-12.69	-18.46	-18.68
Western Cape	9.7	9.3	40.41	45.82	46.31

most likely scenario. This is because of the government's commitment to the servicing of international debt and the focus of the Reconstruction and Development Programme on infrastructural development.

AN APPROPRIATE METHODOLOGY FOR CONSTRUCTING A FORMULA

Division of the Existing National Budget Into Service Categories

Budget information provided by the provinces may be analysed according to institutional categories (first column, Box 3). By using information from selected studies and applying several assumptions, we converted expenditure information on institutional categories into expenditure information on service categories (second column, Box 3). Service categories are more useful for planning purposes and amenable to manipulation by a formula, as will become clear in subsequent paragraphs. The conversion necessitated three sets of calculations.

The Calculation of the National Allocation for Training, Education and Research (NATER)[6]

Information on the extra costs to academic hospitals of accommodating teaching, education and research activities was available from the Western Cape (Strachan, 1994). We used this information to calculate a cost per student (undergraduate medical, surgical and dental): this cost was then used to calculate the extra costs to hospitals in other provinces. This approach assumes that the Western Cape level of expenditure per student is appropriate and that all provinces should enjoy this level of expenditure.[7] This is of course not necessarily so, and we return to this issue later.

---

[6] We use the term NATER as opposed to NITER to emphasise the fact that it is conceptualised entirely differently and that it is, after all, an allocation rather than an increment.

[7] It also assumes that the distribution of expenditure on other categories of student is similar to that of medical, surgical, and dental students. We were unable to test this assumption, given data constraints.

BOX 3
CONVERSION OF INSTITUTIONAL INTO SERVICE CATEGORIES

Institutional categories	Service categories
DOH	DOH
-	NATER
Nurse training	Nurse training
Academic/tertiary hospitals	-
Regional hospitals	-
District hospitals	-
-	Level III hospital services
	Inpatients
-	Outpatients
-	Level II hospital services
-	Inpatients
-	Outpatients
-	Level I hospital services
-	Inpatients
-	Outpatients
PHC : personal	PHC : personal
PHC : non-personal	PHC : non-personal
Specialist psychiatric hospitals	Specialist psychiatric hospitals
TB hospitals	TB hospitals
Ambulance services	Ambulance services
Administration	Administration

The Allocation of Expenditure in Academic/tertiary, Regional and District Hospitals to Level I, Level II and Level III Care

Government surveys in hospitals in three provinces had estimated the proportion of patient days at each of the three possible levels of care (there is no information on Level IV care in South Africa at present, and expenditure on this level is included *de facto* in the NATER allocation) (Brown and van den Heever, 1994; personal communication with Dr. R. Broekmann, 1995; Provincial 1995/96 budgets). These estimates were extrapolated to all provinces, with some of care. Because of methodological constraints, these calculations probably underestimated expenditures on Level III care which, for the purposes of a formula, is more acceptable than an overestimation. This is because of the need to re-distribute resources from higher to lower levels of care. Sensitivity analyses performed suggested that even fairly large errors in our estimates of relative expenditure on different levels of care would not result in large changes to target provincial allocations.

The Separation of Costs for Each Level of Care into Outpatient and Inpatient Costs

Some South African data suggest that the cost of an outpatient visit in a district hospital is 43% of the cost of an inpatient day, while in regional and academic/tertiary hospitals it approximates 70% (Lombard *et al.*, 1991). We extrapolated this information to calculate the national costs associated with inpatient versus outpatient care at each level of care.

Calculation of the "Top-Slice"

The procedure for converting institutional categories into service categories allowed us to estimate provincial and thus total national expenditure on each sort of category. The next step was to decide which part of the national budget would be redistributed by means of a formula, and which part would be reserved as a "top-slice," representing national functions. In contrast to the DOH approach, we argue that Level III care should be included in the top-slice. This is because Level III care is presently concentrated in a few provinces, and it is unclear at the present time whether the government will attempt to decentralise these services to the remaining provinces or focus on improving the access of patients in such provinces to highly specialised services. Also, a political decision still needs to be made on whether total Level III expenditure should be cut and how to manage such cuts, especially in terms of the effect on personnel.[8] Thus, according to our

---

[8] This is particularly important given the fact that academic hospitals have experienced widespread strikes in the recent past, and that many disaffected staff in key positions are being attracted into the private sector.

recommendations the top-slice consists of expenditure on the DOH, nurse training, NATER, and Level III care. NATER and Level III expenditures are distributed between provinces currently engaging in these activities, on an equitable basis as described above.

Redistribution of the "Bottom-Slice"

Our methodology for calculating the formula by which the bottom-slice is re-distributed differs from that of the DOH. First, we believe that it is inappropriate to use the base-year population as the denominator in per capita estimates. This is because of changes in the relative distribution of the population over time, due to differential growth rates and migration. In our calculations we use the projected population for 2000/01, for the sake of comparison with the DOH formula.

Secondly, we believe that the purpose of the public health budget is primarily to provide services to people unable to pay for services (either in the public or private sector). This is said in the context of recent government proposals to introduce a form of social health insurance which would extend health care coverage for employed people. We use the average of medical scheme membership (including dependents) and the number of employed people (including dependents) to estimate the number of people able to afford their own health care.[9] This number is subtracted from the total population in each province.

Thirdly, we believe that the population should be weighted by indicators that reflect in considerable detail the relative need for health care of people of different sex, age and health status. Table 4 summarises the indicators we use to weight the denominator population used in calculating the relative distribution of national expenditure on each service category between the provinces. This approach allows us to re-distribute current expenditure on different service categories more equitably. It does not yet address the issue of re-distributing expenditure between levels of care, an issue considered later in this paper.

Two aspects of our methodology for weighting for relative need for health care require explanation. In terms of age-sex utilisation information, while South

---

[9] We use an average because not all people who can afford their own health care belong to medical schemes, whereas some employed people earn such small wages that they cannot afford their own health care.

**Table 4 Mechanisms for Weighting Populations for Differences
in Demographic Structure and Health Status, By Service Type**

Service Type	Weighting Mechanism to Reflect Demographic Structure	Weighting Mechanism to Reflect Health Status
Inpatient Services		
Acute, non-psychiatric, non-tuberculosis services	United Kingdom age-sex utilisation rates	Provincial to national ratio of PYLLs per death due to preventable causes
Psychiatric hospitals	Not weighted for demographic structure	Not weighted for health status due to insufficient data
TB Hospitals	Not weighted for demographic structure	Provincial to national ratio of PYLLs per death due to respiratory diseases
Outpatient Services		
Personal PHC services	Age-sex utilisation rates and costs of an essential PHC package as estimated by the Need Norms Project (Rispel *et al.*, 1996)	Provincial to national ratio of PYLLs per death due to preventable causes
Non-personal PHC services	Not weighted for demographic structure	Provincial to national ratio of PYLLs per death due to preventable causes
Emergency Services	Not weighted for demographic structure	Provincial to national ratio of PYLLs per death due to accidents, poisonings, and violence
Administrative Services	Not weighted for demographic structure	Not weighted for health status

African rates for primary health care services have recently been calculated (Rispel *et al.*, 1996), for hospital inpatient services we were forced to use rates from the United Kingdom. Bourne *et al.* (1990) found that the use of rates from developed countries affects the final outcome of calculations only very slightly, compared to the use of local rates.

Our choice of potential years of life lost (PYLL) as the indicator of health status is justified because it avoids the problem in South Africa of incorrect mortality rates due to under-reporting of deaths, especially in areas inhabited by disadvantaged populations. To calculate PYLLs one simply needs to know at what age reported deaths have occurred.[10]

CONCLUSION

The overall structure of the formula we propose is reflected in Figure 1. Table 5 summarises the degree to which our formula conforms to the principles for an appropriate needs-based formula as derived from the international literature (Doherty and van den Heever, 1996).

AN ALTERNATIVE FORMULA: APPLICATION

We believe that while the needs-based formula can be used to set hypothetical provincial resource targets, annual allocations should be determined by a combination of several factors which reflect the macro-economic context and organisational constraints within which the public health sector operates. These are:

1. the annual growth of the national health budget;
2. policies to shift resources into high priority services (such as primary health care services and district hospitals);
3. a 6% ceiling, in real terms, on the annual growth of provincial budgets and a 3% floor, in real terms, on the annual cutting of budgets;
4. the convergence of all provinces towards equity of expenditure on service categories such as Level II hospital care, Level I hospital care and primary health care services, as indicated by the bottom-slice; and
5. the actual expenditure by a province (as opposed to its budgeted expenditure).

The allocations for different scenarios in Table 3 are a result of modeling what changes are possible over a five-year period within the constraint of the overall size of the health budget (assuming a 2%, 0.5% and zero growth in the health budget

---

[10] We assume that deaths due to different causes and different ages are under-reported to the same degree in an area.

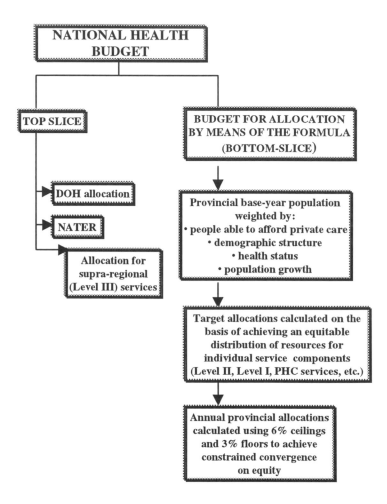

Figure 1 The Structure of an Alternative Formula

**Table 5 Conformity of Our Methodology to the Principles for an Appropriate
Needs-Based Formula Derived from the International Literature**

Principle	Extent to Which Our Methodology Conforms to This Principle
A formula should be simple, clear, and uncontroversial	While not as simple as the DOH formula, our formula more clearly defines different sorts of allocations and makes explicit assumptions on the basis of real data. This may promote a more objective debate concerning the merits of the formula, but could lead to controversy over changes in target allocations for provinces.
A formula must be robust (that is, not too sensitive to changes in data and assumptions)	Unfortunately, it is difficult to create a robust formula given the paucity of data. However, we have consistently used actual data rather than make unfounded assumptions and have shown that one of the most rough calculations (that is, the level of spending on Level III care) is not very sensitive to changes in assumptions. Likewise, we have documented our assumptions and calculations to allow other researchers to perform sensitivity analyses on our work (Doherty and van den Heever, 1996). Of course, our assumptions need to be reviewed as new data become available.
A formula should avoid indications which reflect existing supply of services	This our methodology does with respect to the bottom slice, especially regarding our choice of a mortality indicator and the exclusion from the denominator of the population able to afford its own health care.
A formula should make use of indicators that are well and frequently recorded	This our methodology does, especially with respect to our choice of a mortality indicator.
A formula should correlate well with health risks and the need for health care	This we believe our methodology does, especially with respect to our choice of a mortality indicator, the use of age and sex utilisation rates, the exclusion from the denominator of the population able to afford its own health care, and the use of population figures projected to 2000.

(Continued)

Table 5 (Continued)

Principle	Extent to Which Our Methodology Conforms to This Principle
A formula should take account of:	
Demography;	This our methodology does by using age and sex-specific utilisation rates.
Health Status;	This our methodology does by using Potential Years of Life Lost as a proxy indicator.
Cross-Boundary Flows;	This our methodology does to some extent through allocating Level III care to the top-slice, as this care is only provided by four of the nine provinces. However, more research is needed to find mechanisms for compensating provinces for the treatment of Level II and Level I patients from other provinces. Also, proper referral policies that guarantee under-resourced provinces access to well-resourced provinces for specialist services are required.
The costs of teaching and research;	This our methodology does through the NATER estimate.
The Special costs of delivery in different areas.	This our methodology does not address. This is because there are no clear data on what these special costs are in different provinces. More research and policy is required in this regard.

per annum in real terms). Within the overall budget constraint resources are steadily shifted to relatively poorly resourced provinces as well as to high priority services. In other words, we go further than the formula proposed in the previous section by allowing the national level of expenditure on different service categories to reflect new national priorities. The shift of resources is constrained by a 6% ceiling on budget growth and a 3% floor on budget cuts, in real terms. Thus, our model includes four of the five factors listed above: the fifth one -- the extent to which provinces conform to their annual budgets -- is obviously dependent on expenditure data which become available on a year by year basis.

We estimate how shifts will occur between different service categories by making assumptions regarding the degree to which changes will occur in the number of students trained as well as per capita expenditure on each sort of service category. These assumptions are guided by our interpretation of national priorities (see Box 4) and, as we have already explained, are constrained by overall budget growth as well as ceilings and floors on the rate of change of individual allocations. As national priorities are translated into plans it will be possible to replace our intuitive assumptions with concrete information.

BOX 4
ASSUMED PRIORITIES FOR THE RESTRUCTURING OF HEALTH SERVICES WITHIN CURRENT RESOURCE CONSTRAINTS

The strengthening of *primary health care* services is a central objective of the government.

Hospital services are of lower priority than primary health care, and are targeted for rationalisation and efficiency improvements.

Within hospital services, *highly specialised* services are targeted for re-prioritisation.

As high costs are associated with the *training of medical doctors* and with *specialised medical research*, these activities are likewise targeted for re-prioritisation.

The country requires more *primary health care nurses*. This could be achieved through the re-training of professional nurses. The annual costs of re-training are not necessarily very high.

Current levels of *nurse training* are probably acceptable and could be maintained at existing levels. If there is any re-prioritisation of training expenditure, nurse training must be protected as nurses represent the foundation of the health system.

Existing levels of expenditure on *emergency services* are acceptable. If possible, these services should be protected from major expenditure reductions.

Current spending on *TB hospital services* is inadequate and should be increased if possible.

Specialist psychiatric services are regarded as important but probably there should be no growth in expenditure levels in real terms.

The *national Department of Health* is relatively well funded and could be subjected to cuts if necessary.

Our model predicts that provinces will not reach equity in the next five years, especially under the scenario of zero real growth in the national health budget which we believe to be very likely.[11] Of course, every effort needs to be made to encourage provinces to move towards equity. We believe that requiring realistic annual changes in budgets will serve as considerable encouragement. In addition, a variety of policies other than the needs-based formula should be implemented to support the attainment of equity. Most obvious amongst these, and relatively achievable in the short term, are mechanisms for ensuring access for patients from under-resourced provinces to highly specialised services which are only available in well-resourced provinces. For example, strict referral protocols and obligations could be enforced, and under-resourced provinces could be allocated the funds to purchase Level III services from other provinces. This would mitigate one of the most glaring inequities of the present system, namely, geographic differences in access to specialist care.

THE ROLE OF THE FORMULA IN A FEDERAL SYSTEM

As mentioned at the start of this paper, the government will distribute the 1997/98 national budget on a consolidated basis (Financial and Fiscal Commission, 1995). Under this system, provinces will receive a bloc grant to fund an array of sectors (such as housing, education, and health care). In future years, a few conditional grants may be preserved for services that are a high national priority (such as district health care). While this approach may be consistent with the level of provincial autonomy suggested by a federal system, we believe it is inappropriate to introduce it before the gross distortions within the health system are ameliorated. This is because, under this approach, the health department of each province will have to negotiate for its allocation with other sectors within the province. In an

---

[11] It is important to note that our figures assume that there are practical constraints on expanding and cutting back budgets by more than 6% and 3% in real terms, respectively. The slow shift in real resources (such as personnel and facilities) over the past two years bears this assumption out. However, it is possible to achieve large cuts in some areas if planning is thorough, purposeful and decisive. For example, some highly specialised units in some academic hospitals could be closed, as could wards in hospitals with very low occupancy rates. If this were to become the case, equity could be achieved more rapidly. Nevertheless, budget allocations should reflect these planned changes, rather than attempt to achieve them through the formula itself.

ideal world, provinces would allocate budgets to sectors on the basis of priority needs. However, in the real world, it is unlikely that provincial health departments will be able to capture large parts of the budgets formerly allocated to other sectors, even if health priorities demand this. This is because of the entrenched interests of each sector as well as the difficulty of transforming large bureaucracies. There is thus no guarantee of either the desired level of funding for health care, or of equitable inter-provincial allocations to health for services not subject to conditional grants. This is particularly so in some of the poorest provinces, such as the Eastern Cape, which have extremely poor health services but very costly bureaucracies due to the inclusion of former "homeland" administrations.[12] In such provinces there is likely to be enormous resistance to trimming the size of the bureaucracy in favour of service delivery, and therefore great difficulty in achieving the growth in health budgets originally envisaged by the DOH formula.

Thus, we argue for the maintenance, especially in the short to medium term, of a modified health services formula (remembering that this formula should attempt to achieve equity over a longer period of time than envisaged by the DOH formula). In other words, we argue that initially the entire provincial budget for health care should be made a conditional grant and be calculated on the basis of a health formula. In effect this would mean that a minimum standard for expenditure on health would be set for each province on an annual basis, shifting provinces towards equitable health expenditure over time. Such a compromise would protect the interests of the public health service and support provincial and national departments in their planning activities and motivation for more resources. Over time alternative standards could be developed which relate more directly to the types of services that should be delivered (for example, a package of PHC services or staffing guidelines). Provinces would remain free to spend at levels higher than the minimum standard but would have to do so through extra-budgetary sources (such as user fee collection at hospitals).

---

[12] "Homelands" were rural areas in which, under the apartheid government, the majority of Africans were required to live. People were designated to these areas on the basis of ethnicity.

CONCLUSION

We have discussed our methodology for the development and application of a formula, and have demonstrated that it is possible to devise an explicit and rational process even within the constraints placed by incomplete, inaccurate and inappropriate data. We stress that it is our methods, rather than our results, that are of importance. As new data become available our assumptions and figures can easily be adjusted within the overall framework. It is important that efforts to improve data are planned for the coming years.

We have also hinted at the role of a health services formula in moving provinces towards equity and shifting services towards high priority activities. We believe that our approach supports these twin objectives more effectively than the formulae proposed by government, and will result in a real shift of resources -- such as personnel, drugs, supplies, facilities and equipment -- on the ground. Box 5 summarises the value of our approach in supporting reform.

Nevertheless, we stress that it is foolish to rely on a formula as the main instrument of change. A whole range of decisions that complement and augment the virtues of a health care formula are required. Amongst these are policies addressing the re-prioritisation of services, plans to operationalise policies to ensure the transformation of service provision on the ground, and policies that support equity through other mechanisms (such as social health insurance and equitable referral protocols).

We appreciate that our message that equity cannot be achieved as rapidly as expected is not a welcome one. However, we have argued that practical and political constraints will make it very difficult to progress at the rapid pace envisaged by the Department of Health. On the other hand, we believe that it is possible to promote the reallocation of resources in a more planned and speedy manner than implied by the Financial and Fiscal Commission's proposals for consolidated budgets. We argue that both sets of government proposals could hinder progress towards equity and hope that our research will prompt the development of a process which is better equipped to support the health objectives of the new government. This process will require extensive consultation with crucial actors in the budgeting system (among them, national and provincial heads of finance and service departments, national and provincial parliaments, and the Financial and Fiscal Commission), culminating in legislation.

We believe that the issues raised, and lessons learned, by the South African experience of resource re-allocation are of relevance to other countries which strive

---

BOX 5
CONTRIBUTION OF OUR PROPOSED APPROACH TO
SUPPORTING THE REDISTRIBUTION OF RESOURCES

Need is estimated more fairly and accurately, even within the existing data constraints

The disaggregation of expenditure data by service category allows low priority activities to be targeted for cuts

Changes in the annual budgets are achievable

A sustainable mechanism for ensuring long-term convergence towards equity is provided

Instability in the health system will be limited

The integrity of the budgeting process will be restored

The re-distribution of resources within the public health sector will remain consistent with overall changes to the provincial budgeting system

Progress towards change will be measurable against national guidelines

Provinces will still retain considerable flexibility around what services they provide, and how they provide them

The re-distribution of real resources (such as personnel), as opposed to financial resources, will be facilitated

---

towards redressing inequity and promoting primary health care, whether these countries operate under a centralised or decentralised budgeting system.

REFERENCES

Brown, M. and van den Heever, A. (1994) Report by the consultants on the existing expenditure trends and functional costs to support the function analysis and rationalisation programme in terms of the National Health Plan and the RDP. Unpublished report prepared for the PWV Strategic Management Team.

Bourne, D.E., Pick, W.M., Taylor, S.P., *et al.* (1990) A methodology for resource allocation in health care for South Africa. Part III. A South African Resource Allocation formula. South African Medical Journal 77:456-9.

Doherty, J. (1994) *The distribution of health expenditure between levels of care: a literature review. National Health Expenditure Review,* Technical Paper No.2. Durban: The Health Systems Trust.

Doherty, J., McIntyre, D., Bloom, G., and Brijlal, P. (1996) Value for money in South African health care: findings of a review of health expenditure and finance. *Central African Journal of Medicine* 42(1):21-24.

Doherty, J. and van den Heever, A. (1996) *Issues in resource allocation: an inter-provincial formula in support of equity. A report to the Health Systems Trust.* Johannesburg: Centre for Health Policy.

Financial and Fiscal Commission. (1995) *The allocation of financial resources between the national and provincial governments: recommendations for the fiscal year 1996/97.* Midrand: Financial and Fiscal Commission.

Hospital Strategy Project. (1995a) *Defining hospitals by level of care: towards a consensus position.* Johannesburg: Hospital Strategy Project.

Hospital Strategy Project. (1995b) *The distribution of resources and services within academic hospitals: a pilot study. Draft research protocol.* Johannesburg: Hospital Strategy Project.

Lombard, C.J., Stegman, J.C., and Barnard, A. (1991) Modeling net expenditure of hospitals in the Cape Province. *South African Medical Journal* 80:508-510.

Owen, C.P. and van den Heever, A. (1995) *The inter-provincial allocation formula for the health budget: an analysis, and recommendations for a change towards equity.* Johannesburg: Health Policy Co-ordinating Unit.

Rispel, L., Price, M., Cabral, J., et al. (1996) *Confronting need and affordability: guidelines for PHC services in South Africa.* Johannesburg: Centre for Health Policy.

Strachan, B. (1994) *Recommendations and guidelines for allocating the health budget to provinces (first draft).* Prepared for the Health Care Financing Committee Advising the Department of Health. (Unpublished).

12

Equity in Managed Competition

CLAUDE SCHNEIDER-BUNNER
LATEC
Université de Bourgogne
21000 DIJON - France

ABSTRACT

The equity objective in European health care systems is clearly an egalitarian one. However, under the pressure of financial constraints, achieving greater efficiency is the main aim of the managed competition reforms. But what are their consequences for equity? This paper is based on the definition of three conceptions of equity — liberal, egalitarian, Rawlsian — applied to health and health care. While the reforms attempt to safeguard the egalitarian dimension (public funding), liberal equity is introduced (quest for efficiency and greater freedom). The consequences of the strategic behaviours (financial selection, cream skimming) entail protective measures for the worst-off. But how does this defense truly correspond to Rawlsian equity?

Health, Health Care and Health Economics: Perspectives on Distribution
Edited by Morris L. Barer, Thomas E. Getzen, and Greg L. Stoddart
Copyright 1998 John Wiley & Sons, Ltd.

INTRODUCTION

Since the early 1970s health economics and social justice studies have developed in parallel, the latter primarily in political philosophy but also in economics. However, the overlap between these two fields is a relatively under-explored area of research despite -- or perhaps precisely because of -- the fact that from the outset one of the primary aims of European health care systems has been to guarantee equal access to health care.

In the current context of containment of health spending at a time when countries throughout Europe have engaged in reforms aimed primarily at improving efficiency it is worthwhile comparing health economics and theories of justice. What concepts of justice can be envisaged with regard to health or access to health care? Which of these concepts lie behind the health system reforms?

In this chapter I shall be looking more particularly at the consequences -- in terms of equity -- of those reforms that foster competition among health care providers and/or purchasers, which are new strategies in the quest for efficiency that are being tried out or contemplated in Europe. On which concept of equity is the managed competition model based? To answer this question we need first to ascertain from contemporary theories of social justice which concepts of equity are applicable to health and health care. Then the criteria for equity thus defined can be used to elucidate those concepts of equity that underpin the quasi-market model.

EQUITY IN HEALTH AND HEALTH CARE

Contemporary thinking provides a striking contrast between the importance attached to the notions of justice and injustice and the difficulty involved in defining them. Health is no exception: while in Europe equal access to health care is viewed as one of the main goals of health systems, it remains unclear quite what is really meant by this. This contrast can be largely explained by the complexity of the notion of justice, which complexity is illustrated by the diversity among theories of justice whether propounded by political philosophers or by economists underscoring the "ethical approach" of their discipline.[1]

To impose some sort of order on this diversity, two organizing principles are

---

[1] As opposed to the "engineering approach." These expressions are taken from Sen (1987).

used to identify three theoretical standpoints. The first principle is based on the distinction between outcome and procedure: some argue that justice should apply to the outcome or consequences of actions, while for others justice is a matter of procedure or deontology. The second organizing principle makes use of the link between theories of justice and the concepts of equality, freedom and efficiency which more commonly crop up in analyses of health systems.

The combination of these two principles leads us to the following three standpoints:

- an egalitarian standpoint uniting consequentialist theories for which the justice of a situation is measured by the equal distribution of a specific outcome;
- a liberal standpoint grouping deontological theories where the fairness of a situation depends on the transactions that contributed to its development and is based on the respect of individual freedom and the efficiency of market mechanisms;
- a Rawlsian standpoint combining aspects of both ends and means while seeking to combine equality, freedom and perhaps to a lesser extent efficiency.

Each of these theoretical standpoints can be applied to health -- the ultimate objective of health systems -- and to health care -- the intermediate objective (Table 1).

Table 1 Criteria of Equity for Health and Health Care

	Health	Health Care
Egalitarianism		
Negative	Equal health	Equal access
Positive	Equal right to health	Equal treatment for equal need
Liberalism		
Libertarianism	Health =Initial endowment	Access according to market rules
"Redistributive" liberalism	Special good	Mixed: market + distributive principle
Rawlsism	Equity as choice	Free access + responsible
Equality of opportunity		attitude through funding
	Fair equality of opportunity	Access to minimum
Equality of resources		level of care
	Selected outcome	Differential criterion

EGALITARIAN EQUITY

Although pure egalitarianism has lost much of its relevance (wouldn't a society where individuals were equal in *every* respect be both undesirable and unachieveable?), the egalitarian view of equity still remains the most widespread conception, as is obvious from the way equity and equality are commonly assimilated. Egalitarianism reappears in the shape of *specific egalitarianism*[2] propounding equality for certain aspects only of distribution, such as the enjoyment of property or fundamental rights or again the satisfaction of certain needs. Health is obviously one of the prime areas in which to apply egalitarianism of this kind.

Contemporary egalitarianism is based on two types of argument. A first set of arguments is derived from egalitarian justifications of the welfare state. On the one hand, the welfare state is founded on an egalitarian ideal that prioritizes the fight against inequalities in people's conditions. It is not a matter of imposing perfect equality but more pragmatically of tending towards this by *reducing inequalities*. On the other hand, in a more positivist version based on the concept of human rights, the egalitarian criterion of justice is one of *equal rights*: showing equal consideration to every individual for the respect of his human dignity also means respecting his social rights, *i.e.*, material living conditions, education, health or culture.

A second type of egalitarian argument picks up on the theme of *equal satisfaction of needs*, derived from the communist ideal. Although the idea of distributing all commodities according to the needs of each is no longer really applicable nowadays, the principle of "to each according to his needs," borrowed from utopian socialism and advocated by Marx for communist society, remains a distributive principle of primary importance for certain special goods such as health.

These egalitarian justifications have inspired many interpretations for health or access to health care. With regard to state of health first, three egalitarian criteria can be made out. With regard to health care, two further criteria can be envisaged.

---

[2] The term is from Tobin (1970).

Equality for Health

The criterion of **equality of health** can be defined within the logic of the egalitarian ideal. Since the purpose of health systems is to produce health, it is to this end result that equality should apply. But as it is impossible to attain this ideal, in keeping with the negative and more pragmatic version of egalitarianism, the criterion becomes one of reducing inequalities with regard to health. This is how, for instance, the WHO objective of equity is formulated in the "Health for All" programme set up in 1985: inequalities in health between countries and between social groups in the same country should be reduced by 25% by the year 2000. The scope of a health policy including the objective of equal health encompasses a vast area: from food to housing and working conditions, not omitting health care. This all-round approach to health is both the strong point of the criterion —inclusion of all the factors that influence health -- and its weak point -- the health system cannot influence all the factors.

A. Wagstaff (1991) suggested **social welfare maximization** as a criterion, which has the advantage of effecting a synthesis between equal health and efficiency, understood as the maximization of health. For this he defines a social welfare function (SWF)[3] inspired by the works of Atkinson (1970) on the measurement of inequalities. This criterion may be likened to the previous one insofar as it explicitly recommends a reduction in health inequalities through a coefficient of aversion to inequality.

A positive definition of equality with regard to health can be derived from the concept of social entitlements: the criterion of equity is then one of **equal entitlement to health**. American workers dealing with health entitlement[4] have generally construed it as a negative right. In this sense, I am entitled to have no-one damage my health, just as my right to individual freedom implies that no-one is allowed to interfere with this freedom. It is, however, a liberal right. In Europe, by contrast, the right to health is more commonly understood in the egalitarian sense of a positive right. Everyone should be able to enjoy a satisfactory standard

---

[3] SWF takes the following form: $W = (\tau - 1)^{-1} [\alpha.h_A)^{1-\tau} + (\beta.h_B)^{1-\tau}]$ where h_A and h_B are measures of the health of two individuals or groups of similar individuals A and B, α and β are weightings associated with the health of A and B, and τ indicates the degree of aversion to inequality in health outcomes. See also their contribution to this volume.

[4] See for example Lee and Jonsen (1974), Beauchamp and Faden (1979), Siegler (1979), Daniels (1985).

of health, meaning in particular that the community has a duty towards each individual to implement the necessary resources to respect this fundamental right.[5]

All these criteria -- equal health, social welfare maximization and equal entitlement to health -- fail to constitute as such an adequate criterion of equity. They need to be supplemented by criteria for access to health care. The two approaches consisting in defining equity for health or for access to health care are, from this point of view, complementary.

Equality for Health Care Distribution

In health care, two separate interpretations of the egalitarian requirement can be made out: on the one hand, individuals should have the same opportunities to obtain care (equal access) and on the other hand individuals should enjoy identical care if they have the same needs (equal treatment).

According to the negative version of egalitarianism the objective is to prevent impediments to acquiring health care from arising: **equal access to health care** must be guaranteed. Le Grand (1982) suggests a first definition of equal access: two individuals have equal access to a good if they have to pay the same "price" -- in money terms and also in terms of distance and time -- to obtain it. This definition is weakly egalitarian because two individuals with different incomes would have to face the same outlay. A second definition by Olsen and Rogers (1991) stipulates that "people have equal access to a good if and only if they are able to consume the same quantity of that good." This definition is more egalitarian as it reduces the sacrifice (in terms of consumption of other goods) that individuals with low purchasing power must make when they have to consume health care. To eradicate inequalities in the standard of living caused by sacrifices related to health care consumption, Olsen and Rogers' definition should be supplemented by a condition of free health care. It is in this third and most egalitarian sense that equal access is understood in countries with national health services.

According to the positive version of egalitarianism, it is not just a matter of equalizing opportunities for access to health care but also of equalizing the

---

[5] Notice that this criterion could also be met by extending the Rawlsian principle of equal freedom to health. In this case, health should be considered as a basic right, whose equalization for all is required by this first principle.

exercise of this possibility. The criterion of **equal treatment for equal need** fulfills both of these conditions: equal access but above all equal use depending on needs. As Mooney (1992, p. 104) emphasizes, equal utilization depends on both supply and demand whereas equal access is solely a supply-side phenomenon. Culyer and Wagstaff (1993) presented different interpretations of need. Without going into detail it should be emphasized that these different interpretations lead to the same distribution pattern if formulated simply in terms of horizontal equity (equal treatment for equal need), but the implications are different with vertical equity (how can unequal needs be treated unequally). If practice needs can be measured in terms of morbidity, health care spending represents treatment, in this way the distribution of standardized expenditure among different income groups serves as an indicator of equality (or inequality).[6]

LIBERAL EQUITY

The common ground among liberal investigators is their faith in market forces: it is the rule for the smooth running of society as it is the only mode of coordination of individual actions that respects the two fundamental values of liberalism: individual freedom and private property. It is therefore commutative justice that is defended here: justice lies in voluntary exchange. Freedom and efficiency are ensured by this fair procedure. Inequalities, which are not unfair as long as the freedom/property pairing is respected, may be diminished by individual and charitable initiatives dictated by a sense of moral duty, pity or hope that help will be forthcoming if one finds oneself in the same situation, or even by collective action authorized by a social contract.

Two liberal currents can be distinguished: the intransigent liberalism of libertarians is illustrated by the theories of Hayek (1960, 1976) and Nozick (1974); the more moderate "redistributive" liberalism can be traced to contractualist theories such as those of Buchanan and Kolm. The specific feature of the second current --acceptance of redistributive intervention by the state -- has earned it the name of "redistributive" liberalism, the inverted commas being needed because it is at best restricted redistribution given that it remains

---

[6] This criterion and this method have been adopted in the European COMAC project for assessing equity in the health care system (Van Doorslaer, Wagstaff, and Rutten, eds., 1993). See also the contribution of A. Williams in this volume.

subordinated to the voluntary agreement of every individual.

Libertarianism

The application of the libertarian conception of justice to health and health care leads to two rules. First, **health is an initial endowment**, just like real property or money and other qualities of human capital. The distribution of this endowment cannot be challenged: inequalities of health are not unfair. By Hayek's conception of fairness, considering such inequalities as unfair would mean that someone can be held responsible for them, which would run counter to the fact that the social order is a spontaneous order.[7] In a Hayekian perspective of responsibility, each individual is responsible for his own state of health, which does not mean he could necessarily do something so as not to be ill or that he is necessarily meritworthy for enjoying good health. Awareness of their responsibility must lead individuals to modify the way they set about prevention and obtaining medical care regardless of whether they are really able to exercise their responsibility when they are ill.

Thus, if health is an ordinary good, it is clear that **access to health care** must **obey market forces**, *i.e.*, individual preferences, the attitude towards risk, and financial resources. For Nozick (1974) the advantage of the market lies in the fact that the market respects individual freedom. No health entitlement can be justified if not acquired by a transaction in keeping with the principle of voluntary exchange. The production of health care does not come within the remit of the minimal state. Hayek (1960) resorts to a utilitarian argument to justify allocation of resources by market principles: in accordance with the market principle of remuneration by productivity, those individuals for whom disease or infirmity causes the greatest loss (the most productive members of the active population) may receive priority treatment since they attribute a higher market value to health care.

A system of private insurance is more efficient than case by case payment, especially because of the marked concentration in expenditure. This system is private as everyone must be free to use their resources as they wish. Thus anyone who sets little store by his health, if he is prepared to take the risk, is free to elect

---

[7] For Hayek social justice is meaningless: as the notion of justice applies only to actions (or by extension to their perpetrators) and as social order is a spontaneous order, that is too complex to be the intentional result of one or even several deliberate actions, the idea of social justice means personifying society so as to judge its actions and therefore to deny its nature as a spontaneous order.

not to take out insurance or to choose inexpensive insurance contracts and to concentrate his resources on other things which, for him, have greater utility. A compulsory insurance system is unfair -- in the libertarian sense -- as people are no longer entirely free to use their own resources as they wish. The only transfers of resources authorized for aid to those excluded from health care are private and voluntary donations that are consistent with the donor's freedom of choice. For libertarians, needs can in no event be a pretext for claiming entitlements.

"Redistributive" Liberalism

The liberal conception that accepts redistributive intervention by the state can be distinguished from the libertarian position if individuals all agree to recognize that **health is a special good** requiring collective action that they will entrust to the state. While the market remains the general rule for acquiring most goods, partial aid may be awarded to individual beneficiaries for certain goods. The application of Buchanan's (1986) contractualist analysis to health would entail accepting that individuals are not responsible for unequal health due to birth but that such inequalities should be corrected.[8] For Kolm (1985) technical features of the health good could lead participants in the liberal social contract to authorize (limited) state intervention.

In this light, the libertarian position on access to health care may also be modified and **access to health care** will be governed partly by market forces and partly by **another distributive rule** decided in accordance with the wishes of individuals. However a question mark remains about which rule to use: the advocates of "redistributive" liberalism are divided about the justification of redistribution. Whether collective donations or compulsory insurance mechanisms (Kolm, 1985), or correction of unequal starting positions (Buchanan, 1986), redistribution would remain limited in any case, for example, to the form of minimum care of the "safety net" type. In addition, social transfers authorized by a liberal social contract are legitimate not because of any social entitlement of the beneficiaries but through the exercise of the freedom of choice of those who engage in the transfers.

---

[8] Subscribers to the constitutional contract would agree, according to Buchanan, on the necessity to equalize the starting positions. Inequalities caused by effort, choice, and chance, by contrast, do not warrant correction.

RAWLSIAN EQUITY

The publication of John Rawls' *Theory of Justice* (1971) fueled the debate on social justice not only in political philosophy but also among economists. While the theory has attracted libertarian responses and contractualist liberal responses, it has also fostered thinking on collective justice. The theories we include under the Rawlsian standpoint seek to reconcile freedom and equality and to combine procedure and end results. Like the theories of the liberal standpoint, they are procedural as the principles of justice apply to social institutions and not to concrete situations, and like those of the egalitarian standpoint they are consequentialist in that the principles of justice are selected from the end result of this procedure.

In Rawlsian theory, the principles of justice that should be applied to the basic social institutions are determined in the original position, a hypothetical situation in which anyone can place himself at any time to simulate impartial reasoning regardless of his personal interest or, in Rawlsian terms, by placing himself behind a "veil of ignorance." Rational and mutually disinterested individuals would agree, under the conditions of the original position, on the following principles of justice: first the principle of equal freedom (1) concerning public liberties and second, applying to socio-economic inequalities, the principle of fair equality of opportunity (2a) and the difference principle (2b).[9]

Two trends are found among the extensions of Rawls theories: on the one hand supporters of equality of resources (Dworkin, 1981a, 1981b; Van Parijs, 1990, 1991, 1995) and on the other hand the supporters of equality of opportunity (Sen, 1980, 1985, 1987; Arneson, 1989; Cohen, 1989). Fleurbaey's (1995) recent approach borrows from both forms.

Rawls avoids health-related issues.[10] Despite this, Rawlsian applications for health and access to health care can be envisaged. Two approaches have been suggested: that of Le Grand (1991) can be linked to the equal opportunity trend

---

[9] These principles of justice are arranged in lexical order (order of precedence). Principle 1 takes precedence over principle 2: this is the rule of precedence of freedom, which means in particular that basic freedoms cannot be restricted even on the pretext of improving the position of the worst-off. Then principle 2a takes precedence over principle 2b, which means for Rawls that the focus must fall on the chances of those who have least.

[10] He assumes, to simplify the analysis, that "everyone has normal physical needs so that the problem of special health care does not arise" (Rawls, 1974, p. 142).

while that of Daniels (1982, 1985) starts from equal opportunities and leads to equal resources. This paper propounds an application of the difference principle that is more akin to equality of resources.

Le Grand: Equity as Choice

Le Grand, like Arneson, starts from the idea that inequalities in welfare resulting from freely consented actions cannot be unfair (Le Grand, 1991). Arneson (1989) deduces from that the criterion of equal opportunity for welfare which is respected when individuals have an equivalent set of opportunities for living their lives. Cohen (1989) supports a similar view -- with the equal access to advantage criterion -- arguing that all involuntary disadvantages should be eliminated, *i.e.*, the negative effects "for which the sufferer cannot be held responsible" (Cohen, 1989, p. 916).[11]

Transposed to the case of health, this equal opportunity approach asserts that "disparities in health states that arise from fully-informed individuals exercising autonomous preferences facing the same range of choices over health and health-related activities are not inequitable; but disparities in health that can be directly related to differences in the constraints facing those individuals are inequitable" (Le Grand, 1991, p. 116). Implications in terms of health policy vary depending on the extent of individual responsibility. For illnesses related to uncontrolled factors, health care should be free for patients and paid for either by society or by whoever was responsible for the disease or infirmity if the origin can be clearly identified (*e.g.*, accident or contamination). For illnesses resulting from voluntarily accepted risks (sports, cigarettes, etc.) the application of the responsibility principle should, however, be tempered. If the illness arises for x% of people adopting this risky behaviour, anyone behaving this way is liable for x% of the costs arising from such risks, whether the risk was realised for that individual or not. Therefore, contribution to costs cannot be made at the time of care but must

---

[11] The idea of responsibility used by Arneson, Cohen and Le Grand is that of "responsibility by control" (Individuals are responsible for what they control fully) and not "responsibility by delegation" (whatever the extent of control) adopted in equality of resources by, for example, Rawls or Dworkin inasmuch as individuals are liable for their preferences (Fleurbaey, 1997). Equality of opportunity based on this strict view of responsibility is consequently somewhat egalitarian, as opposed to the liberal equality of opportunity (*e.g.*, the equality of starting positions of Buchanan (1986) where individual responsibility is extended to variables they do not necessarily control.

be made beforehand by a compulsory insurance for risky activities and taxes on risky products. All told, Le Grand recommends a health system providing **free care and responsible financing** combining progressive contributions (so as to equalize choice sets) and contributions for risky activities.[12]

Daniels: Fair Equality of Opportunity and Minimum Health Care

Daniels (1982, 1985), who proposes to apply Rawls' theory, first questions the nature of the state of health as a "good." How can the special attention it is afforded be accounted for? Rather than considering that normal functioning is a condition of happiness (it is possible to be happy although "diminished"), Daniels argues that good health is necessary for individuals so they can pursue their objectives or their "life plans." Health institutions make up part of the basic institutions that guarantee fair equality of opportunity (cf. Rawls' principle 2a) conserving for everyone the opportunity range open to them in society.[13]

This analysis may be likened to the idea of "capabilities" developed by Sen (1985, 1987) based on criticism of Rawls' idea of primary goods. For Sen, individual freedom cannot be guaranteed by simply making the same quantity of primary goods available: the true exercise of freedom depends not only on the resources available to an individual but also on his capability to transform those resources into achievements (which he terms "functionings"). Enjoying good health is part of the basic capabilities which Sen recommends should be equalized, just as Daniels considers health as a factor of fair equality of opportunity.

Daniels goes on to deduce from his conception of health a criterion of equity for organizing access to health care. The basic institutions should allow everyone to accede to **minimum health care**. The scale of this minimum comprises the "services needed to maintain, restore, or compensate for the loss of normal functioning" (1982, p. 73).[14] Therefore, the health system should satisfy as a

---

[12] These egalitarian implications (free care and progressive financing) were criticized by Pereira (1993) who judged that equity as choice should lead to more liberal implications. The disagreement is based in fact on the extent of individual responsibility (cf. preceding note).

[13] Daniels understands equal opportunity among equals (people with the same talents). Acknowledging that talents may be underdeveloped for social reasons, he recommends that such inequalities should be the subject of special policies (*i.e.*, education) as the health services are not intended to eradicate *all* inequalities.

[14] Note that this minimum level is more extensive than the liberal minimum, which is envisaged only to attenuate market forces.

priority those health needs that have a substantial impact on the range of opportunities. Daniels considers the possibility of a multi-tier health system: the minimum level, corresponding to needs that are judged important because of their impact on the opportunity range, includes the care that must be provided socially; the other levels, corresponding to subsidiary needs or wants, may also need to be covered by society but for other reasons.

Daniels starts from a concept of equal opportunity and finishes by recommending equal resources. In this he concurs with the approach of Van Parijs (1991, 1995) based on the principle of maximizing "real freedom for all." To ensure maximum real freedom, Van Parijs claims, everyone must be guaranteed a standard of living through unconditional redistribution in the shape of a universal allowance.

Differential Criterion

Finally a third Rawlsian approach may be contemplated through the difference principle (principle 2b) by which economic and social inequalities are only acceptable if they are to the advantage of the least well-off members of society. This approach is justified if it is considered that health is one of the selected outcomes in the sense of Fleurbaey (1995). For Fleurbaey only certain outcomes should be taken into account by redistributive social institutions. These outcomes are termed "primary functionings" for which society has been delegated responsibility. Fleurbaey further recommends that, for greater efficiency, equality of selected functionings be interpreted as a maxim in, just like the Rawlsian difference principle.

Generally, the necessity to compensate "handicaps" -- leading to some individuals being underprivileged -- is a common concern in Rawlsian theories. For Dworkin (1981b), for example, to bring about equal resources, the authorities must make transfers similar to those of a virtual market where individuals, aware of their preferences and their ambitions but unaware of their talents, guarantee themselves against the weakness of their internal resources, *i.e.* against lack of talent or the occurrence of handicaps. Van Parijs (1990) includes in his principle of justice a constraint of "undominated diversity," which implies compensation for individuals with special needs related to unfavourable internal endowments.

The third Rawlsian criterion requires a definition of the worst-off. In Rawls' theory, the worst-off are those individuals who have few social primary goods (including income and wealth[15]). The worst-off are, therefore, people whose health is threatened and the poorest. This third criterion, which may be termed the differential criterion, recommends then **different treatment for the poorest and the most seriously ill**: access to health care must be organized in their favour.

By way of conclusion to this outline of the criteria of equity, it is important to emphasize that the three groups of theories of social justice and the criteria they imply in the area of health do not purport to reply directly to the concrete questions asked by those involved in health systems. They nevertheless form a framework for analysis adapted to the evaluation of health systems. It is therefore on the basis of these three sets of equity criteria — egalitarian, liberal and Rawlsian — that in the second part of this paper I shall analyse equity in the model of managed competition as applied or envisaged in European health systems.

FORMS OF EQUITY ON QUASI-MARKETS

The difficulties encountered in exercising lasting control over health spending with the conventional means of regulation have led to the implementation of measures that are more incentive than coercive. The uncontrolled spiraling of health expenditure can be analysed as the result of malfunctions in a non-market economic set-up where the collective dimension of production and funding creates inefficiencies by altering the responsibilities of the various agents. The quest for efficient allocation of resources means introducing or bolstering certain market factors so as to change the rules of the game among the players. Managed competition on quasi-markets is part of such a strategy. The Netherlands and the United Kingdom have headed along this path and aroused interest in many other European countries, including France. Figure 1 shows a simplified diagram of these models of managed competition.

The creation of competition at the supply side is intended to encourage producers to cut health costs by making them responsible while leaving them greater scope for independent action. Competition is instigated by one (or more) purchaser(s) with whom the suppliers —whether public or private— negotiate contracts as to price, quantities and the quality of health care. In the UK, for

---

[15] In Rawls' classification, the primary social goods are income and wealth, but also the basis of self-respect, fundamental rights and freedoms, opportunity for access to different social positions and the power that goes with them.

example, independent public hospitals, which should in time be the only form of public hospital, are in competition with each other and with private clinics. This competition is fostered by two types of purchaser: the District Health Authorities, which have been transformed from passive paymasters into active health care purchasers, and the large medical practices which have the possibility of becoming fund holders (GPFHs) and buying the care required for their patients (except emergency care and highly specialized care that are still in the hands of the local authorities) from the different suppliers they choose depending on the value for money on offer.

Figure 1 Managed Competition in Health Care :
Examples from the Netherlands and the United Kingdom

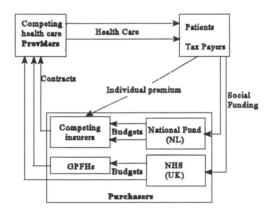

The creation of competition among health care purchasers completes the competition among suppliers. Thus the amount assigned to health care is no longer fixed externally by the authorities but by interaction with ultimate demand. Competition among purchasers is created by consumers through an individual premium paid to the insurer of their choice. This premium represents to some extent a market price because it varies with the individual preferences of the person insured (depending on his choice of any additional cover) and depending on the efficiency of the insurer (depending on its ability to manage its clients and negotiate contracts with health care providers). In the Netherlands, the reform has led to a double funding arrangement: one part is taxed and repaid by the national fund to each approved insurer depending on the risk its clients represent and the other part is paid by each individual to the insurer of his choice and includes a mandatory all-inclusive part for compulsory basic insurance and possibly an optional part corresponding to any additional cover opted for.

The inclusion of market mechanisms in health systems does not necessarily imply that a liberal conception of justice is in operation. While the creation of competition is part of a liberal approach it is still controlled and organized within the framework of health systems constructed around egalitarian logic. What is the concept of equity underlying these new health systems? It will become clear that the three dimensions are mixed: while the maintenance of some degree of egalitarianism is the stated objective where equity is concerned, the introduction of competition enhances factors of liberal inspiration, but specific measures for protecting the worst-off stem -- at least in part -- from Rawlsian logic.

EQUALITY THROUGH SOCIAL FUNDING

If there is any area in which equality is popular and considered as paramount, it is certainly that of health. Even the very liberal Margaret Thatcher stressed in the foreword to the White Paper that the National Health Service (NHS) should remain accessible to all regardless of income (Department of Health, 1989). As proof of this intention her government did not alter the arrangements for NHS funding: taxation remains the main source and free access to care provided by the public sector remains the general rule.

In the Netherlands the insurance market is a quasi-market. On the one hand insurance is compulsory to prevent free rider behaviour. On the other hand funding is socialized in part so everyone can be covered: part of the individual's health insurance contribution is paid from a common fund paid for out of income-related taxation. The distribution between the different sources of funding was modified by the Simons government which implemented the Dekker plan: the socialized share of funding was increased from 75% to 85%, reducing the individual share collected directly by the insurers to 15% instead of 25%. In addition, the setting up of a single social funding arrangement -- contributions proportional to income are payable to a single central fund -- supersedes the piecemeal funding system that was in place before the reform.[16] Thus, the introduction of a single and identical basic insurance system for all is steering the system towards greater equality in terms of entitlement to health, as the earlier distortions related to the dual private and public structure of protection against risk are done away with.

The maintenance of social funding should make it possible to conserve egalitarianism. This reasoning is based on the argument that runs "if the state (or compulsory health insurance) replaces individuals for the purchase of health care, then the arguments for rejecting the market related to externalities, incomplete information and *unequal access* are no longer founded" (Mougeot, 1993, p. 122, my italics). Consequently, the main threat for egalitarian equity as exercised by free market operation, namely unequal access to health care for those who cannot afford adequate cover -- because of insufficient resources or excessive needs -- would be eradicated through a collective agent purchasing health care for individuals. The separation of payment and consumption would guarantee egalitarian equity.

FREEDOM THROUGH COMPETITION ...
AND ITS ANTI-EGALITARIAN EFFECTS

The fostering of competition is also part of the liberal logic of equity in the sense that these reforms enhance the criteria of efficiency and freedom and propose using a fair procedure -- the market -- to satisfy both criteria at the same time. It is obviously still too early to assess the *efficiency* of the new incentive mechanisms, as they have been set up only recently. It seems though that the conditions required for success in terms of efficiency are not necessarily met in practice: question marks concern essentially the ability of health care purchasers to promote real competition, to maintain the standard of health care and to limit the size of transaction costs (see Culyer *et al.*, 1990; Le Grand and Bartlett, 1993). The *freedom* of agents is by contrast clearly favoured :

---

[16] Employees whose income was less than a fixed ceiling and beneficiaries of social allowances were affiliated on a compulsory basis to a public health insurance fund, paying income-related contributions; others were covered by private insurers and paid nominal contributions, increasingly differentiated by age and risk; finally, a compulsory special scheme covered the population as a whole against serious risks.

- the freedom of health care consumers covers the choice of doctor, even if he still acts as "gatekeeper" (in the UK patients still need to be registered with a GP, although it is easier to change) and on the choice of health care purchaser (choice of insurer in the Netherlands, and more limited choice —as it is not applicable to all health care— between the various GPHFs in the UK);

- the freedom of health care producers, especially price fixing and negotiation of quantities for contracts;

- health care purchasers enjoy not only the freedom to choose the health care providers with whom they wish to contract (this freedom is the basis of competition among suppliers) but also a margin for manoeuvering that allows them to some extent to choose the insurance subscribers or patients whose budget they manage.

However, this freedom that guarantees liberal justice has a downside, in a real context of imperfect competition marked by the existence of incomplete information among agents, in the form of certain strategic behaviour patterns that are contrary to egalitarian justice.

Risk selection or "cream skimming" is a first illustration of this (Van de Ven and Van Vliet, 1990; Matsaganis and Glennerster, 1994). Even if common effort in funding involves the NHS or the National Fund, hesitation about certain profiles is possible if the budget allocation arrangements do not make fine enough distinctions. Fundholders and approved insurers will prefer risks for which the budget received is higher than expected costs and will avoid patients in need of expensive treatment. Obviously for reasons of reputation or professional ethics the most direct forms of risk selection will not be used. There are, however, more subtle forms that should not be overlooked. Budget administrators could, for example, abstain from making contracts for particularly expensive care, implicitly diminishing the array of risk they cover, or conversely, achieving a good reputation for specialist care (*e.g.*, that related to maternity) in order to attract the least expensive age groups. The danger of risk selection is amplified in the Netherlands for two reasons. On the one hand because it can be anticipated that the ethical barrier of private insurers is not as good a guarantee as that of doctors. And on the other hand because insurers technically have more scope for exercising risk selection: by targeting their advertising or by specialization of their operations, they can attract the more solvent social categories (through contracts for the per-diem compensation of the self-employed) or good risks (additional contracts on specific leisure activities, such as winter sports or water sports, which would procure them a young and active client base, *a priori* in good health and relatively well-off).

The phenomenon of risk selection is compounded by that of **financial selection**, especially in the Netherlands.[17] Competition among insurers is based on the individual premium that each person insured pays to the insurance organization of his choice. This premium depends on the additional rate of cover and the insurer's activity (the price and quality of health care are negotiated with the providers). While everyone has the possibility of deciding on additional cover, they still need the financial resources to choose the adequate cover. The smaller the share of social insurance, the more difficult it will be to prevent people on low incomes from "choosing" the most restrictive forms of cover or even opting for cheap contracts regardless of the quality of care.

Thus, even if individuals all have in theory the same opportunity to accede to health care, the position may in practice contradict the two egalitarian criteria for access to health care: "poor risk" individuals do not enjoy equal access to health care if they are discriminated against, as risk selection is an obstacle for them; and for equal needs, the poorest will be unable to enjoy the same treatment if financial selection and the lack of supplementary cover that it entails prevent them from obtaining the necessary care.

PROTECTING THE WORST-OFF: RAWLSIAN EQUITY ?

In the UK as in the Netherlands the lawmakers have endeavoured to counteract these inegalitarian tendencies by resorting to Rawlsian type measures so that the least-favoured are not left on the sidelines in the quest for efficiency. A number of measures can be listed aimed at protecting those who are most seriously ill and/or present the highest risks against risk selection and at protecting the poorest from financial selection.

In the UK the danger of risk selection has been restricted in that the fund holding practices receive special financing for particularly expensive care.

---

[17] In the UK a link between financing and access to health care is introduced through a tax cutting arrangement for private insurance premiums for the elderly paid by them or by members of their family. Although the effects of this measure should remain restricted, the orientation towards the private sector is made explicit.

Treatment in excess of £5,000 is not included in the fund holders' budget but is covered directly by the NHS (Le Grand, 1992). This system means high risk patients are not threatened with being ousted... but on the other hand it does encourage doctors to increase the prescriptions of certain patients to reach the £5,000 threshold or no longer to limit costs once it is exceeded.

The Dutch reform has introduced two rules against the exclusion of "poor" risks that the insurance organizations must comply with to be entitled to manage the health risk. It is prohibited, first, to refuse to insure an individual, and, secondly, to adjust the additional premium depending on the risk the insured represents. These rules are justified in particular by the fact that the annual health contribution paid to the insurer from the National Fund already takes into account the characteristics of sex and age that are supposed to represent the risk, which, borne socially, no longer need be borne individually.

Finally, to limit the danger of financial selection, the Dutch government has extended basic insurance to dental care and medicines covering 97% of the health services instead of 85% as recommended by the Dekker commission. This extended basic insurance may be construed as the minimum level of care for all defended by Daniels. The basic level has been defined as encompassing "everything that can ensure each person independence and a place in society, or even more simply anything that protects the existence of members of a society" (Pomey, 1993, p. 34).

Despite these protective measures, two problems remain. Is the defense of the worst-off, as exercised, appropriate? And more fundamentally does this defense truly correspond to Rawlsian equity?

1. There is a willingness to protect the least-favoured but are these measures adequate for the task? First, in the face of financial selection, although the problem is more conventional (to what extent does the lack of additional cover entail foregoing the necessary care?) the solution is no simpler for all that. The solution also depends on factors that extend beyond the health system, especially the extent of social inequalities and the degree of poverty. If the proportion of the population liable to give up useful health care is small, a system of efficient social aid may be adequate, which is not necessarily the case when this proportion of the population increases. From this standpoint, the increase in relative and absolute poverty in the UK during the last ten years (Boyle and Le Grand, 1995) combined with the development of privately funded health care must inspire watchfulness despite the current weakness of financial selection mechanisms.

It is by no means certain that risk selection can be avoided by financial incentives as in the UK (selection is carried over to risk within a certain limit) or by regulations as in the Netherlands, as the financial interests of the insurers encourage them to get round such obstacles (how can the more subtle forms of selection be prevented?). Furthermore, two changes to the fundholding terms in the UK have increased the danger of cream skimming by reducing the sharing of risks: the minimum required size to become a GPFH has been lowered from 11,000 to 7,000 patients registered with the practice and the range of care covered by the fund holding has been extended too. To reverse this trend, Matsaganis and Glennerster (1994, p. 56) suggest setting up "risk sharing arrangements between practices [...] such as the establishment of a large contingency fund financed by contributions from the practices." For the Netherlands, where the problem is more worrying, one possible solution —that has been considered— is to change the status of health insurers to a non-profit making mutual insurance type of organization (Hamilton, 1992).

2. Are these measures for protecting the worst-off truly Rawlsian? Is it not rather "redistributive" liberalism that has been implemented in the guise of Rawlsian justice? True, it is difficult in practice to draw a dividing line between what is "redistributive" liberalism (decent minimum, assistance for the worst-off) and what would correspond to the introduction of new community support along the lines of a "Rawls-type" social contract. The many attempts at recuperation of Rawlsian theory are evidence of its ambiguity. If all that is borrowed from Rawls is the "maxim in" principle (maximization of the position of the worst-off) it is certain that this comes close to the liberal version of equity for which social effort focuses, in assistance logic, on the worst-off.

It is debatable, though, whether that is the most faithful interpretation (or the most promising) of Rawlsian theories, for which it is less a matter of maximizing the situation -- in terms of results -- of the worst-off, but of the resources or opportunities they can take avail of in order to achieve their ends. Construed in terms of equal resources or equal opportunities, Rawlsian justice is a more exacting and more egalitarian standard of justice which, when applied to health and access to health care, can open up new pathways for European health systems seeking to safeguard the egalitarian model that presided over their creation and development.

REFERENCES

Arneson, R.J. (1989) Equality and equal opportunity for welfare. *Philosophical Studies* 56: 77-93.

Atkinson, A.B. (1970) On the measurement of inequality. *Journal of Economic Theory* 2:244-263.

Beauchamp, T.L. and Faden R.R. (1979)The right to health and the right to health care. *The Journal of Medicine and Philosophy* 4(2):118-31.

Boyle, S. and Le Grand, J. (1995) Le financement de l'assurance maladie au Royaume-Uni. *Revue d'Économie Financière* 34:281-305.

Buchanan, J. (1986) *Market, Liberty and the State.* Hassocks:Harvester Press.

Cohen, G.A. (1989) On the currency of egalitarian justice *Ethics* 99:906-944.

Culyer, A.J., Maynard, A., and Posnett, J., editors (1990) *Competition in Health Care. Reforming the NHS.* London:Macmillan Press.

Culyer, A.J. and Wagstaff, A. (1993) Equity and equality in health and health care. *Journal of Health Economics* 12:431-57.

Daniels, N. (1982) Equity of access to heath care: some conceptual and ethical issues. *Milbank Memorail Fund Quarterly / Health and Society* 60(1):51-81.

Daniels, N. (1985) *Just Health Care* Cambridge:Cambridge University Press.

Department of Health (1989) *Working for Patients* London:HMSO.

De Jong, G.A. and Rutten, F. (1983) Justice and health for all. *Social Science and Medicine* 17(16):1085-95.

Dworkin, R. (1981a) What is equality? Part I: equality of welfare. *Philosophy and Public Affairs* 10(3):185-246.

Dworkin, R. (1981b) What is equality? Part II: equality of resources. *Philosophy and Public Affairs* 10(4):283-345.

Enthoven, A.C. (1988) *Theory and Practice of Managed Competition in Health Care Finance.* Amsterdam: North-Holland.

Fleurbaey, M. (1995) Equal opportunity or equal social outcome? *Economics and Philosophy* 11:25-55.

Fleurbaey, M. (1997) Equality and responsability. *European Economic Review.* 39:683-689.

Green, D., editor (1988) *Acceptable inequalities ? Essays on the pursuit of equality in health care.* IEA Unit, Paper n° 3, London: The Institute of Economic Affairs - Health Unit.

Hamilton, G.J. (1992) Assurance maladie: l'expérience hollandaise. *Chroniques de la SEDEIS* 7:261-267.

Hayek, F.A. (1960) *The Constitution of Liberty.* London:Routledge & Kegan.

Hayek, F.A. (1976) *Law, Legislation and Liberty, Vol. 2: The Mirage of Social Justice.* London:Routledge & Kegan.

Kolm, S.-C. (1985) *Le contrat social libéral. Philosophie et pratique du libéralisme.* Paris:Presses Universitaires de France.

Lee, P.R. and Jonsen, A.R. (1974) The Right to Health Care. *American Review of Respiratory Disease* 109:591-593.

Le Grand, J. (1982) *The Strategy of Equality. Redistribution and the Social Services* London:George Allen and Unwin.

Le Grand, J. (1992) Market-oriented health care reforms: impact on equity and efficiency. *Actes du Colloque Européen "De l'analyse économique aux politiques de santé", Atelier 3: La dimension sociale,* CREDES, CES, Paris, pp 19-35.

Le Grand, J. (1991) *Equity and Choice, An Essay on Economics and Applied Philosophy.* London:Harper and Collins Academic.

Le Grand, J. and Bartlett, W., editors (1993) *Quasi-markets and Social Policy,* London:Macmillan Press.

Matsaganis, M. and Glennerster, H. (1994) The threat of 'cream skimming' in the post-reform NHS. *Journal of Health Economics* 13(1):31-60.

Mooney, G. (1992) *Economics, Medicine and Health Care,* (1st ed.: 1986), Brighton:Harvester Wheatsheaf.

Mooney, G. (1994) *Key Issues in Health Economics.* Brighton:Harvester Wheatsheaf.

Mougeot, M. (1993) Concurrence et incitations dans le système hospitalier. *Revue Française d'Économie* 8(2):109-31.

Nozick, R. (1974) *Anarchy, State and Utopia.* New-York:Basic Books Inc.

Olsen, E.O. and Rogers, D.L. (1991) The welfare economics of equal access. *Journal of Public Economics* 45:91-105.

Pereira, J. (1993) What does equity in health mean ? *Journal of Social Policy* 22(1):19-48.

Pomey, M.-P. (1993) *La Réforme du Système De Santé Aux Pays-bas.* Paris: Institut La Boétie.

Rawls, J. (1971) *A Theory of Justice.* Cambridge, MA: Harvard University Press.

Rawls, J. (1974) Some reasons for the maximin criterion. *American Economic Review* 64:141-146.

Rawls, J. (1977) The basic structure as a subject. *American Philosophical Quarterly* 14(2):149-165.

Schneider-Bunner, C. (1994) Justice sociale et régulation des systèmes de santé européens. *Journal d'Économie Médicale* 12(4):195-213.

Schneider-Bunner, C. (1995) La justice sociale dans les systèmes de santé européens. *Futuribles* 201:5-25.

Schneider-Bunner, C. (1997) Santé et justice sociale L'économie des systèmes de santé face à la l'equité. Paris: Economica.

Sen, A.K. (1980) Equality of what ? In Sen, A.K., editor, *Choice, Welfare and Measurement*. Oxford:Basil Blackwell, pp 353-369.

Sen, A. K. (1985) *Commodities and Capabilities*. Amsterdam:North Holland.

Sen, A.K. (1987) *On Ethics and Economics*. Oxford:Basil Blackwell.

Siegler, M. (1979) A right to health care: ambiguity, professional resposnability, and patient liberty. *The Journal of Medicine and Philosophy* 4(2):148-157.

Tobin, J. (1970) On limiting the domain of inequality. *Journal of Law and Economics* 13:263-278.

Van de Ven, W. and Van Vliet, R. (1990) How can we prevent cream skimming in a competitive health insurance market ? The great challenge for the 90's. Second World Congress of Health Economics, Zürich, 31 p.

Van Doorslaer, E., Wagstaff, A. and Rutten, F., editors (1993) *Equity in the Finance and Delivery of Health Care. An International Perspective.* Oxford:Oxford Medical Publications.

Van Parijs, P. (1990) Equal endowments as undominated diversity. *Recherches Économiques de Louvain* 56(3-4):327-355.

Van Parijs, P. (1991) *Qu'est-ce Qu'une Société Juste ?, Introduction À La Pratique De La Philosophie Politique*. Paris:Le Seuil.

Van Parijs, P. (1995) *Real Freedom for All*. Oxford:Oxford University Press.

Wagstaff, A. (1991) QALYs and the equity-efficiency trade-off. *Journal of Health Economics* 10(1):21-41.

Williams, A. (1988) Priority setting in public and private health care, A guide through the ideological jungle. *Journal of Health Economics* 7:173-183.

Wood, A. (1981) Marx and equality. In Mepham, J. and Rubin, D.H., editors, *Issues in Marxixt Philosophy*, vol 4, Brighton: Harvester Press, pp 283-303.

World Health Organisation (1985) Les buts de la Santé pour tous, *Copenhague: Bureau régional de l'Europe, Série européenne de la Santé pour tous n°1.*

13

If We are Going to Get a Fair Innings, Someone will Need to Keep the Score!

ALAN WILLIAMS
Centre for Health Economics
University of York, England

The somewhat enigmatic title of my talk is meant to convey the message that if we wish to explore the efficiency-equity trade-off in the context of *reducing inequalities in health*, then we should take up and explore the folk-lore concept of a "fair innings." For those of you who are even more averse to competitive sport than I am, I should perhaps explain that the notion of a "fair innings" is based on the view that we are each entitled to a certain level of achievement in the game of life, and that anyone failing to reach this level has been hard done by, whilst anyone exceeding it has no reason to complain when their time runs out. It manifests itself colloquially in phrases such as "having a good run for your money" or "having a good knock" or, the one I shall employ here, "having a fair innings." In Biblical times a fair innings was held to be three-score-years-and-ten, though I doubt whether many people in those times actually achieved that

Health, Health Care and Health Economics: Perspectives on Distribution
Edited by Morris L. Barer, Thomas E. Getzen, and Greg L. Stoddart
Copyright 1998 John Wiley & Sons, Ltd.

target.   Things are probably not much different today for the majority of the world's population, but in the richer countries we expect more.

I want you to note some important characteristics of the "fair innings." First of all, it is a notion of equity that is *outcome based*, not process-based or resource-based. Secondly, it is about a person's *whole life-time experience*, not about their state at any particular point in time. Thirdly, it reflects an *aversion to inequality*. And fourthly, it is *quantifiable*, and even in common parlance it has strong numerical connotations.   Death at 25 is viewed very differently from death at 85, and age at death is the key variable most often focussed upon.   In my view, age at death should be no more than a first approximation, because the *quality* of a person's life is important as well as its length, as I will indicate shortly.   In the philosophical literature I have not found much scholarly analysis of this concept. The most extensive discussion of it that I know about is by John Harris. He particularly dislikes the supposedly "ageist" bias of QALY-maximisation as an objective of health care, but in groping for some compromise which would prevent the elderly from gobbling up a large chunk of GNP in the vain pursuit of immortality (which is my way of putting it, not his) he makes this observation:

> What the fair innings argument needs to do is to capture and express in a workable form the truth that while it is always a *misfortune* to die when one wants to go on living, it is not a *tragedy* to die in old age; but it is on the other hand both a tragedy and a misfortune to be cut off prematurely.

Without telling us what is the key distinction between a "misfortune" (a person's judgement about themselves?) and a "tragedy" (a social judgement that separates one misfortune from another?), nor how one is to decide when a death is "premature" (back to the "three-score-years-and-ten"?), he ends up accepting as "a reasonable form of the fair innings argument" one in which

> people who had achieved old age or who were closely approaching it would not have their lives further prolonged when this could only be achieved at the cost of the lives of those who were not nearing old age[1]

That is all I need for my immediate purpose, however, which is to explore ways of *quantifying* the concept of a "fair innings," thereby making it "workable," that is, making it a suitable tool for policy analysis in health care (or, better still, for

---

[1] John Harris *The Value of Life*, Routledge & Kegan Paul, London, 1985, pages 91-94.

social policy more generally).

In pursuit of that goal, let me turn to some primitive bits of economics, upon which I intend to build a crude empirical superstructure, in the hope that this will stimulate others to develop and extend it in a more sophisticated way. Here I shall merely offer a starting point and a few direction-indicators.

My starting point is the analytical framework for looking at equity issues in health care that has been presented by Culyer and Wagstaff.[2] They approach these matters with commendable clarity, and are careful to distinguish the different meanings that can be given to the concepts used in the common rhetoric about efficiency and equity. They have laid out analytically the complex relationships between them, and the reasons why some of these concepts may not lead where their propounders imagine (or wish). They also show that in the *provision* of health care, it is possible to define equity and efficiency (quite plausibly) such that no conflict occurs between them. If "efficiency" simply means operating somewhere on the production possibility frontier for health (given the resources and technologies available), then any equity criterion that is applied in order to choose a particular distribution of health *on* that frontier will automatically satisfy the efficiency criterion too. All that remains is a conflict *between different equity objectives*. So is this all much ado about nothing?

I think not. Suppose we take a different view as to what efficiency means in the provision of health care, namely maximising health gain as measured in some standardised way, e.g. in life-years or in quality-adjusted-life-years (QALYs). With the type of production possibility frontier that is normally assumed, standardised health-gain maximisation will define a single point on such a frontier, where it is tangential to a Social Welfare Function in which all units of health are equally valued no matter who gets them. Figure 1 is a modified version of the NE Quadrant of the Culyer/Wagstaff diagrammatics, in which the production possibility curve represents what *health services* can do to affect the health prospects of A and B. On it are identified three key points to which I shall return later. The point labelled "equal" is where the health prospects of A and the health of B are identical (the scale on each axis is different, for reasons which will become apparent shortly). It is the preferred position for a pure egalitarian. The point labelled "maximum" is where the aggregate prospective health of the two

---

[2] Culyer AJ & Wagstaff A, "Equity and equality in health and health care", *Journal of Health Economics* 12 (1993) 431-457, and Culyer AJ "Equality of *What* in Health Policy? Conflicts Between the Contenders" *Disc. Paper 142* Centre for Health Economics, University of York, England, 1995.

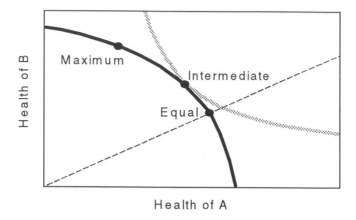

Figure 1 Health Production Possibilities with Social Welfare Function

individuals (measured, say, in life years) is as great as possible, and this would be the preferred position of a pure efficiency maximiser (in the meaning of efficiency that I am using). For those wishing to pursue *both* efficiency *and* equity, some "intermediate" position will be preferred, depending on the precise shape of their social welfare function. It is this "intermediate" position that is my focus of interest today. From *this* perspective, the equity-efficiency trade-off becomes the estimation of the number of (equally-valued) units of health that would be sacrificed by moving from the "maximum" point to any other point on the frontier.

One immediate problem is that we do not know precisely where the frontier is, and we strongly suspect that most of our health care systems are well inside it. One only has to look at data such as those in Figure 2, which compare potential life years lost (on the vertical axis) with real per capita expenditure on health care (on the horizontal axis) to see that very few systems are likely to be close to the efficiency frontier (those furthest to the SW ...like Japan ... are doing best, and those furthest to the NE ... like the USA... are doing worst). But for my purposes, this does not matter too much, because my argument is that *as we move towards the frontier from wherever we are*, we shall also wish to *move towards the most equitable point on it*, rather than in some quite other direction. Only in the unreal situation in which the redistribution of health prospects were costless would it be sensible to argue that efficiency should come first, and equity can be left until later. If you are really committed to equity, the two should be pursued simultaneously. So I shall concentrate on the properties of a social welfare function that might guide us towards where we want to be on the frontier, accepting that we may currently be well within it.

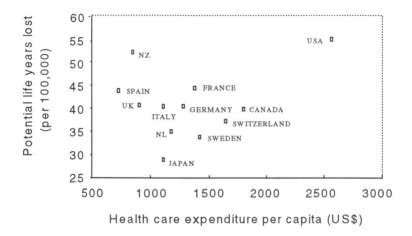

Figure 2 Technical Efficiency of Health Care: A Comparison of Systems

Let me introduce some empirical reality into the argument. Figure 3 is the same as Figure 1, except that it now shows the actual situation in the UK with respect to male life expectancy at birth, with Social Classes 1 & 2 (broadly professional and managerial people) on the vertical axis, and Social Classes 4 & 5 (broadly semi-skilled and unskilled workers) on the horizontal axis. The former have a life expectancy at birth of 72 years, whereas the latter can expect only 67 years, a 5 year difference.

But let me now strip away the production possibility frontier, which I do not need, and concentrate on the social welfare function (Figure 4). It is obvious that the current UK situation is some way off the locus of points representing perfect equality. Now suppose we conducted a society-wide experiment to find out how big a sacrifice, in terms of life expectancy, we would be willing to make in order

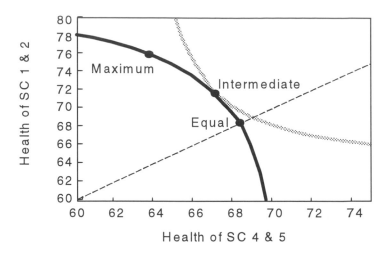

Figure 3 Life Expectancy at Birth -- Males: By Social Class

to eliminate this 5 year discrepancy.[3] Let us suppose that the answer came out to be 6 months. The arithmetical midpoint between 67 and 72 is 69.5, but we have just discovered (hypothetically) that equality at 69 is regarded as of equal social value to the situation we are actually in (i.e., it is on the same social welfare contour). If we may further suppose that our aversion to inequality is perfectly symmetrical between these two groups (meaning that we would be equally concerned if it were SC4&5 who were doing well and SC1&2 who were doing badly), then we have 3 points fixed on the social welfare contour that passes through our current situation. I have fitted a CES-type function to these three points, and when I do so the gradient of the social welfare contour at the current situation is approximately -2, which means that adding a year to the life expectancy of social classes 4&5 has twice the social value of adding one to the life expectancy of social classes 1&2.

---

[3] Note that in this experiment it would have to be made clear that it is not implied that it will actually be possible to eliminate these differences.   What we are seeking is the "price" each individual would be willing to pay (in terms of own health prospects) to equalise people's life chances.   It may also turn out to be the case that people feel that some people (e.g., smokers) do not deserve the same "innings" as other people, i.e. there are different "fair" innings for different classes of person.

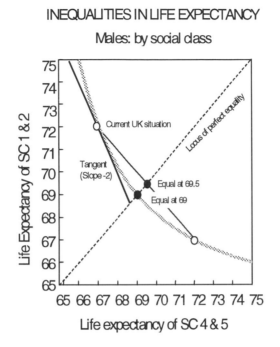

Figure 4 Inequalities in Life Expectancy -- Males: by Social Class

The situation gets worse if, instead of looking at life expectancy at birth, we look at *quality-adjusted* life expectancy at birth, because, as Figure 5 shows, the health-related quality of life of surviving members of SC4&5 is persistently below that of SC1&2, meaning that at all ages they suffer more mobility problems, more pain, and so on.[4] If these data are used to estimate *quality-adjusted* life expectancy

---

[4] These health-related quality-of-life data are based on the EuroQol instrument as applied to a representative sample of over 3000 members of the adult population of Great Britain.

at birth for the two groups (measured in QALYs), the result turns out to be that SC1&2 can expect 66 QALYs over their lifetime, but SC4&5 can only expect 57, a difference of 9 QALYs.   If we take the mean value (61.5 QALYs) to be a "fair innings," then a surviving member of SC1&2 should achieve this by the age of 65, but a surviving member of SC4&5 would not make it until the age of 71.   But their respective survival rates are such that whereas 76% of SC1&2 should get there, only 46% of SC4&5 will do so.

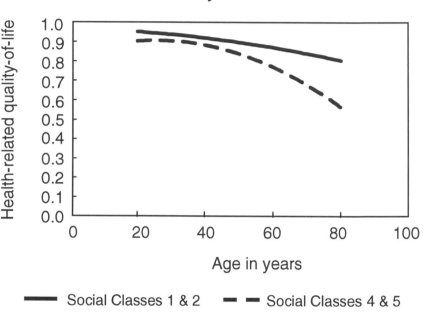

Figure 5 Health Related Quality of Life -- Males: by Social Class

So if we think (as I do) that a fair innings should be defined in terms of *quality adjusted life expectancy at birth,* and that we should be prepared to make some sacrifice to reduce that inequality, it is quite feasible to calculate a set of weights representing the differential social value of improvements in quality-adjusted life years delivered to different sorts of people in our current situation. And those of you with a strong sense of solidarity with your less fortunate fellow-citizens should be doing these calculations for your country, and encouraging your governments to work, formally or informally, with the kind of equity weights that emerge from whatever degree of inequality-aversion emerges. It is a large, but potentially very rewarding, research agenda.

But while your sense of solidarity is still highly aroused, as I hope it is when contemplating this manifest unfairness, I should add that the difference in life expectancy at birth *between men and women* in the UK is even greater than that between the social classes! The difference is 6 years, compared with the 5 identified earlier. But *health-related quality-of-life* differences are *not* so marked between males and females (indeed in the later years the surviving men are actually better off than the surviving women), so the difference in *quality-adjusted* life expectancy is nearer 5 QALYs, and less than the QALY difference between the social classes (which was about 9 QALYs). But again, whereas nearly 80% of women will survive long enough to enjoy a fair innings (which in this case I have taken to be 60 QALYs), less than 60% of men will do so. We males are not getting a fair innings!

But whatever social group we belong to, the survivors will slowly improve their chances of achieving a fair innings, and as their prospects improve, the equity weights attached to them should decline. Thus the age-related weights for surviving males and females in the UK might be as shown in Figure 6. It will be noted that since females are always expected to be on the favoured side, the equity weights applying to them are always low, but they get steadily lower for survivors as their prospects slowly improve still more. But males start out on the unfavoured side, with high weights (around 2.0) initially, which decline with age and reach 1.0 for those who survive into their early sixties, and thereafter become less than one when their *prospects* are that they will exceed the "fair innings." Thus there would be generated a set of age weights to apply *within* each relevant subgroup of the population. When I started on these calculations I had hoped that what I was going to lose in the equity-weights as a 70-year-old member of SC1&2, I might get back by way of compensation for the misfortune of having been born male. Unfortunately it is not so. My current weight as a member of SC1&2 is about 0.6, and as a male about 0.9, so I am in deep trouble in the inequality aversion stakes.

By any reasonable count I have had a "fair innings," and I would not deny it. My immediate death could not be said to be *unfair*, and it might not even be *efficient* to keep me going if anything serious struck ..... but just think what the

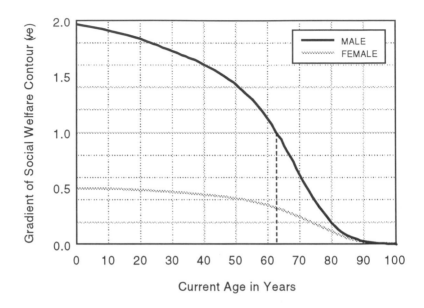

Figure 6 Survival and Gradient of SWF: "Fair Inning" = Expected Death at 74.5

world would have lost!   It looks as if I am going to have to rely on some other equity principle to bail me out ..... desert perhaps?   After all, I have always been kind to animals, my grandchildren think I'm great, and I am even nice to women ... though it appears that this has not really been at all necessary.   I shall have to devote my next paper to the measurement of desert!

Meanwhile .....

This consideration of equity alongside efficiency was motivated by two different desires. The first was to relate discussions of social justice, as typically conducted by non-economists, more closely to ways of thinking that are natural to economists, so as to encourage other economists to pick them up and run with them. The second was to impose some quantitative rigour upon the assertions made by non-economists about what is equitable, so that whenever it is argued that more weight should be given to one class of persons, it has to be acknowledged that this means that some identified other class of person is going to suffer. There is a regrettable tendency for equity arguments to be conducted within a rhetorical framework in which it appears possible to "do good" at no opportunity cost whatever. It generates a great deal of righteous self-satisfaction for the romantic escapists, and it puts economists back in the role of the dismal scientists always stressing the sacrifices that will have to be made. But romantic escapism does not help the hard-pressed decision-makers who grapple with these issues in real-life every day.

This is a first attempt to take one such equity principle, the "fair innings" argument, and subject it to empirical manipulation. The term "manipulation" is used advisably, because the empirical data that I have employed are stretched to the limits (some would doubtless say "beyond their limits") in order to stimulate thought, and to indicate what could be done if we chose to go down that route. I must confess I have always found the notion of a "fair innings" intuitively appealing, and having now worked through it in more detail I still find it intuitively appealing. But considering what an apparently simple idea it is, it seems to lead us into deep water rather quickly, concerning how we are to define it, how we are to measure it, and to what subgroups in society we should apply it. Yet it does capture a great deal of the concerns that people express when resisting the single-minded pursuit of efficiency in health care priority-setting.

If the nature and implications of particular positions are to be clarified in a policy-relevant way, this discussion has to move on to seek quantification of what are otherwise often quite vacuous assertions (e.g., that access should be determined by need, without "access" or "need" being defined in an operationally meaningful manner, and without making any attempt to estimate the costs, in terms of other benefits foregone). Only with some quantification will it be possible to devise rules that can be applied in a consistent manner with a reasonable chance of checking on performance (i.e. holding people accountable). At present, although reassurance is frequently offered that equity considerations have been taken into account, there is no way of establishing what bearing, if any, those principles actually had upon the outcomes. Judging by the persistence of health inequalities, and the almost universal agreement that they are deplorable, it is tempting to conclude that the rhetoric is not matched by any real commitment to do anything effective. Quantification thus has potential for clarification, for performance measurement, for accountability, and for policy analysis and reappraisal. The quest for greater quantification of equity considerations seems worth pursuing on those grounds alone, despite the hostility that it is likely to engender from those who mistakenly equate precision with lack of humanity.

For a long time I have been of the view that the best way to integrate efficiency and equity considerations in the provision of health care would be to attach equity-weights to QALYs. QALYs measure benefits of health care in standard units, and equity-weights allow benefit valuation to become person-specific to the extent that that is policy-relevant. But there has always been a danger that such personalised weights become arbitrary and capricious, and come to be used to fudge outcomes in ways that would not be acceptable if their basis were exposed. One safeguard against this is to have some "over-arching" general principle enunciated, whose implications can be estimated quantitatively, and the outcome of which can be confronted with evidence. From this standpoint, the fact that it is possible to move from a general notion of a "fair innings," to specific numerical weights reflecting the marginal social value of health gains to different people, seems to me to be an important break-through.

Finally I think that the focus on outcomes-with-equity-weights-attached, has great advantages over other approaches to the reduction of health inequalities, because it rules out the giving of priority to things that do no good, which is the danger with equalising policies that concentrate on process (including access) or on resources. It also sets clear limits on how far we are willing to go in helping the disadvantaged, for a weight of (say) 2 indicates that we are willing to spend twice as much as the norm to provide one extra QALY for such a person, but that is the limit. This is far preferable to the vague notion of "priority groups" whose champions are left to struggle on unclear terms with more powerful competitors in the annual scramble for resources.

So I commend the "fair innings" argument as a promising way forward for economists interested in the equitable provision of health care. But if we are to know whether or not people are getting a "fair innings," somebody has to keep the score! That is a challenge to researchers and practitioners alike, and one that will involve collaboration between many disciplines. But we health economists are well placed to drive it, and I hope that some of you will be inspired to do so. If so, go to it!

14

Health Utility Indices and Equity Considerations

HAN BLEICHRODT

iMTA
Erasmus University
Rotterdam
The Netherlands

ABSTRACT

The aim of this paper is to propose methods that incorporate equity concerns into cost utility analysis. The focus of the paper is on QALYs, but the results apply to health utility indices in general. Two interpretations of QALYs are considered: QALYs as (von Neumann Morgenstern) utilities and QALYs as measures of health. A justification is provided for aggregating consistently scaled "QALYs as utilities" over individuals. The conditions underlying unweighted aggregation of QALYs are identified. These conditions exclude two common types of equity concern. Algorithms are proposed that take into account equity concerns and that are relatively easy to apply.

Health, Health Care and Health Economics: Perspectives on Distribution
Edited by Morris L. Barer, Thomas E. Getzen, and Greg L. Stoddart
Copyright 1998 John Wiley & Sons, Ltd.

INTRODUCTION

Utility indices for health care programs, such as QALYs, have been criticized for being primarily concerned with efficiency, while ignoring equity implications[1]. The importance of incorporating equity considerations into cost utility analysis has been widely acknowledged by researchers in the field (*e.g.* Williams, 1993). However, despite statements of intent, few attempts have been made thus far to actually develop methods by means of which equity considerations can be taken into account in cost utility analysis. One of the few exceptions is Wagstaff (1991), who suggested combining equity and efficiency considerations in cost utility analysis by means of the social welfare function underlying Atkinson's (1970) index of inequality. However, Wagstaff did not pursue this idea any further, in particular he did not indicate how the parameters of this social welfare function can be assessed by experimental methods.

The aim of this paper is to derive functional forms that allow trading off the efficiency gains of a health care program against their equity implications. Given that QALYs are the most frequently used outcome measure in cost utility analysis, we will refer to the gains of a health care program as the number of QALYs gained. However, it should be emphasized here that all results derived in the sequel of the paper apply to other utility based outcome measures as well. It is also important to realize that this paper is concerned with equity concerns over consistently scaled QALYs, consistent in the sense that QALYs are comparable over individuals. This distinguishes this paper, for example, from the paper by Gafni and Birch (1991) in which the influence of equity considerations on the scaling of the von Neumann Morgenstern utility function is shown and in which algorithms are developed to ensure consistent scaling. However, the two approaches are not completely independent. We briefly return to this issue in the section on *Ex Ante Versus Ex Post Equity.*

The functional derivations presented in this paper are based on the tools of multi-attribute utility theory. Multi-attribute utility theory has been developed as a procedure to make explicit the trade-off between conflicting objectives. Two interpretations of QALYs that have been distinguished in the literature are considered: QALYs as von Neumann Morgenstern (vNM) utilities and QALYs as measures of health.[2] It has been claimed that the QALYs as utilities approach lacks a theoretical foundation, since utilities cannot be interpersonally compared in a meaningful way. This problem is addressed in the sections on *Aggregation of Utilities* and *von Neumann Morgenstern Utilities.*

---

[1] Cf *e.g.* Lockwood (1988); Harris (1988); Smith (1987); Broome (1988); Broome (1993)

[2] These two interpretations are not necessarily mutually exclusive.

The structure of the paper is as follows. The section immediately following this one discusses the two interpretations of QALYs, while the next sections provide a rationale for aggregating consistently scaled "QALYs as utilities" over individuals. In the section on *Aggregation of Utilities* it is argued that if we want to incorporate equity considerations in cost utility analysis, full interpersonal comparability of utilities is needed. The following section presents the argument that vNM utilities can meaningfully be interpersonally compared. In the next section, entitled *QALY Utilitarianism*, the conditions are identified under which the aggregation of QALYs over individuals takes the form of "QALY-utilitarianism," *i.e.*, the unweighted summation of QALYs over individuals. The section on *Ex Ante Versus Ex Post Equity* shows that these conditions inhibit the inclusion of two common types of equity concern: a concern for the fairness of the allocation process, generally referred to as *ex ante* equity, and a concern for the (final) distributional implications, referred to as *ex post* equity. Replacing the relevant conditions by alternative conditions allows the inclusion of *ex ante* and *ex post* equity concerns. Subsequent sections propose three procedures by means of which equity concerns can be captured in cost utility analysis. The procedures described in the section on *Ex Post Equity Algorithms for QALY Aggregation* address *ex post* equity, while the section that comes next describes a procedure that simultaneously takes into account *ex ante* equity and *ex post* equity. The paper concludes with a summary and discussion of the main findings of the paper. The appendix contains proofs of results presented in the main text of the paper.

INTERPRETATION OF QALYs

The definition of the number of QALYs for an individual, as given by Pliskin, Shepard, and Weinstein (1980), is the following:[3]

$$QALY = \sum_{t=1}^{T} u(q_t)$$

where T stands for the remaining number of periods the individual still has to live, q_t stands for the quality of life level attained in period t and $u(q_t)$ is the utility of living in health state q_t at period t. At least two interpretations have been distinguished in the

---

[3] One may object that this formulation is unnecessarily simple and that, for example, discounting should be allowed for. However, this simple representation does not imply a loss of generality in terms of the results of this paper: all results carry over straightforwardly if a more general expression is substituted.

literature[4] as to what the number of QALYs represents: *QALYs as vNM utilities* and *QALYs as measures of health*. According to Torrance (1986): "In one approach health state utilities are claimed to be utilities obeying the axioms of von Neumann Morgenstern utility theory......In the other approach...health state utilities are claimed to measure the overall quality of life" [p.27].

With respect to the first interpretation, QALYs as vNM utilities, conditions have to be imposed on the individual preference relation to ensure that a QALY is a valid vNM utility. Criticism that decision making based on QALYs may not accurately reflect individual preferences is based on the presumption that ideally a QALY should be a vNM utility. In the interpretation of QALYs as vNM utilities, we abstract from the discussion whether the conditions that equate QALYs and vNM utilities are reasonable and it is simply assumed that the individual preference relations satisfy these conditions.[5] It should be noted though that if the preference conditions underlying the QALY measure are not satisfied, another utility based outcome measure can simply be substituted. As remarked already in the introduction, all results presented in the remainder of the paper apply to other utility based measures as well.

The second interpretation, QALYs as measures of health, is rooted in the extra-welfarist tradition that originates from Sen (1979) and has been applied to health by Culyer (1989). Wagstaff (1991) notes: "Though utility theory is frequently used in the derivation of quality of life scores, it is used simply to measure people's health rather than the utility they derive from it" [p.23]. Part of the appeal of this latter approach stems from the fact that the comparability of "QALYs as utilities" across individuals may be problematic.

It is not an aim of this paper to decide which of these two interpretations is most appropriate. The equity algorithms presented in the sections on *Ex Post Equity Algorithms for QALY Aggregation* and *Algorithms Incorporating Both Ex Post and Ex Ante Equity* have been developed with the intention of being applicable under both interpretations. However, equity considerations relate to comparisons between individuals and therefore it must first be established whether QALYs can be aggregated in both interpretations. The common way to aggregate QALYs is by unweighted summation. Because of this, the QALY approach has been criticized as embodying a return to classical, or Benthamite, utilitarianism. Wagstaff (1991) has argued that in the interpretation of QALYs as measures of health this criticism does

---

[4] Nord (1994) provides a third interpretation: QALYs as a social value. We will not consider this interpretation for the obvious reason that in this interpretation aggregation plays no role.
[5] For a critical evaluation of these conditions cf. *e.g.* Mehrez and Gafni (1989); Loomes and McKenzie (1989).

not stand scrutiny. Classical utilitarianism focuses on the aggregation of utilities whereas the QALYs as measure of health approach mainly sees QALYs as reflecting characteristics of people without being concerned with the utility they derive from these characteristics. The idea behind this line of argument is that characteristics do not face problems of measurability and comparability across individuals. In the remainder of this paper this view is taken for granted. It is assumed that in the interpretation as a health measure, QALYs can indeed be aggregated across individuals and that the equity algorithms to be developed later can be applied to QALYs as measures of health.

The assertion made in this paper that QALYs as vNM utilities can also be meaningfully aggregated requires clarification. The question whether vNM utilities are interpersonally comparable and have a meaning in social welfare analysis has provoked much debate over the past five decades. In the next section we will establish that to incorporate equity considerations into cost utility analysis full interpersonal comparability of utilities is necessary. In the section on *von Neumann Morgenstern utilities* a rationale is given why QALYs as vNM utilities can be considered to be fully interpersonally comparable.

AGGREGATION OF UTILITIES

Under classical utilitarianism, social welfare was set equal to the sum of intuitively measurable and comparable individual utilities. These individual utilities were simply assumed to exist, no attention being paid to their origin. This concept of utility and social welfare was challenged by the Pareto school, which claimed that utility is an ordinal concept, reflecting only the individual ordering of outcomes and being incomparable across individuals. Arrow's work on social choice lies within this Paretian tradition. In deriving his celebrated impossibility theorem,[6] Arrow defined a social welfare function (SWF) as a functional relation specifying a social ordering for any given n-tuple of individual orderings. By using only ordering information Arrow deliberately limited the informational framework, excluding all information on preference intensities. Arrow showed that if the number of individuals is finite and if the number of social states is greater than two, no SWF can satisfy the following four conditions: *(i) unrestricted domain:* the SWF should work for all logically possible individual orderings; *(ii) weak Pareto:* if every individual strictly prefers allocation *x*

---

[6] See Arrow (1950, 1951a, 1963). In Arrow (1950, 1951a) the domain restriction was not defined tightly enough as was pointed out by Blau (1957). The version in Arrow (1963) is the best known version.

to allocation *y* then society should strictly prefer *x* to *y*; *(iii) non-dictatorship:* there is no individual such that social preference is completely determined by the preferences of this individual regardless of the preferences of all other individuals in society; *(iv) independence of irrelevant alternatives:* social preference between two allocations should be independent of all other allocations. The requirement of independence of irrelevant alternatives excludes all information about other allocations and thereby inhibits the use of any information other than the individual orderings over *x* and *y*. Using information on cardinal utility depends on the scaling of the utility function and this necessarily involves taking into account other alternatives.

Various attempts have been undertaken to escape from Arrow's impossibility theorem by weakening his conditions. In this paper we consider the enrichment of the informational base of Arrow's social choice approach, *i.e.* a relaxation of Arrow's fourth condition, independence of irrelevant alternatives. A social welfare functional (SWFL) is defined as a rule that specifies exactly one social ordering for any given n-tuple of real-valued individual utility functions. Let L_i be defined as the set of individual utility functions that are informationally equivalent, *i.e.* that provide the same information on individual preferences. For example, given Arrow's assumptions, all individual utility functions that are positive monotonic transformations are informationally equivalent. If individual utility is cardinally measurable, then elements of the set L_i of informationally equivalent utility functions are positive linear transformations of each other: $U_i = a + bU'_i$, $a \in \mathbb{R}$; $b > 0$; $U_i, U'_i \in L_i$.

A measurability set L is defined as the set of all possible combinations of the n-tuples of informationally equivalent individual utility functions. Depending on the assumptions about interpersonal comparability, the measurability set can be restricted. Combining the measurability assumptions about individual utilities with the assumptions about interpersonal comparability defines the measurability-comparability set L^*. In Arrow's framework of social choice, where no interpersonal comparability is assumed and only the information revealed by individual orderings is incorporated, L^* consists of all individual utility functions that are positive monotonic transformations of each other. Sen (1970b, 1977b) distinguishes several other measurability-comparability combinations:

- *cardinal non-comparability-L^** consists of all individual utility functions that are unique up to positive linear transformations;
- *ordinal level comparability-L^** consists of all individual utility functions that are unique up to similar positive monotonic transformations;
- *cardinal unit comparability-L^** consists of all individual utility functions that are

unique up to location and common scale, i.e. $U_i = a_i + bU_i^*$, $a_i \in \mathbb{R}$ (the set of real numbers), b>0,

- *cardinal full comparability-L** consists of all individual utility functions that are unique up to common location and common scale, i.e. $U_i = a + bU_i^*$, $a \in \mathbb{R}$, $b>0$.

Lemma 8*2 in Sen (1970) shows that assuming cardinal non-comparability is not sufficient to solve Arrow's impossibility result. However, the other three informational frameworks are sufficient to remove the dilemma posed by Arrow's theorem. Clearly, it is interpersonal comparability that is crucial in enriching the informational basis of social choice.

In cost utility analysis the calculation of the net advantage of one program over another is of interest. For such an analysis to be relevant, units should be comparable. Location need not necessarily be common to all individuals, since in calculating net advantages the individual-specific locations are subtracted away and play no role in determining the relative effectiveness of programs. Suppose for example that for a particular n-tuple of individual utility functions program x is preferred to program y. That is, $\Sigma\ [U_i(x_i)-U_i(y_i)]>0$, but also $\Sigma\ [a_i + bU_i(x_i)-a_i-bU_i(y_i)]=b\Sigma\ [U_i(x_i)-U_i(y_i)]>0$, $a_i \in \mathbb{R}$ and $b>0$, and thus adding individual specific constants does not influence the relative effectiveness of programs. If b would be individual specific, which corresponds with cardinal non-comparability, x might no longer be preferred to y. This suggests that in cost utility analyses we need only impose cardinal utility functions that have their scale in common, *i.e.*, cardinal unit comparability. It seems not necessary to assume level comparability. However, several authors[7] have shown that if cardinal unit comparability is assumed rather than cardinal full comparability, slightly strengthened versions of Arrow's conditions imply that the only possible SWFL is the utilitarian one. In such an informational framework, simply aggregating the number of utilities/QALYs over the relevant population is unobjectionable. This result was to be expected. The notion of equity involves special consideration being given to the badly-off and this necessarily involves bringing in comparisons of utility levels. Given that the starting point of this paper was a concern for the equity consequences of utility-based decision making, a framework has to be imposed that allows such concerns to be justified. That is, a rationale must be given for assuming cardinal full comparability.

---

[7] *E.g.*, d'Aspremont and Gevers (1977); Sen (1977b); Deschamps and Gevers (1978).

Von Neumann Morgenstern Utilities

If the vNM axioms hold then individual utility functions are cardinal, *i.e.*, unique up to positive linear transformations. A possibility is, therefore, to use individual vNM utilities as an input in the social welfare functional. Taking individual vNM utilities as the basis from which social welfare judgements are to be derived was first proposed by Harsanyi (1955). Harsanyi's position has been severely criticized. The essence of the criticism was that vNM utilities are inextricably bound to situations involving risk. Arrow (1951a, p.10): "....it [vNM utility theory] has nothing to do with welfare considerations, particularly if we are interested primarily in making a social choice among alternative policies in which no random elements enter. To say otherwise would be to assert that the distribution of the social income is to be governed by the tastes of individuals for gambling."

One can respond to such criticism in one of two ways. The first type of answer acknowledges that vNM utilities are only relevant in the context of risk, but asserts that health decision making typically involves risk and that, therefore, vNM utilities do have relevance in this context (*e.g.*, Ben-Zion and Gafni [1983]). The second type of response challenges the assertion that vNM utilities only have relevance in the context of risk. According to this line of reasoning, cardinal utility has a meaning independent of risk. That cardinal utility has a meaning independent of risk has been criticized by Arrow (1951b) who writes about cardinal utility under certainty: "...which is a meaningless concept anyway [p.425]." Similar views have been expressed by Savage (1954), Ellsberg (1954), Luce and Raiffa (1957), and Fishburn (1989). Harsanyi (1987) on the other hand asserts that: "In fact, people's vNM utility functions are an important piece of information for welfare economics and ethics because they are natural measures for the intensity of people's desires, preferences and wants (pp.546-547)." Wakker (1994) provides a defense for a unified notion of utility that does not need risk for its existence, but that has relevance for risk. Wakker observes that the development of expected utility theory by von Neumann and Morgenstern was motivated by their desire to obtain a cardinal utility that is relevant to game theory. The same cardinal utility, the expectation of which represents individual choices over lotteries over outcomes, is used as a unit of exchange between players in a game. Wakker (p.8): "I think the applicability of risky utility as means of exchange between players is as questionable as its applicability to welfare theory, or any other case of decisions under certainty." It cannot be excluded that vNM had in mind one notion of utility for the entire economic science. This viewpoint, that vNM utilities do indeed have relevance in other contexts than risk, underlies the discussion of QALYs as vNM utilities in this paper.

Having provided a rationale for using cardinal (vNM) utilities as the foundation of social welfare judgements, the question remains how interpersonal comparability can be ensured given that individual utilities are unique only up to positive linear transformations and given that scaling up the utility of one individual, while keeping the utilities of the other individuals constant, may alter the outcome of the social choice problem. Hildreth (1953) suggested considering two specially defined outcomes X and Y, such that everyone prefers X to Y, and to assign predefined real values to these social states. This makes individual utility functions interpersonally comparable. In fact this approach is typically used in cost utility analysis. The general approach to aggregation, as outlined, for example, by Williams (1981) and Torrance (1986), is to assign a utility of zero to death and a utility of one to normal or full health and to regard a year of healthy life as being of equal intrinsic value to everyone. Torrance and Feeny (1989) have argued that it may be more in line with existing practice to assume that a life in full health has equal value for everyone. Applying this scaling, moreover, avoids the problem that utilities have to be assigned to health states without specifying the time dimension of the health states. Gafni and Torrance (1984) have argued that health states have a time dimension inextricably bound to them and that it is impossible to measure utilities for health without specifying a time dimension. Gafni and Birch (1991) have argued that the common way to measure vNM utilities is inconsistent with the criterion that a life in full health is of equal value to everyone. They have provided an algorithm to measure utilities that are consistent with this criterion. In their approach the vNM utility function is scaled such that a life in full health receives utility one and immediate death utility zero. This approach guarantees that individual utilities are consistently scaled and interpersonally comparable. A disadvantage of the method proposed by Gafni and Birch is that two rather than one standard gamble questions are necessary to determine health state utilities. The measurement task therefore becomes more involved.

Summarizing, the above discussion establishes a rationale for aggregating QALYs as (vNM) utilities. The section on *Aggregation of Utilities* showed the need for cardinal fully comparable utilities if we are to allow distributional considerations to play a role in cost utility analysis. vNM utility theory establishes cardinality of the individual utilities. Following Wakker's argument a case can be made for the assertion that vNM utilities do indeed have relevance in the context of welfare judgments. Finally, by Hildreth's approach, which is typically followed in cost utility analysis, a consistent scaling procedure emerges, which ensures that individual vNM utilities can be interpersonally compared in a meaningful way.

QALY UTILITARIANISM

Notation and Structural Assumptions

This subsection introduces notation and structural assumptions. Denote the set of QALY allocations by X. A typical element of the set X is a vector $x=(x_1,....,x_n)$ representing an allocation of QALYs resulting from the implementation of a health care program with each x_i indicating the number of QALYs received by individual i and n being the number of individuals affected by the program. Assume without loss of generality that for each individual the possible number of QALYs is non-negative, *i.e.*, $X \in \mathbb{R}_+$. We are interested in the social preference relation $\gtrsim$ over the set of QALY allocations, meaning "at least as good as". Let $\succ$ and $\sim$ denote its asymmetric and symmetric part respectively. Throughout $\gtrsim$ is assumed to be a weak order. That is, $\gtrsim$ is complete, either $x \gtrsim y$ or $y \gtrsim x$ or both, and transitive, if $x \gtrsim y$ & $y \gtrsim z$ then $x \gtrsim z$. Moreover, $\gtrsim$ is assumed to be continuous. Continuity of the preference relation guarantees that if a real-valued function is defined over X, this function has an interval as its image.

Denote by $x_{-i}v_i$ the vector x with coordinate i (the number of QALYs individual i receives) replaced by v_i: $x_{-i}v_i = (x_1,x_2,..., x_{i-1}, v_i, x_{i+1},..., x_n)$. Let A be a subset of the individuals affected by a health care program: $A \subset I = \{1,2,...,n\}$. Then $x_{-A}v_A$ denotes the vector x in which for all individuals in subset A x_i is replaced by v_i. For example if $A=\{1,2,3\}$, then $x_{-A}v_A = (v_1,v_2,v_3,x_4,...,x_n)$. Denote by $\gtrsim_i$ the individual preference relation "at least as good as". As before, $\succ_i$ and $\sim_i$ are defined as the asymmetric and symmetric parts of $\gtrsim_i$ respectively.

Let Z be a set of probability distributions over the set of QALY allocations X. A typical element of Z is $(p^1,x^1;....;p^m,x^m)$ where allocation x^j occurs with probability p^j and m can be any natural number. Let $\gtrsim_Z$ be a social preference relation defined on Z. Throughout the paper it is assumed that individual preference relations over probability distributions satisfy the von Neumann Morgenstern (vNM) axioms. In the formulation by Jensen (1967), a preference relation $\gtrsim'$ satisfies the vNM axioms if: (i) $\gtrsim'$ is a weak order; (ii) vNM independence holds: $P \gtrsim' Q \Leftrightarrow (\mu P + (1-\mu)R) \gtrsim' (\mu Q + (1-\mu)R)$ $\forall 0 < \mu < 1$ and $P, Q, R \in Z$; (iii) Jensen continuity holds: $(P \succ' Q, Q \succ' R) \Rightarrow \kappa P + (1-\kappa)R \succ' Q$ and $Q \succ' \rho P + (1-\rho)R$ for some $\kappa, \rho \in (0,1)$. If a preference relation satisfies the vNM axioms, a cardinal real-valued utility function exists, the expected value of which represents the preference relation.

Derivation of QALY Utilitarianism

We will derive (QALY) utilitarianism by adding a condition to the axiomatic framework of Harsanyi (1955) in which a partial characterization of utilitarianism is given. The method of proof differs from the proof given by Harsanyi in that use is made of a result developed by Fishburn (1965). Further, by using a theorem from Maas and Wakker (1994) the utility function is shown to be continuous. Continuity is important to establish. If QALYs (real numbers) are added up across individuals the social utility function is implicitly assumed to be continuous. However Harsanyi's result does not imply this.

Harsanyi not only required *individual* preferences to satisfy the vNM axioms, as has been assumed in subsection 5.1, but also required *social* preferences to satisfy the vNM axioms. According to Harsanyi the vNM axioms are essential requirements of rationality, much in the same spirit as Arrow considered weak ordering to be a basic requirement of rationality of social preferences. Further, Harsanyi imposed the following condition:

Condition H: *If two alternatives, defined by probability distributions over the set of outcomes, are indifferent from the standpoint of every individual, then they are also indifferent from a social standpoint.*

As shown by Harsanyi (theorem V), these three conditions allow the derivation of the SWFL as a weighted sum of the individual utilities:

$$U(x) = \sum_{i=1}^{n} \lambda_i U_i(x_i) \qquad (2)$$

This is not a full characterization of QALY-utilitarianism, given that the scaling factors λ_i may differ between individuals and the utility functions are individual-specific. QALYs are assumed to be similar across individuals. Therefore a condition has to be added to ensure this similarity.

A permutation π of the n individuals is a function specifying a rearrangement of the individuals. Denote by $\pi(i)$ the permuted value of i. Now consider the following condition:

Condition A (anonymity): *$(U_i)\sim_z(U_{\pi(i)})$ for all $(U_i) = (U_1,...U_n)$ and permutation functions π on $I = \{1,...,n\}$.*

Condition A asserts that social indifference should hold between a utility/QALY allocation x and any utility/QALY allocation y which is a permutation of x. Condition A ensures that social preference is independent of who gets which utility/QALY. For example, in the hypothetical situation that there is one additional QALY to be divided between two individuals with a similar endowment of QALYs,[8] by condition A, society should have no preference as to which individual will receive this additional QALY. However, condition A is weaker than what is referred to in the cost utility literature as "a QALY is a QALY no matter who gets it." According to the latter, society should in every situation be indifferent with respect to who gets a QALY. Condition A only says that in case one QALY allocation is a permutation of another, indifference should hold. For example, suppose a program has resulted in a QALY allocation $(3,1)$, i.e., individual a has received three QALYs and individual b has received one QALY, and one more QALY is to be allocated. Then by the argument that "a QALY is a QALY no matter who gets it" society should be indifferent between allocations $(4,1)$ and $(3,2)$. However, condition A does not provide guidance with respect to social preference between $(4,1)$ and $(3,2)$. Condition A asserts that if society prefers $(3,2)$ to $(4,1)$ then it should also prefer $(2,3)$ to $(1,4)$ when the initial allocation is $(1,3)$: by condition A $(2,3)_{\sim_z}(3,2)$; we know that $(3,2)\succ_z(4,1)$; applying condition A once again gives $(4,1)_{\sim_z}(1,4)$ and thus by transitivity $(2,3)\succ_z(1,4)$. Imposing condition A on top of Harsanyi's conditions is necessary and sufficient for QALY utilitarianism.

Theorem 1: *The following two statements are equivalent:*
(i) The social preference relation $\gtrsim_z$ can be represented by QALY utilitarianism:

$$U(x) = \sum_{i=1}^{n} U(x_i) \qquad (3)$$

(ii) both individual and social preferences satisfy the vNM axioms and moreover conditions H and A hold. Furthermore U is continuous and unique up to positive linear transformations.

---

[8] Note that the impact of other endowments, *e.g.*, income, is ignored by condition A. These could be incorporated by making health utilities dependent on these endowments. For example, if health state utilities are income dependent, condition A has implications for income-dependent health utilities.

A proof of this result can be found in the appendix.

Ex Ante Versus *Ex Post* Equity

Theorem 1 has been derived by imposing four conditions: that individual preferences satisfy the vNM axioms, that social preferences satisfy the vNM axioms, condition H and condition A. In the remainder of the paper we continue to require that individual preferences satisfy the vNM axioms. Particularly during the last two decades much empirical evidence has been presented that descriptively individual preferences frequently violate these axioms. Normatively the axioms still have considerable force and are appealing enough to adhere to. We will also continue to assume that condition A holds. Condition A asserts that the identity of a QALY recipient should play no role in health decision making. Condition A ensures that the principle that a life in full health should be equal for all individuals holds, and thereby allows consistent scaling of the utility functions according to the equity principles developed by Gafni and Birch (1991). Moreover, as the example in the previous section shows, condition A does not predict choice with respect to every allocation and therefore allows additional equity principles to be imposed.

The remainder of the paper examines the consequences of relaxing the two remaining conditions, that social preferences satisfy the vNM axioms and condition H. The restrictiveness of these assumptions can be illustrated by means of an example. Consider two individuals (or equivalently two groups of individuals) and two possible states of the world, X and Y, each with a probability of occurrence of 0.5. This probability is known to both individuals. Consider the following three health care programs each resulting in different QALY allocations:

Program	State X	State Y	Expected Utility
1	(1,0)	(1,0)	1
2	(1,0)	(0,1)	1
3	(1,1)	(0,0)	1

Under the assumptions being made, by theorem 1, social indifference should hold between the three health care programs, given that the expected utilities of the three programs are equal. However, it is conceivable that the decision maker will prefer programs 2 and 3 to program 1 given that the former two programs offer both individuals a possibility of receiving a QALY, whereas program 1 denies the second individual the possibility of receiving a QALY. Diamond (1967)[9] has argued that it is essentially vNM independence that requires indifference to hold in the above example. This is most easily seen by comparing programs 1 and 2. Under condition A, the decision maker is indifferent between the outcomes of the two programs when state Y occurs. However, under state X, the outcomes of the two programs are equal and therefore, by vNM independence, overall indifference should prevail. On the other hand, if the decision maker is concerned with the fairness of the allocation process, generally referred to as *ex ante* equity, program 2 should be chosen, because this offers both individuals a possibility of obtaining a QALY. Incorporating *ex ante* equity concerns implies dismissing the requirement that social preferences satisfy the vNM axioms. Incorporating *ex ante* equity considerations can be ensured by imposing the following *ex ante* equity condition on the social preference relation:

Condition E: *If $p_k=q_k$ for all $k \in I \backslash \{i,j\}$; $p_i+p_j=q_i+q_j$ and $|p_i-p_j|<|q_i-q_j|$ then $P \succ_z Q$.*[10]

where P and Q are lotteries over X and the $p_i's$ and $q_i's$ are marginal probabilities, indicating the probability that individual i receives a given amount of QALYs, Q^c. In words condition E says the following. Suppose all individuals, other than i and j, have the same marginal probability of receiving Q^c under two health care programs (in the above example Q^c is equal to one). Taken together i and j have the same marginal probability of receiving Q^c, but in one program this marginal probability is more equally divided between the two individuals (in the situation described by condition E this is the program giving rise to probability distribution P). Then, by condition E, the program with the more equal distribution of marginal probabilities over i and j is to be preferred to the one that leads to a less equal distribution of marginal probabilities over i and j. Condition E is not incompatible with condition H. Condition E dictates how differences in marginal probabilities should affect social preference, whereas condition H dictates how equality of marginal probabilities should affect social preference.

It is also conceivable that, in choosing between programs 2 and 3, a social decision maker prefers program 3 to program 2, given that program 3 guarantees an equal distribution of QALYs under both states of the world, whereas program 2 necessarily leads to a situation of inequality. This preference is determined by a

---

[9] See also Sen (1976); Broome (1982); Ulph (1982). For a counterargument, see Harsanyi (1975).

[10] Condition E is comparable to Fishburn's (1984) axiom of risk-sharing equity in the context of public risk evaluation. See also Fishburn and Straffin, (1989).

concern for the final distribution of QALYs, often referred to as *ex post* equity. Let p_{i-j} denote the probability of the event that only individual i gets a QALY and let p_{i+j} denote the probability of the event that both individual i and individual j receive a QALY. In the example above, p_{i-j} is *0.5* for program 2 and 0 for program 3, whereas p_{i+j} is *0* for program 2 and *0.5* for program 3. Incorporating a concern for *ex post* equity can be established by imposing the following condition on the social preference relation:

Condition P:
If $P=Q$, $P,Q \in Z$ apart from $p_{i-j}=q_{i-j}-\gamma$, $p_{j-i}=q_{j-i}-\gamma$, $p_{i+j}=q_{i+j}+\gamma$, with $\gamma>0$, then $P \succ_z Q$ [11].

It can easily be seen that condition P is incompatible with condition H. In the situation described by condition P, $p_i=q_i$ for all individuals, so by condition H, $P\sim_z Q$. However, probability distribution P offers a greater probability of individuals i and j both receiving a QALY. Therefore, by condition P, $P\succ_z Q$. Thus, incorporating *ex post* equity considerations in health care decision making means rejection of condition H. Condition H, innocuous as it may appear, has the effect of making social choice dependent on individual preferences only. The condition leaves no room for supra-individual interests. Incorporating distributional concerns therefore means relaxing the condition that social choice depends only on individual preferences and allowing complementarity between individual utility/health levels. In the next section two approaches are discussed to incorporate such complementarity.

---

[11] This condition is the converse of Keeney's (1980) assumption of catastrophe avoidance. Fishburn (1984) and Fishburn and Straffin (1989) have developed similar "common fate equity" axioms for the context of public risk evaluation.

EX POST EQUITY ALGORITHMS FOR
QALY AGGREGATION

A Multiplicative Social Utility Function

As has been observed in the proof of theorem 1, condition *H* is equivalent to additive independence (Fishburn, 1965, 1970). Therefore, a way to introduce complementarity is to translate generalizations of additive independence, known from the literature on multi-attribute utility theory, to the context of social choice. One possibility is to impose the analogue of mutual utility independence on the social preference relation.[12] Mutual utility independence is a preference condition that is entirely formulated in terms of lotteries on outcomes. I deviate slightly from this approach by making as little use of lotteries as possible in the conditions imposed on the social preference relation. The main motivation underlying my approach is that lotteries are highly artificial constructs that are typically not available in real world health decision situations. This does not imply that lotteries have no role to play in health decision making. They are for example necessary in standard gamble measurements. The reason I have avoided the use of conditions that are formulated in terms of lotteries is that in my opinion such conditions are harder to understand than conditions that are formulated in terms of certainty. The ultimate aim of characterizations is to clarify what assumptions a particular representation depends on. The easier the preference conditions are to understand the easier it is to assess the appeal of representations. An additional motivation to use the independence condition *SE* stated below is that this condition is more common in social choice theory and that a justification for imposing it has been given.[13]

Condition SE: *The social preference relation* $\succeq$ *satisfies condition SE if for all QALY allocations* $x, x', y, y' \in X$, *for all subsets of individuals* $A \subset I = \{1,...,n\}$:
$$[v_{-A}x_A \succeq v_{-A}y_A] \Leftrightarrow [w_{-A}x_A \succeq w_{-A}y_A]$$

By condition *SE*, individuals who are indifferent between two QALY allocations, the individuals who are not in subset *A*, exert no influence on social preference. Condition *SE* is the analogue of the "sure thing principle" in decision making under uncertainty

---

[12] For a definition of mutual utility independence, see for example, Keeney and Raiffa (1976, p.289).
[13] For a defense, see Fleming (1952); Deschamps and Gevers (1978); and Sen (1976, 1977b).

[Savage, 1954] and of "complete strict separability" in consumer theory [Blackorby *et al.*, 1978]. Condition *SE* underlies the current practice of using incremental analysis in cost utility analysis [cf. *e.g.*, Drummond *et al.*, 1987]. Incremental analysis prescribes how to calculate the net advantage of one program over another. The implication of this is that if two programs produce the same amount of QALYs for certain individuals, then these individuals do not influence the outcome of the analysis. This is exactly what condition *SE* asserts.

Condition *SE* is entirely formulated under conditions of certainty. However, because we seek a representation for the social preference relation under conditions of risk, we have to impose a condition which is defined with respect to preferences under risk. Consider the following condition:

Condition UI: *Let B be a subset of individuals, i.e. $B \subset I = \{1,...,n\}$, let y be a particular constant QALY allocation, $y \in X$, and let $\gtrsim_{z|y}$ be the preference relation defined over probability distributions on $\mathbb{R}^B_+$ by fixing the values of those individuals outside subset B (I-B) at levels identical to those of y. B is utility independent if $\gtrsim_{z|y}$ is independent of the constant value at which y is fixed.*

In the special case where all probability distributions are degenerate, *i.e.* one outcome results with probability one, condition *UI* is equivalent to condition *SE*. If condition *UI* holds for all subsets of individuals *B*, mutual utility independence holds. However, in combination with condition *SE* it is not necessary to impose condition *UI* for all subsets of individuals. It is sufficient to impose that *UI* holds for *one* individual. Thus, if all other *n-1* individuals are indifferent between two QALY allocations, then social preferences for lotteries on these two allocations are governed by the preferences of this particular individual. Denote this condition as UI^1. Condition UI^1 only holds when all other individuals are indifferent. The relevant individual can therefore not be considered to be a dictator in Arrow's sense. Condition UI^1 is an artificial condition, because situations like the one described in the condition will rarely occur and this makes it hard to assess the condition. However, condition UI^1 is not very restrictive in terms of the social preference relation. If the one individual for who condition UI^1 holds, is the individual who is worst off in terms of health, then it seems defensible to impose that, in case all other individuals are indifferent, social preferences under risk should be governed by the preferences under risk of this individual.

A second theorem can now be given:

Theorem 2: *The following two statements are equivalent:*
(i) the social preference relation can be represented by:

$$U(x) = (1/\lambda)\prod_{i=1}^{n}\left[\lambda U(x_i) + 1\right] - (1/\lambda) \qquad (4)$$

*where U(**x**) is a continuous social utility function, unique up to positive linear transformations and scaled between 0 and 1, the U(x_i) are identical additive utility functions, that can be interpreted as (re-scaled) QALYs and λ is a scaling constant, that is not equal to zero.*
(ii) both individual and social preferences satisfy the vNM axioms; social preferences satisfy conditions A, SE and UI[1].
If condition P also holds then λ>0.

A proof of this result can be found in the appendix.

The scaling parameter λ reflects the influence of complementarity. For example, for two individuals equation (4) reduces to:

$$U(\boldsymbol{x}) = U(x_1) + U(x_2) + \lambda U(x_1)U(x_2) \qquad (5)$$

If λ>0, complementarity increases social utility, which is the effect of imposing condition P.

Consider the example of the two individuals[14] and the three health care programs described above. Recalculating the social utility of health care programs 1, 2 and 3 gives 1, 1 and 1+0.5λ respectively. Thus, under condition P, program 3 is now preferred, which is consistent with the (imposed) preference for *ex post* equity. Indifference still holds between programs 1 and 2, because they have the same distributional implications. Indifference between programs 1 and 2 reflects the fact that *ex ante* equity has not been taken into account.

The value of λ reflects views on equity. These views can either be those of a policy maker or those of the general public. The question whose views are more appropriate is not the subject matter of this paper. Views on equity can partly be expressed by conditions such as condition P, but to determine the relative weight given to aggregating the individual QALYs (the efficiency side) and to complementarity between individual QALYs (the *ex post* equity side) require explicit choices with

---

[14] To be formally correct, for two individuals a stronger condition than SE has to be imposed: the analogue of Wakker's (1989) hexagon condition which will be discussed later in this paper.

respect to the equity-efficiency trade-off. Trading off attributes is common practice in multi-attribute utility theory and the tools of multi-attribute utility theory can be of great help in eliciting preferences between efficiency and equity in health care.

Under condition A one trade-off question is sufficient to determine λ. As an illustration, consider again the example of two individuals. In theorem 2, the $U(x_i)$ are re-scaled QALYs (for more details see the proof of theorem 2 in the appendix): $\lambda_i U'(x_i)$ where all λ_i are equal and positive and $U'(x_i)$ indicates the number of QALYs each individual receives. For the purpose of the theorem this was no problem given that vNM utility functions are unique up to positive linear transformations. However, to calculate λ we need to determine λ_i. This can be done by asking for the indifference probability p in the choice between $(1,0)^{15}$ with certainty and a gamble with outcomes $(1,1)$ with probability p and $(0,0)$ with probability $(1-p)$. Suppose the indifference probability is 0.4. Scale $U(x)$ such that $U(1,1)=1$. Then, substituting values in equation 5, $1 = 0.4*1 + 0.4*1 + \lambda*0.4*1*0.4*1$. This gives $\lambda=1.25$. It is conceivable that exact values for λ cannot be specified in every situation, but only a range of values. In that case it seems sensible to include this range of values for λ in sensitivity analyses.

Finally, the multiplicative social utility function, as derived above, only incorporates equity concerns to a limited extent. By condition SE, indifferent individuals do not exert an influence on social preference. In a situation where the non-indifferent individuals are already in a good health state but the indifferent individuals are in an appalling health state, it may be preferred that the non-indifferent individuals do not receive more QALYs in order to prevent a more unequal distribution of health (utility). Such equity concerns cannot be accommodated by the proposed multiplicative social utility function. In the next section we propose a social utility function that is able to embrace *ex post* equity concerns in a more comprehensive way.

A Two Component Social Utility Function

Continue to assume that social preferences satisfy the vNM axioms. Therefore, as in section, *QALY Utilitarianism*, and in the subsection on *A Multiplicative Social Utility Function*, the social preference relation is defined over probability distributions. We propose a method that allows the decision maker to simultaneously consider the

---

[15] Or $(0,1)$ which is under condition A equivalent to $(1,0)$.

maximization of QALYs, that can both be interpreted as health and utility, and the distribution of these QALYs, that is *ex post* equity. The idea is to assess a two component social utility function $U(y) = U(y_1, y_2)$, the components of which are the total number of QALYs (y_1) and a real valued summary index reflecting the *ex post* distribution of these QALYs (y_2). The set of outcomes, Y, is assumed to satisfy certain structural assumptions.[16] The assessment of such a two component multi-attribute utility function becomes much easier if the following assumption can be accepted:

Condition TCI (two component independence): *If two lotteries induce the same probability distribution over Y_1 (total number of QALYs gained) and the same probability distribution over Y_2 (the summary index reflecting the ex post distribution), then these lotteries are indifferent.*

This condition is similar to additive independence (and to condition H for the special case of two individuals) and guarantees, in combination with the assumption that the social preference relation satisfies the vNM axioms, by theorem 2 in Fishburn (1965) that $U(y)$ is additive:

$$U(y) = \lambda_1 U_1(y_1) + \lambda_2 U_2(y_2) \qquad (6)$$

where U, U_1 and U_2 are scaled vNM utility functions, and λ_1 and λ_2 are scaling constants that reflect views on the trade-off between "efficiency" in the sense of the maximization of QALYs and *ex post* equity.

The summary index defined over the *ex post* distribution should satisfy certain properties. For example, it should be sensitive to a transfer from an individual who is relatively well off in terms of the number of QALYs received from the implementation of a health care program, to an individual who receives less QALYs from this program. An example of such a summary index is Theil's entropy measure [cf. Sen, 1973]:

$$y_2 = \sum_{i=1}^{n} x_i \ln(nx_i) \qquad (7)$$

where x_i denotes the share of the total amount of QALYs received by individual i. y_2 increases with inequality in the QALY distribution, therefore, under condition P, $\lambda_2 U(y_2)$ must have a negative sign.

---

[16] Y is assumed to be a Cartesian product of Y_1 and Y_2, $Y_1 \in I\!R_+\backslash\{0\}$ and $Y_2 \in I\!R_+$.

Assume that condition *TCI* holds. Assume further that the utility function for the amount of QALYs is linear[17] and that the utility function for the *ex post* distribution is equal to Theil's entropy index. Then for the example in the section on *Ex Ante Versus Ex Post Equity* we obtain: $U(program\ 1) = U(program\ 2) = \lambda_1 + \lambda_2 \ln 2$; $U(program\ 3) = \lambda_1$. Under condition P $\lambda_2 < 0$, and thus program 3 is preferred, consistent with a preference for *ex post* equity.

Only one trade-off question has to be asked to determine the scaling constants, λ_1 and λ_2. Suppose that a program yields benefits for two groups of individuals and that the maximum amount of QALYs the program can generate is 100. Then the best possible outcome is (50,50): the number of QALYs is maximized and there is no inequality. Scale $U(.)$ such that $U(50,50)=1$. The worst outcome is $(x,0)$ in which x is infinitesimally small: the number of QALYs is minimized and there is complete inequality. Let $U(x,0)$ be zero. Now λ_1 can be determined by eliciting the indifference probability in a choice between $(100,0)$, *i.e.* the number of QALYs is at its maximum, but inequality is complete, for certain and a gamble giving (50,50) with probability p and $(x,0)$ with probability $(1-p)$. Suppose $p=0.85$. Substituting in equation (6) gives: $U(100,0)=\lambda_1 * 1 = p$. Thus $\lambda_1 = 0.85$ and λ_2 is by consequence equal to 0.15.

If condition *TCI* does not hold, complementarity between y_1 and y_2 has to be introduced in the model. For example, if the social preference relation does not satisfy condition *TCI*, but does satisfy a somewhat stronger condition than *SE*,[18] and does satisfy *UI_1*, then the term $\lambda \lambda_1 \lambda_2 U_1(y_1) U_2(y_2)$ should be added to the additive form, reflecting complementarity. In this case one additional trade-off question has to be asked to determine the scaling constants.

ALGORITHMS INCORPORATING BOTH *EX POST* AND *EX ANTE* EQUITY

In the section on *Ex Ante Versus Ex Post Equity* it was argued that if a concern for *ex ante* equity is to be incorporated in social preference, the vNM utility function can no longer be used. Therefore, in this section, rather than taking a preference relation over

---

[17] This assumption may appear restrictive. However, it reflects the impact of the efficiency side in the decision making process: one of the arguments in the overall utility function is the maximization of the amount of QALYs. To represent the efficiency side of the decision making process the total amount of QALYs seems a good indicator. If the linear function is not believed to be appropriate, alternative functional forms can simply be substituted.
[18] The hexagon condition.

probability distributions as primitive, a representation is sought for a preference relation under certainty. In this section we consider a three component social value function $V(y) = V(y_1, y_2, y_3)$, where y_1, y_2 and y_3 denote the number of QALYs gained, which can be both utilities and health, and real valued summary indices reflecting the *ex post* equity and the *ex ante* equity of the QALY allocation process respectively. More specifically, we will derive á representation for the value function $V(y_1^{ce}, y_3)$[19] in which y_1^{ce} denotes the certainty equivalent amount of QALYs gained, with the *ex post* equity index held fixed, for probability distributions over y_1 and y_2. Under the assumption that social preferences increase monotonically with the number of QALYs, which seems reasonable and typically is assumed in cost utility analysis, the equivalent number of QALYs will consistently rank order lotteries, a higher number corresponding to more preferred. $V(y_1^{ce}, y_3)$ is equivalent to $V(U(y_1, y_2), y_3)$ in which U is a vNM utility function defined over y_1 and y_2. By means of the social value function the certainty equivalent number of QALYs of a gamble can be traded off against its *ex ante* equity implications. Thus we continue to assume that social preferences with respect to lotteries over y_1 and y_2 while holding y_3 fixed satisfy the vNM axioms. vNM utility functions are still used to evaluate attributes y_1 and y_2, because *ex ante* equity is defined in the context of risk and therefore utility functions that are applicable in the context of decision making under risk are called for. Social policy making is essentially a normative decision problem, and to date there is no theory that challenges expected utility theory as a normative theory of decision making under risk. Diamond's objection against vNM utility theory concerned its implications for *ex ante* equity. Diamond's argument does not conflict with the use of vNM utility functions to evaluate y_1 and y_2. We will describe the preference conditions that make it possible to represent $V(Y)$ by the following simple expression:

$$V(y) = \kappa_1 V_1 [\lambda_1 U_1(y_1) + \lambda_2 U_2(y_2)] + \kappa_3 V_3(y_3) \qquad (8)$$

where U_1 and U_2 are (scaled) vNM utility functions, and V_1 and V_3 are (scaled) value functions.

Consider the following preference condition:

---

[19] The set Y is again assumed to be a Cartesian product set. It is assumed that $Y_1 \in I\!R_+ \backslash \{0\}$; Y_2, $Y_3 \in I\!R_+$. In combination with the assumption that $\geq$ on Y is a weak order, this guarantees the existence of V(Y). If $\geq$ on Y is moreover assumed to be continuous, then V(Y) will be continuous.

Hexagon condition:

$$\text{if } [(y_1^{ce'}, y_3) \sim (y_1^{ce}, y_3') \ \& \ (y_1^{ce''}, y_3) \sim (y_1^{ce'}, y_3') \ \& \ (y_1^{ce'}, y_3') \sim (y_1^{ce}, y_3'')] \text{ then}$$
$$(y_1^{ce''}, y_3') \sim (y_1^{ce'}, y_3'').$$

Suppose $y_1^{ce''} \succ y_1^{ce'} \succ y_1^{ce}$ and that $y_3'' \succ y_3' \succ y_3$. By the first two indifferences in the hexagon condition, both the utility difference between $y_1^{ce'}$ and y_1^{ce} and the utility difference between $y_1^{ce''}$ and $y_1^{ce'}$ are just sufficient to compensate the utility difference between y_3' and y_3. Then the third and the (implied) fourth indifference assert that if the utility difference between $y_1^{ce'}$ and y_1^{ce} is also just sufficient to compensate the utility difference between y_3'' and y_3', then the utility difference between $y_1^{ce''}$ and $y_1^{ce'}$ should also be just sufficient to compensate the utility difference between y_3'' and y_3'. The hexagon condition is, under transitivity of the indifference relation, implied by the Thomsen condition, which has been more commonly used as a characterizing condition for an additive two attribute utility function [*e.g.*, Debreu, 1960].

Given that the hexagon condition holds, a preference relation $\succeq_A$ can be defined over probability distributions on y_1 and y_2, while fixing y_3 at some constant reference value. This preference relation is assumed to satisfy the vNM axioms and condition *TCI* (two component independence).

Then the following result can be stated:

Theorem 3: *The following are equivalent:*
(i) $V(Y)$ can be represented by equation (8)
(ii) the social preference relation on Y is a continuous weak order that satisfies the hexagon condition, and $\succeq_A$ satisfies the vNM axioms and condition TCI.
Furthermore, V, U_1, U_2, V_3 are continuous and unique up to positive linear transformations. The λ_i's are scaling constants.

A proof of this theorem can be found in the appendix.

The summary index y_3, reflecting *ex ante* equity, should be sensitive to changes between individuals in the marginal probability of obtaining a given amount of QALYs, Q^c. The following index has this property:

$$y_3 = (1/n) \sum_{i=1}^{n} (q_i - q_m)^2 \qquad (9)$$

where q_i denotes the marginal probability of individual i receiving Q^c and q_m denotes the mean probability of receiving Q^c. A more equal distribution of marginal probabilities leads to a lower value for the summary index. Therefore, under condition E, $\kappa_3 V_3(y_3)$ should be negative. The amount of QALYs with respect to which q_i and q_m are defined should be chosen according to what it is believed that individuals are entitled to. For example, if the conviction exists that every individual should have an equal probability of receiving a life in full health then q_i denotes the individual probability of obtaining a life in full health.

Suppose with respect to the example of *Ex Ante Versus Ex Post Equity* that the conditions of theorem 3 hold and that U_1, U_2, V_1 and V_3 are identity functions, *i.e.* $U_i(y_i)$ $= y_i$, with y_2 and y_3 as in equations (7) and (9) respectively. Then *V(program 1)*$=\kappa_1(\lambda_1 + \lambda_2 \ln 2) + 0.25\lambda_3$; *V(program 2)*$=\kappa_1(\lambda_1 + \lambda \ln 2)$; *V(program 3)*$= \kappa_1 \lambda_1$. Imposing conditions E and P has the effect of making λ_2 and λ_3 both negative. Therefore, under conditions E and P the resulting ranking of the health care programs is: $3 \succ 2 \succ 1$.

The assessment of the scaling constants follows from a procedure similar to the one outlined at the end of the subsection on *A Two Component Social Utility Function*. The only difference is that in this case two trade-off questions have to be asked given that there is one additional scaling constant (one of the κ's) to assess. The additive value functions V_1 and V_3 can be assessed along the lines sketched in section 3.7 in Keeney and Raiffa (1976).

Condition *TCI* is a restrictive condition. Complementarity between $U(y_1)$ and $U(y_2)$ can be introduced by replacing condition *TCI* by the weaker condition of mutual utility independence between y_1 and y_2. If condition *TCI* is replaced by mutual utility independence, but the other conditions of theorem 3 still hold, $V(y)$ can be represented by the following equation:

$$V(y) = \kappa_1 V_1 [\lambda_1 U_1(y_1) + \lambda_2 U_2(y_2) + \lambda \lambda_1 \lambda_2 U_1(y_1) U_2(y_2)] + \kappa_3 V_3(y_3) \qquad (10)$$

This follows from theorem (6.1) in Keeney and Raiffa. In equation (10) three trade-off questions have to be asked to determine all the scaling constants: λ_1, λ_2 and one of κ_1 and κ_3.

SUMMARY AND DISCUSSION

The aim of this paper was to derive equity algorithms for utility based decision making. Because QALYs are the most commonly encountered utility based measure in the health economics literature, the paper focused on QALY based decision making. However, it should be emphasized once again that the results of the paper are entirely general: they apply to other utility based outcome measures as well. Two interpretations of QALYs were considered: QALYs as (vNM) utilities and QALYs as measures of health. In the interpretation of QALYs as utilities, an important issue that has to be resolved is the question whether utilities can be interpersonally compared. The possibility of aggregating utilities over individuals has been heavily debated within the economic science. The sections on *Aggregation of Utilities* and *von Neumann Morgenstern Utilities* provide a justification for aggregating QALYs as consistently scaled vNM utilities over individuals.

The section *QALY Utilitarianism* provided a characterization of unweighted aggregation of QALYs. It was shown that two of the conditions underlying the common practice of unweighted aggregation of QALYs over individuals are at variance with two types of equity concerns: a concern for the final distribution of the number of QALYs (*ex post* equity) and a concern for the fairness of the QALY allocation process (*ex ante* equity). By relaxing these two conditions, alternative aggregation procedures were derived that take into account (some of the) equity considerations. Even though these alternative aggregation procedures are less restrictive than unweighted QALY aggregation, they still impose restrictions on social preferences that may not be tenable in every decision context. Further generalizations of these alternative aggregation procedures are possible. One road to explore is whether results from rank dependent utility theory, currently the most popular alternative for expected utility theory in decision making under risk and uncertainty, can be translated to the context of social decision making. The idea underlying rank dependent utility theory is that different outcomes/ individuals get assigned different weights. This is basically the idea underlying the equity principles proposed in this paper.

The paper further shows that incorporating equity concerns can be achieved at relatively low cost: two additional trade-off questions are in general sufficient. Obviously, trade-offs between efficiency and equity considerations are not always easy to make. However, this can be no excuse for not making this trade-off explicit. As shown in this paper, multi-attribute utility theory can be of great help here.

APPENDIX

Proof of theorem 1:

Condition H is in fact equivalent to the condition of additive independence, which is familiar in multi-attribute utility theory. Additive independence asserts that preferences with respect to lotteries over alternatives depend only on the marginal probability of each outcome occurring and not on the joint probability distribution. Given that it has been assumed that $\succeq_z$ has been defined over a set of (simple) probability distributions, and satisfies the von Neumann Morgenstern axioms, theorem 11.1 in Fishburn (1970)[20] can be applied. According to this theorem:

$$U(x) = \sum_{i=1}^{n} U_i(x_i) \qquad (A1)$$

where the $U_i(x_i)$, called additive individual utility functions, are defined from the expected utility of the degenerate lottery that gives outcome x_i with probability 1. Given the fact that the additive individual utility functions $U_i(x_i)$ are unique up to similar positive linear transformations, it follows that the λ_i's in Harsanyi's theorem are positive. This guarantees positive association between individual and social preferences, one of Arrow's (1951a) conditions.

Imposing condition A on top of the other conditions, leads to the QALY utilitarian representation. If $(U_1, U_2,..., U_n)$ is an array of representing additive individual utility functions, then by *condition A* so are $(U_2, U_3,..., U_n)$, $(U_3, U_4,...,U_1, U_2)$,..., $(U_n, U_1,...,U_{n-1})$. Then $\{(1/n)\Sigma_i U_i, (1/n)\Sigma_i U_i,...,(1/n)\Sigma_i U_i\}$ is representing as well and so, by the uniqueness properties of the U_i, is $(\Sigma_i U_i,...,\Sigma_i U_i)$. This shows that the additive individual utility functions can be chosen identical. Set U equal to one of these additive individual utility functions and this gives the desired result.

Continuity follows from the continuity of $\succeq$ and from theorem 3.2 in Maas and Wakker (1994). Additive independence implies utility independence, which in turn implies independence. The structural assumptions made in the subsection on *Notation and Structural Function* ensure that the other conditions in Maas and Wakker (1994) are fulfilled. Weak order has been assumed. Restricted solvability and the Archimedian axiom follow from the fact that $X_i=\mathbb{R}_+$ and $X=\mathbb{R}^n_+$. $\mathbb{R}_+$ is endowed with the usual Euclidean topology, which is connected and separable. $\mathbb{R}^n_+$ is endowed with the product topology and, by theorem 5.3 in Fishburn (1970), is connected and

---

[20] See also theorem 4 in Fishburn (1965).

separable. By the proof of theorem 6.14 in Krantz, Luce, Suppes and Tversky (1971), continuity of $\succeq$ with respect to a connected product topology implies restricted solvability and the Archimedean axiom.

Proof of theorem 2:

By Maas and Wakker (1994, theorem 3.2) conditions *SE* and *UI'* are equivalent to utility independence for all subsets of $I=\{1,.....,n\}$ and U is continuous. Then by theorem 6.1 in Keeney and Raiffa (1976), if $\lambda \neq 0$, $U(x)$ can be written as:

$$\lambda U(x) + 1 = \prod_{i=1}^{n} \left[\lambda \lambda_i U_i(x_i) + 1 \right] \qquad (A2)$$

where $U(x)$ and the U_i are scaled between 0 and 1. Suppose the U_i are scaled according to the algorithm proposed by Gafni and Birch (1991). Then a life in full health has utility 1 for all individuals. If $\lambda=0$, it follows from equation (6.12) in Keeney and Raiffa (1976) that $U(x)$ can be written as equation (A1), which in combination with condition *A* gives QALY-utilitarianism.

Suppose without loss of generality that $(0,0,..,0)$ is the worst social allocation and set $U(0,0,...,0)=0$, which is allowed by free scaling of the utility function. By *condition A*: $(x,0,0,..,0) \sim_z (0,x,0,...,0) \sim_{z'} ... \sim_z (0,0,...,0,x)$. Substitute this in equation (A2) to give: $\lambda \lambda_1 U_1(x) = \lambda \lambda_2 U_2(x) = ... = \lambda \lambda_n U_n(x)$. Thus all $\lambda_i U_i$ are equal. Set these equal to $U(x_i)$. Rearranging terms gives equation (4).

Denote by $[p,x;(1-p),y]$ a program that gives allocation x with probability p, and allocation y with probability $(1-p)$. By condition P, $[0.5,(x,x,0,..,0);0.5,(0,0,..,0)]$ is preferred *to* $[0.5,(x,0,...,0);0.5,(0,x,0,...,0)]$. Calculating the expected utility of these two programs making use of equation (4) gives:

$$0.5*[(1/\lambda)*(\lambda U(x)+1)^2 - (1/\lambda)]$$
$$> 0.5*[(1/\lambda)*(\lambda U(x)+1)-(1/\lambda)]+0.5*[(1/\lambda)*(\lambda U(x)+1)-(1/\lambda)] \qquad (A3)$$

Under the assumption that a QALY is a vNM utility, *i.e.* $U(x)=x$, eq. (A3) can be rewritten as

$$(1/2\lambda)*(\lambda x+1)^2-(1/2\lambda) > (1/\lambda)*(\lambda x+1)-(1/\lambda) \qquad (A4)$$

which, after rearranging terms, gives $\lambda x/2 > 0$. Given our assumption that x is non-negative and in this particular case cannot equal zero, it follows that $\lambda > 0$.

Proof of theorem 3:

Given that Y is assumed to be a Cartesian product, that the one-attribute subsets are intervals in the real numbers, that it is implicitly assumed that the decision maker thinks both attributes of $V(Y)$ should influence social preference (*i.e.*, both attributes are essential), and that $\gtrsim$ on Y is a continuous weak order that satisfies the hexagon condition, by theorem III.4.1. in Wakker (1989), $V(Y)$ can be represented by:

$$V(y) = \kappa_1 V_1(y_1{}^{ce}) + \kappa_3 V_3(y_3) \tag{A5}$$

with V and the additive value functions V_i scaled between 0 and 1, continuous and unique up to similar positive linear transformations. The κ_i are scaling constants.
    Equivalently equation (A5) can be written as

$$V(y) = \kappa_1 V_1[U(y_1,y_2)] + \kappa_3 V_3(y_3) \tag{A6}$$

Given that condition *TCI* is equivalent to additive independence for two attributes, theorem 2 in Fishburn (1965) can be applied to give:

$$V(y) = \kappa_1 V_1[\lambda_1 U_1(y_1) + \lambda_2 U_2(y_2)] + \kappa_3 V_3(y_3) \tag{A7}$$

where the U_i are scaled between 0 and 1, unique up to similar positive linear transformations and are continuous given continuity of V_1.
    Finally, it remains to be shown that $y_1{}^{ce}$ can always be determined. By continuity of the vNM utility function it is possible to find a certainty equivalent for every lottery over y_1 and y_2. Furthermore, given continuity of $V_1 \gtrsim_A$ restricted to degenerate probability distributions is continuous. By the vNM axioms $\gtrsim_A$ is a weak order. Finally y_1 and y_2 are elements of intervals in the real numbers. Thus, by Lemma III.3.3. in Wakker (1989) $\gtrsim_A$ satisfies restricted solvability. Suppose (y_1,y_2) denotes the certainty equivalent of a lottery. By restricted solvability if $(a_1,x) \succ_A (y_1,y_2) \succ_A (c_1,x)$ where x denotes the value at which the *ex post* equity index is held fixed, then there exists (b_1,x) such that $(b_1,x) \sim_A (y_1,y_2)$. If we fix x at the value corresponding to no inequality then there will exist such (a_1,x) and (c_1,x) and thus y can always be determined.

ACKNOWLEDGMENTS

I am grateful to Peter Wakker, Eddy van Doorslaer, Christophe Gonzales and Magnus Johannesson for helpful comments.

Reprinted from *Journal of Health Economics*, Vol. 16, No. 1, Bleichrodt H, Health utility indices and equity considerations, 1997, with kind permission from Elsevier Science - NL, Amsterdam, The Netherlands.

REFERENCES

Arrow, K.J. (1950) A difficulty in the concept of social welfare. *Journal of Political Economy* 58:328-346
Arrow, K.J. (1951a; Second Edition, 1963) *Social Choice and Individual Values* New York:Wiley.
Arrow, K.J. (1951b) Alternative approaches to the theory of choice in risk-taking situations. *Econometrica* 19: 404-437.
Atkinson, A.B. (1970) On the measurement of inequality. *Journal of Economic Theory* 2: 244- 263.
Ben-Zion and Gafni, A. (1983) Evaluation of public investment in health care: Is the risk irrelevant? *Journal of Health Economics* 2: 161-165.
Blackorby, C., Primont, D., and Russell, R.R. (1978) *Duality, Separability, and Functional Structure: Theory and Economic Applications.* New York:Elsevier.
Blau, J. H. (1957} The existence of a social welfare function. *Econometrica* 25: 302-313.
Broome, J. (1982) Equity in risk bearing. *Operations Research* 30: 412-414.
Broome, J. (1988) Goodness, fairness and QALYs. In: Bell, M. and Mendus, S., editors., *Philosophy and Medical Welfare.* Cambridge:Cambridge Univ. Press.
Broome, J. (1993) Qalys. *Journal of Public Economics* 50: 149-167.
Culyer, A.J. (1989) The normative economics of health care finance and provision. *Oxford Review of Economic Policy* 5: 34-58.
d'Aspremont, C. and Gevers, L. (1977) Equity and the informational basis of collective choice. *Review of Economic Studies* 44: 199-208.
Debreu, G. (1960) Topological methods in cardinal utility theory. In, Arrow, K.J., Karlin,S., and Suppes, P., editors, *Mathematical Methods in the Social Sciences.* Stanford, CA:Stanford University Press.

Deschamps, R. and Gevers, L. (1978) Leximin and utilitarian rules: A joint characterization. *Journal of Economic Theory* 17: 143-163.

Diamond, P.A. (1967) Cardinal welfare, individualistic ethics and interpersonal comparisons of utility: (Comment) *Journal of Political Economy* 75: 765-766.

Drummond M.F., Stoddart, G., and Torrance, G.W. (1987) *Methods for the Economic Evaluation of Health Care Programs.* Oxford: Oxford University Press.

Ellsberg, D. (1954) Classic and current notions of "measurable utility." *Economic Journal* 64: 528-556.

Fishburn, P.C. (1965) Independence in utility theory with whole product sets. *Operations Research* 13: 28-45.

Fishburn, P.C. (1970) *Utility Theory for Decision Making.* New York: Wiley.

Fishburn, P.C. (1984) Equity axioms for public risk. *Operations Research* 32: 901-908.

Fishburn, P.C. (1989) Retrospective on the utility theory of von Neumann and Morgenstern. *Journal of Risk and Uncertainty* 2: 127-158.

Fishburn, P.C. and Straffin, P. (1989) Equity considerations in public risk evaluation. *Operations Research* 37: 229-239.

Fleming, M., (1952) A cardinal concept of welfare. *Quarterly Journal of Economics* 66: 366-384.

Gafni, A. and Birch, S. (1991) Equity considerations in utility-based measures of health outcomes in economic appraisals: an adjustment algorithm. *Journal of Health Economics* 10: 329- 342.

Gafni, A. and Torrance, G.W. (1984) Risk attitude and time preference in health. *Management Science* 30: 440-451.

Harris, J. (1988) More and better justice. In, Bell, M. and Mendus, S., editors. *Philosophy and Medical Welfare.* Cambridge University Press: Cambridge, pp. 75-96.

Harsanyi, J.C. (1955) Cardinal welfare, individualistic ethics, and interpersonal comparisons of utility. *Journal of Political Economy* 63: 309-321.

Harsanyi, J.C. (1975) Non-linear social welfare functions, or do welfare economists have a special exemption from Bayesian rationality. *Theory and Decision* 6: 311-332.

Harsanyi, J.C. (1987) von Neumann Morgenstern utilities, risk taking and welfare. In: Feiwel, G.R., editor, *Arrow and the Ascent of Modern Economic Theory.* London: McMillan.

Hildreth, C. (1953) Alternative conditions for social ordering, *Econometrica* 21: 81-89.

Jensen, N.E. (1967) An introduction to Bernoullian utility theory. I. Utility functions. *Swedish Journal of Economics* 69: 163-183.

Keeney, R. and Raiffa, H. (1976) *Decisions with Multiple Objectives: Preferences and Value Trade-Offs*. New York:Wiley.

Keeney, R. (1980) Equity and public risk. *Operations Research* 28: 527-533.

Krantz, D.H., Luce, R.D., Suppes, P., and Tversky, A. (1971) Foundations of measurement. Vol.I. *Additive and Polynomial Representations*. New York: Academic Press,

Lockwood, M. (1988) Quality of life and resource allocation. In, Bell, M. and Mendus, S. editors. *Philosophy and Medical Welfare*. Cambridge: Cambridge University Press, pp. 33-55.

Loomes, G. and McKenzie, L., (1989) The use of QALYs in health care decision making. *Social Science and Medicine* 28: 299-308.

Luce, R.D. and Raiffa, H. (1957) *Games and Decisions*. New York:Wiley.

Maas, A. and Wakker, P.P. (1994) Additive conjoint measurement for multiattribute utility. *Journal of Mathematical Psychology* 38: 86-101.

Mehrez, A. and Gafni, A. (1989) Quality-adjusted life years, utility theory and Healthy-years equivalents. *Medical Decision Making* 11: 140-146.

Nord, E. (1994) The QALY-a measure of social value rather than individual utility? *Health Economics* 3: 89-93.

Pliskin, J.S., Shepard, D.S., and Weinstein, M.C. 1980, Utility functions for life years and health status. *Operations Research* 28: 206-224.

Savage, L.J. (1954) *The Foundations of Statistics*. New York, Wiley.

Sen, A.K. (1970) *Collective Choice and Social Welfare*. San Francisco: Holden Day.

Sen, A.K. (1973) *On Economic Inequality*. Oxford: Clarendon Press.

Sen, A.K. (1976) Welfare inequalities and Rawlsian axiomatics. *Theory and Decision* 7: 243-262.

Sen, A.K. (1977) On weights and measures: Informational constraints in social welfare analysis. *Econometrica* 45: 1539-1572.

Sen, A.K. (1979) Personal utilities and public judgements: Or what's wrong with welfare economics? *Economic Journal* 89, 537-558.

Sen, A.K. (1986) Social choice theory. In, Arrow, K.J. and Intriligator, M. editors. *Handbook of Mathematical Economics,* Vol. III Amsterdam: North Holland .

Smith, A. (1987) Qualms about QALYs. *The Lancet* i: 1134.

Torrance, G.W. (1986) Measurement of health state utilities for economic appraisal: A review. *Journal of Health Economics* 5: 1-30.

Torrance, G.W. and Feeny, D. (1989) Utilities and quality-adjusted life years.

International Journal of Technology Assessment in Health Care 5: 559-575.

Ulph, A. (1982) The role of *ex-ante* and *ex-post* decisions in the valuation of life. *Journal of Public Economics* 18: 265-276.

Wagstaff, A. (1991) QALYs and the equity-efficiency trade-off. *Journal of Health Economics* 10: 21-41.

Wakker, P.P. (1989) *Additive Representations of Preferences: a New Foundation of Decision Analysis.* Dordrecht:Kluwer.

Wakker, P.P. (1994) Separating marginal utility and risk aversion. *Theory and Decision* 36: 1-44.

Williams, A. (1981) Welfare economics and health status measurement. In: van der Gaag, J. and Perlman, M. editors., *Health, Economics and Health Economics.* Amsterdam:North Holland, pp. 271-281.

Williams, A. (1993) Priorities and research strategy in health economics for the 1990s. *Health Economics* 2: 295-302.

15

How ought Health Economists to Treat Value Judgments in their Analyses?

A. J. CULYER

Department of Economics and Related Studies
University of York
England

The following three papers exemplify varying degrees of frustration with the ways in which (some) health economists incorporate (or fudge) value assumptions and the hostile reaction from fellow professionals to attempts to liberate themselves from the limitations of Pareto. The value assumptions in question are not, in the main, those concerning the methodology of economics (such as: "what virtues ought a good theory to have?") but value assumptions concerning society (such as: "would such and such a change in current arrangements be better for society than the *status quo*?"). In any event, I am going to focus only on the latter. As will be seen, there are implications for the way we do policy-oriented research. Indeed, how could it be otherwise? Nonetheless, I do not believe that discourse about this class of value judgments is primarily discourse about methodology. Since I have myself struggled over several years with a similar frustration, my story becomes

Health, Health Care and Health Economics: Perspectives on Distribution
Edited by Morris L. Barer, Thomas E. Getzen, and Greg L. Stoddart
Copyright 1998 John Wiley & Sons, Ltd.

inevitably a personal one and I apologise in advance for what would otherwise be an unduly immodestly frequent resort to (sometimes obscurely located) references from my own pen (later, keyboard).

A major part of this frustration arises from the limitations or misuse (Culyer, 1995a, Culyer and Evans 1996) of the Pareto criterion (PC). PC had a commendable objective, which was to minimise the intrusion of personal values into economic analysis, whose intrusion would otherwise at best threaten to bring good positive and empirical analysis into disrepute by giving a false "scientific" authority to values having no such authority or, at worst, turn our trade into a particular form of (essentially Panglossian) special pleading (Culyer, 1984). PC sought to minimise this intrusion by making a fundamental value assumption that was likely (it was hypothesised) to command widespread support: an approach embodying Keynes' plea for economists to act like "humble, competent people, on a level with dentists" (Keynes, 1972). (The attribution to Keynes of a humble competency of any kind boggles the imagination!) But this was a plausible plea for PC. After all, to have assumed that a change harming no one but benefiting at least one was a good change to make seems innocuous enough. When I first began to apply economic theory to problems in social policy, this characteristic of PC was especially useful as a unifying theme in what, at the time, was a highly diverse set of topics. It was also a useful antidote to the politicisation of the analysis of social problems (Culyer, 1971a, 1971b, 1973, 1980). However the edifice of welfare economics erected upon this value assumption requires a number of other demanding analytical and empirical assumptions to hold for its valid application (whose holding is all too rarely investigated in actual policy-oriented papers). In addition, and at least as restricting, is the fact that it is simply inapplicable to the many situations that arise involving uncompensated losses, transfers, and decisions intrinsically involving distributive equity in resource allocation. PC does not require such issues to be resolved in any particular way (conservative or radical); it simply has nothing to say about them.

But this was not all. As the following three contributors make clear, there are numerous other grounds for disquiet with PC. Rice (1998) itemises the possibilities (facts?) that relative "standing" matters to individuals more than absolute, that caring externalities are often either ignored or dealt with through theoretical devices such as lump sum transfers that never achieve empirical fulfilment, and that individual preferences are not only exogenously treated but also treated with unwarranted respect. Mooney (1998) makes similar points, adding to the list the fact that some preferences are manifestly unethical, such as racist or sadistic ones (which raises the issue even to Paretians of which *preferences* ought to count in an individual's welfare function before it may be legitimately embodied in a social welfare function), the idea of a "community commodity" which embodies the value to individuals both of participating acts within a community and of identifying with that community, and the issue (in the context of extra-welfarism rather than Paretianism) of "external judgments" which raises the question of which *individuals'* welfare functions ought to be embodied in the social welfare function (an issue that is also raised implicitly by the way in which "individual" and "consumer" are subtly interchanged in the authors' critiques of the use of PC, with the "individual" being traditionally treated as the relevant unit in traditional welfare economics and the "consumer" only so treated in bastardised forms). Hurley (1998), taking many of these objections to conventional welfare economics for granted, adds a further set of objections to extra-welfarism as a method of overcoming some of these difficulties: consequentialism (the idea that only ultimate outcomes matter), monism (the idea that only health as an outcome matters), and the limitations of a view of equity seen solely in terms of distributional justice.

The question then arises: "is there an alternative procedure in normative economics?" -- a procedure that retains the attractive imposition of political modesty on economists while also liberating us to use our apparatus to address and answer policy questions that PC denies us (and which extra-welfarism may also deny us)? An articulated general approach that seemed to supply what was needed first came to (my) attention in Sugden and Williams (1978). They assigned the economist a relatively humble role in policy analysis and suggested, as a replacement for the potential Pareto improvement version of PC (which Reinhardt has ridiculed anyway as a perversion of the PC), the use of directly obtained or carefully inferred values of "policy-makers" or "decision-makers." These may well take some teasing out. As any good consultant knows, this is usually the first and most crucial task to be undertaken; moreover, it is not over at the start of a project whose progress will, if well done, require constant referral back to check on value assumptions or to introduce new ones (Culyer, 1990b). In this scheme of things, the economist does indeed become a kind of consultant, by contributing to a decision-making *process*. The choice between options is ultimately for the policy "customer" (actual or imagined); the task of the economist is to spell out the consequences of the options and ensure that no reasonable option has been excluded from consideration at an appropriate stage of the analysis.

An entirely separate strand of thought, but one that is complementary, is Sen's (1979, 1980) idea of "basic capabilities" as the metric to replace (or to be used in addition to) "welfare" as economists customarily understand it. I have tried (Culyer, 1989, 1990a, 1992) to develop this in a rather more general way, which I have termed "extra-welfarism," so that, in principle, the analysis of efficiency in systems like health care (including markets for insurance and health care) and in specific projects within systems (like the relative cost-effectiveness of particular medical procedures) may embrace whatever maximand(s) may be given by the customers of research or inferred by diligent enquiry by the analyst to be relevant.

Although Mooney (1998) rightly claims that reliable external sources of this kind are not easily found, an implication of the approach is that it is a part of the analyst's duty to find out from their clients what the relevant values are and, at the broadest level of policy analysis, to seek suitably broad (and non-empty) authoritative value statements. At this broad level, the approach can be illustrated by taking public utterances of the following type seriously and asking what that implies for health economics research methods:

> The purpose of the NHS [National Health Service in England] is to secure through the resources available the greatest possible improvement in the physical and mental health of the people of England by: promoting health, preventing ill-health, diagnosing and treating disease and injury, and caring for those with long term disability and disease; a service available to all on the basis of clinical need, regardless of ability to pay. In seeking to achieve this purpose the NHS, as a public service, aims to judge its results under three headings: equity, efficiency and responsiveness. (Department of Health, 1996)

> The objective of the NHS Research and Development strategy is to ensure that the content and delivery of care in the NHS is based on high quality research relevant to improving the health of the nation. (Department of Health, 1991)

> The knowledge produced by trials, overviews or technology assessment can be regarded as "bullets" of effectiveness. Just like a bullet, they are of little value by themselves,and need to be loaded, aimed and fired to hit their target. (Moore *et al.*, 1994)

These three quotations, all of which come from recent official British sources, bring out successive issues in policy analysis. The first, summarily taken, states health maximisation and equitable distribution as two prime objectives of the NHS (it does not imply that these are the *only* objectives); the second defines a derived demand for health services research and implies that the NHS ought to use effective (even cost-effective) procedures, medical and other; the third implies that information provision in the pursuit of health gain requires supplementation to achieve behaviour change on the part of those at whom the information is directed. Serious economic research can address all of these issues. The first relates to measures of health and health gain as a principal output of the NHS (and other health-affecting activity) well-exemplified in the central role health economists have played in developing methods for measuring healthy, or quality-adjusted, life years (which I date from Culyer, Lavers & Williams, 1971); research into health production functions; research into equity in the distribution of health and health care; research into "responsiveness" and the ways in which consumer values might be traded off against other objectives; and research into allocation criteria such as "clinical need" -- a treacherous terrain but one that some of us have nonetheless invaded (Culyer, 1995b, Culyer & Wagstaff 1993, Williams 1974). The second relates to the cost-effectiveness of technologies and consequential methodologies for cost and outcome measurement and their valuation, while the third relates to research into behaviour change in pursuit of the overarching objectives of the system (presumably to change the behaviour of professionals within the system and patients) and the evaluation of mechanisms designed to achieve desired behaviours.

The economic research implied by these public (value) statements evidently generates only a portion of the research portfolio of health economics. The agenda therein implied is, however, one that can manifestly be more completely researched within the extra-welfarist approach than traditional welfare economics based on the PC. To the aforementioned desirable humility implied for economists in their role might also be added a more useful and policy-relevant role, by virtue of the fact that they would be addressing issues of concern to policy- and decision-makers. Their being addressed by no means requires the jettisoning of the entire economics toolkit. This may be seen readily by recognising that what is chiefly required is the insertion into objective functions of entities that either replace or are additional to the traditional concept of "welfare" or "utility," such as "health" and other characteristics of individuals, distributional concerns, and processes (for a rather standard piece of recognisable economics technology applied in this way see Culyer and Wagstaff, 1993). In fact, I can detect no omission inherent in Paretianism and logged by the authors who follow which cannot be appropriately treated within the extra-welfarist rubric.

Hurley (1998) takes issue with this view of the potential of extra-welfarism. In general, I think he pushes extra-welfarism in a direction I personally would not wish to push it, thus making it something of a straw man and failing to exploit its capacity (or, as he might have seen it, a variation in its capacity) for incorporating some of the factors he plausibly claims should command our attention. One such factor is "consequentialism," which he interprets in such a fashion as to embrace only final outcomes and to exclude processes. However, since processes are also the consequences of decisions, this is to go unnecessarily and, in my view, undesirably far. Moreover, I would want to include, or at least to allow in principle the possibility of including, not only the participation of the public in the processes through which decisions are made, which is an aspect of Mooney's communitarianism, but also the very processes of change and their consequences for individuals as members of society, as employees, and so on. These decisions usually have consequences like *losing one's job* rather than just being unemployed, or *changing one's role in an organisation* rather than just having a new employment contract. Consequences are consequences, whatever their type may be, and any that might affect welfare ought to command the attention of true Paretians let alone those of us who want to go beyond utilities in general as well as beyond the utilities that are to be had from commodities.

Monism -- the idea that a single dimension in potential outcome space is sufficient -- also receives Hurley's disapprobation. I suppose it well might *a priori*. But there are two issues at stake here. One is empirical. If there is to be an empirical grounding for the selection of the values to be embodied in evaluative economics (for example, the values shall be those of a study's clients, or those of a sample of the general public, or those stated by ministers of health) then whether it is appropriate or not to consider a single dimension, such as "health," is an empirical matter (of course, *deciding who is authoritative* in such matters is not merely an empirical matter). One will not know until one asks the relevant judges or seeks out the relevant "authoritative" statements. In practice, I suspect one's conclusions about the adequacy of employing a single outcome will depend also on context (for example, the R&D context implied by the series of official quotations that I cited earlier) and on practicality (if one sort of outcome is judged by those deemed authoritative to do the judging to be of overwhelming significance, little damage may be done by setting others to one side).

The other issue relates to what it is proper to include or exclude *a priori*. Here I side fully with Hurley. Since the great objection to the use of PC is its exclusivity, any replacement must be appropriately inclusive. In principle that means capability of including whatever is deemed relevant. But this is what is done in extra-welfarism. The only reason Hurley adduces for claiming that extra-welfarism is less inclusive than it should be lies in his belief that my own writings "strongly imply that health should be *the* outcome of concern" (Hurley,

1998). He admits that this is never stated unequivocally and there is a good reason for this, namely that it would be an unproductive limitation on what is conceived as a liberating framework of analysis. The fact that I, along with others, have strongly argued for the better measurement of health gain, and for positive predicted health gain as a necessary condition for the existence of a need for health care, and even for health maximisation as a proximate objective of a national health service, does not imply either that I take a monistic position or that I think extra-welfarism entails monism. (For a pugnacious piece that will, I fear, do little to allay Hurley's fears on these matters see Culyer, 1997.) My own view of the priorities for research in this area has been based partly on the sort of empirical consideration I have already mentioned and partly (even mainly) on the belief that progress in the measurement and use of one (important) type of outcome should not have to await the outcome of a deeper and more comprehensive theoretical settlement of all the issues raised in the emerging research programme. These are practical judgments partly to do with the practical business of developing one's own research programme and partly to do with the practical business of offering policy advice in a world of limited and imperfect information.

I see no alternative to the need for practical judgments of this kind. The papers that follow, for example, amply indicate the richness and complexity of the visions of equity that require much greater elaboration at the theoretical level, let alone empirical application. Whatever view anyone else might take, I do not consider it a compromise of principle to hold off the exploration of the policy consequences of using outcome measures that are incomplete, so long as they are significantly different from our conventional measures. I even applaud their elevation to the status of high policy statements of objectives (as in the quotations cited) on the grounds of the clarity they engender and the focus and stimulus they provide for more sophisticated and comprehensive future developments that involve a wider public than just economists.

It is important that these potentially enriching departures from Paretianism are not strangled at birth on the grounds either that the theory is as yet incomplete or that they entail a loss of discretion by economists as to choice of value judgments. And there are, moreover, challenges within the extra-welfarist programme to which the authors in this volume make no reference. One is the sector-specificity of the objective function and the as yet unresolved issue as to its generalisability across the entire scope of economic activity, public and private. There is also a significant advantage of the extra-welfarist approach which the authors do not mention. This is the considerable virtue that it facilitates in a variety of ways interdisciplinary collaboration between economists and others such as epidemiologists, managers, medics and philosophers, few of whom will find the PC approach appealing even if they were fully to understand it. It is a rather good thing for economists to find a language which can be used for talk not only amongst themselves. Fortunately, all the authors here seem agreed (albeit implicitly) on the value of that!

REFERENCES

Culyer, A.J. (1971a) The nature of the commodity "health" and its efficient allocation. *Oxford Economic Papers* 38:295-303 (reprinted as chapter 18 in Ricketts, M., editor (1989) *Neoclassical Microeconomics*, Vol 2, Aldershot:Edward Elgar, pp. 310-318.

Culyer, A.J. (1973) *The Economics of Social Policy*. London:Martin Robertson.

Culyer, A.J. (1980) *The Political Economy of Social Policy*. London:Martin Robertson.

Culyer, A.J. (1984) The quest for efficiency in the public sector: economists versus Dr. Pangloss. In Hanusch, H., editor, *Public Finance and the Quest for Efficiency*. Detroit: Wayne State University Press, pp. 39-48.

Culyer, A.J. (1989) The normative economics of health care finance and provision. *Oxford Review of Economic Policy* 5:34-58 (reprinted with changes in McGuire, A., Fen, A.P., and Mayhew, K., editors. *Providing Health Care: The Economics of Alternative Systems of Finance and Delivery*. Oxford: Oxford University Press, 65-98.

Culyer, A.J. (1990a) Commodities, characteristics of commodities, characteristics of people, utilities, and the quality of life. In Baldwin, S., Godfrey, C., and Propper, C., editors, *Quality of Life: Perspectives and Policies*. London:Routledge pp. 9-27.

Culyer A. J. (1990b) Socio-economic evaluations: an executive summary. In Luce, B., and Elixhauser, A., *Standards for Socio-economic Evaluation of Health Care Products and Services*. Berlin: Springer, pp. 1-12.

Culyer, A.J. (1992) Need, greed and Mark Twain's cat. In Corden, A., Robertson, E., and Tolley, K., editors, *Meeting Needs in an Affluent Society*. Aldershot:Avebury, pp. 31-41.

Culyer, A.J. (1995a) Chisels or screwdrivers? A critique of the NERA proposals for the reform of the NHS. In Towse, A., editor, *Financing Health*

Care in the UK: A Discussion of NERA's Prototype Model to Replace the NHS. London: Office of Health Economics, pp. 23-37.

Culyer, A.J. (1995b) Need: the idea won't do - but we still need it. *Social Science and Medicine* 40:727-730.

Culyer, A.J. (1997) The principal objective of the NHS ought to be to maximise the aggregate improvement in the health status of the whole community. *British Medical Journal* 314:667-669.

Culyer, A.J. and Evans, R.G. (1996) Mark Pauly on welfare economics: normative rabbits from positive hats. *Journal of Health Economics* 15: 243-251.

Culyer, A.J., Lavers, R.J., and Williams, A. (1971) Social indicators - health. *Social Trends* 2: 31-42 (reprinted with the same title in Shonfield, A., and Shaw, S., editors, *Social Indicators and Social Policy* London:Heinemann.

Culyer, A.J. and Wagstaff, A. (1993) Equity and equality in health and health care. *Journal of Health Economics* 12:431-457.

Department of Health (1991) *Research for Health*, London, Department of Health.

Department of Health (1996) *Priorities and Planning Guidance for the NHS 1997/98.* London: Department of Health.

Hurley, J. (1998) Welfarism, extra-welfarism and evaluative economic analysis in the health sector. This volume.

Keynes, J.M. (1972) *The Collected Writings of John Maynard Keynes, Vol ix, Essays in Persuasion* London: Macmillan for the Royal Economic Society.

Mooney, G. (1998) Communitarianism and health care economics. This volume.

Moore, A., McQuay, H., and Gray, M., (1994) *Bandolier: the First Twenty Issues.* Oxford, Bandolier supported by the NHS R&D Directorate.

Rice, T. (1998) The desirability of market-based health reforms: a reconsideration of economic theory. This volume.

Sen, A.K. (1979) Personal utilities and public judgements: or, what's wrong with welfare economics? *Economic Journal* 87:537-558.

Sen, A.K. (1980) Equality of what? In McMurrin, S., editor, *The Tanner Lectures on Human Values*, Vol. 1, Cambridge:Cambridge University Press.

Sugden, R. and Williams, A. (1978) *The Principles of Practical Cost-Benefit Analysis.* Oxford:Oxford University Press.

Williams, A. (1974) "Need" as a demand concept (with special reference to health). In Culyer, A.J., editor, *Economic Policies and Social Goals: Aspects of Public Choice.* London: Martin Robertson, pp. 60-76.

16

Welfarism, Extra-Welfarism and Evaluative Economic Analysis in the Health Sector

JEREMIAH HURLEY

Centre for Health Economics and Policy Analysis
McMaster University
Hamilton, Ontario, Canada

ABSTRACT

The welfarist and extra-welfarist evaluative frameworks differ in important ways, most notably in the types of information admissible in an evaluation. While this difference has a number of wide-ranging implications, in this paper I argue that common elements shared by the two frameworks mean that they also share some important limitations. Both frameworks share consequentialist foundations, which implies that an intervention or policy can have only instrumental value; they impose uni-dimensionality in the outcome space, which restricts the types of information that can be considered in an evaluation; and they can accommodate

Health, Health Care and Health Economics: Perspectives on Distribution
Edited by Morris L. Barer, Thomas E. Getzen, and Greg L. Stoddart
Copyright 1998 John Wiley & Sons, Ltd.

only a limited range of equity concepts.   These limitations often preclude incorporating in a valid way a number of factors potentially important in evaluating health interventions and policies.   I suggest some possible ways forward in developing broader and more flexible evaluative frameworks to reflect better the values in society.

INTRODUCTION

Getting better "value for money" appears to be the mantra of health care planners and policy makers in these cost-conscious 1990s. One prominent means for accomplishing this is to base resource allocation in the health care sector more firmly upon evidence generated by the evaluation of alternative policies, programs, and interventions. The greater reliance on evaluative evidence is manifested in many ways, including the "outcomes" movement and the associated efforts to develop practice guidelines, initiatives to require evidence of efficiency as part of submissions to have a drug listed on public formularies, and efforts to incorporate effectiveness and efficiency evidence as part of structured rationing and priority-setting exercises.[1]

These efforts, however, can achieve greater value for money only to the extent that the evaluative frameworks used to generate the evidence reflect that which we truly value. It is critical, therefore, that we scrutinize the evaluative frameworks employed to ensure that they accord with the concerns of policy makers and the public. One type of scrutiny -- the one that has probably received the greatest attention by economists -- examines the congruence between the empirical methods employed and the conceptual framework of the analysis. The current controversy regarding the properties of alternative utility-based measures of outcome exemplifies this pursuit of internal consistency.[2] A second type of scrutiny appraises the conceptual frameworks themselves (*e.g.*, Sen and Williams, 1982a; Culyer, 1989, 1990; Fox, 1990; Frankford, 1994). This paper, which is in the latter spirit, critically examines two evaluative economic frameworks used in the health sector, the "welfare economic" and "extra-welfarist" frameworks.

---

[1] This is not to say that in all such efforts evidence is actually given primacy, but each signals a new ethos that decisions should be based on evidence.

[2] See *e.g.*, Gafni, 1989; Mehrez and Gafni, 1989; Gafni and Birch, 1992; Johanesson, Plishkin and Weinstein, 1993; Mehrez and Gafni, 1993; Johanesson, 1995; and Bleichrodt, 1995.

"Welfare economic" refers to the framework for normative economic analysis that has developed within the neo-classical economic tradition (see, *e.g.*, Boadway and Bruce, 1984). The welfare economic framework, which is familiar to most economists, rests squarely on notions of individual utility or preference as the foundation for analysis. For applied analysis, the empirical approach derived from the welfare economic framework is cost-benefit analysis, a method in which the costs and benefits of the alternatives being evaluated are measured in commensurate units, usually money. "Extra-welfarist" refers to frameworks for normative economic analysis that reject the conceptual foundations of the neo-classical welfare framework, particularly the exclusive focus on utility-based notions of welfare. Amartya Sen has been a strong advocate for extra-welfarist approaches to evaluation in economics (*e.g.*, Sen, 1985). The health sector has been particularly receptive to extra-welfarist ideas, in part because of features of health care markets that render questionable certain elements of the welfare economic framework and because the role of health care in the health production function provides greater scope for third-party judgements of welfare than is the case for many goods (Evans, 1984). Culyer, who rejects utility-based notions of welfare as inappropriate for normative assessment in the health sector, builds on Sen's ideas to develop an "extra-welfarist" framework that replaces utility with health as the primary outcome of interest for evaluation (Culyer, 1989, 1990). For applied analysis, Culyer advocates using quality-adjusted-life-years (QALYs) as a measure of health, albeit QALYs in which the weights are not necessarily derived from utility values. Extra-welfarist approaches represent an important break with the welfare economic tradition, and Culyer's work represents one of the more sustained, and more successful, efforts in the health sector to develop from first principles an alternative to the welfare economic framework.[3]

Despite the important differences between the welfare economic and extra-welfarist frameworks, in this paper I argue that because they share a number of structural elements, both frameworks suffer from many of the same limitations. The starting point for this judgement is the normative proposition that a framework for normative analysis ought to be congruent with the fundamental values that prevail in society. This does not imply slavish conformity with every expressed whim or preference (even when expressed by a majority of the population), but

---

[3] For the remainder of the paper, when I use the term "extra-welfarist" I use it in a narrow sense to refer to frameworks in the health sector that advocate for health as the outcome of concern rather than utility. I focus particular attention on Culyer's work because it is the most developed.

rather that deeply held values in society are an important reference standard, and indeed, in many cases may be a more important reference standard than an abstract, theoretical standard, regardless of how rigorous, refined, and elegant it is. In some very important respects, both the welfare economic and the extra-welfarist frameworks are not congruent with fundamental values in society. This is obviously not an original observation; indeed, as will be plain, I draw heavily on the work of others.

In addition, some of key features of the frameworks included on pragmatic grounds actually buy surprisingly little, even at a purely conceptual level, towards producing unambiguous rankings of policies (a commonly cited objective for such evaluations). This is particularly true of the welfare economic framework. At the end of all the necessary qualifications, one is left feeling that if one truly takes the framework seriously and follows all its precepts (as we are exhorted to do), frequently one can say surprisingly little about which policies are best from an economic point of view. In addition, where the framework does permit such judgements, one has done so only by imposing methods at odds with common social values.

If we are to move forward, we must be willing to break even more radically from the welfare economic framework than has the extra-welfarist approach. We need break with some of the shared elements of the two frameworks, including the exclusive focus on outcomes, the uni-dimensionality of the outcome space, and the rather limited scope for accommodating equity concerns into the analysis.

In the paper I first briefly outline the central elements of both the welfare economic and the extra-welfarist approaches. I then discuss the shared elements of the frameworks and the limitations engendered by these elements. Finally, I offer some suggestions for directions in which to develop frameworks for the evaluation of social and health policies that can better reflect the fundamental values in society.

THE WELFARE ECONOMIC AND EXTRA-WELFARIST FRAMEWORKS

Neo-classical welfare economics is built on four central tenets: utility maximization, consumer sovereignty, consequentialism, and welfarism. Utility-maximization embodies the behavioural proposition that individuals choose rationally -- that is, given a set of options, an individual can rank the options and choose the most preferred among them according to defined notions of consistency.[4] Consumer sovereignty is the maxim that individuals are the best judge of their own welfare. Any judgement of individual welfare should be based on their own assessment. It rejects paternalism, the notion that a third party may know better than the person what is best for them. Consequentialism holds that any action, choice, or policy must be judged exclusively in terms of the resulting, or consequent, effects. Outcome, not process, is what matters. Welfarism is the proposition that the "goodness" of any situation (*e.g.*, resource allocation) be judged solely on the basis of the utility levels attained by individuals in that situation.

Taken together, these four tenets require that any policy be judged solely in terms of resulting utilities achieved by individuals, as assessed by individuals themselves. Issues of who receives the utility, the source of the utility, or indeed, any non-utility aspects of the situation are ignored. The only data required to evaluate alternative policies within the welfare economic framework are the utilities generated by each policy (Sen, 1979).

Completing the process of evaluation requires a criterion by which to rank alternative policies based on the utility information. Early neo-classical welfare economics was solidly utilitarian: utility was assumed to be cardinally measurable and interpersonally comparable, and the best policy was the one that maximized the sum of utilities in the population. With the development of ordinal utility theory, which dropped the assumptions that utility is cardinally measurable and interpersonally comparable, the criterion of maximizing the sum of utilities was replaced by the criterion of Pareto Optimality. A resource allocation is judged to be Pareto Optimal if and only if it is impossible to increase one person's utility without simultaneously decreasing another's. For applied welfare analysis this shift came with a heavy price. For a given set of resources, each of many possible allocations of those resources can be Pareto Optimal; the Pareto criterion does not lead to a single, best allocation. Second, because nearly all policy changes hurt someone, strict application of the criterion leads to policy paralysis. In an effort to overcome this limitation, attention shifted to the criterion of a Potential Pareto Improvement: a policy is said to produce a Potential Pareto Improvement if benefits that accrue to the gainers are sufficiently large to enable them to (hypothetically) compensate the losers, making the losers no worse off than they

---

[4] Consistency follows from the axioms of choice: (1) completeness; (2) reflexivity; and (3) transitivity (Varian, 1978).

were before the policy, while still retaining some net benefit for gainers. Much practical policy work is conducted on the basis of this principle.[5]

Culyer's extra-welfarist approach for the health sector is rooted in a distinction between things, characteristics of things, people, and characteristics of people. Things are commodities in the usual sense (*e.g.*, automobiles, ice cream cones) and characteristics of things are attributes of those commodities (*e.g.*, styling, horsepower; flavour, fat content). Analogously, characteristics of people refers simply to attributes that describe a person, *e.g.*, hair colour, age, sex, race, height, health sta tus, degree of social isolation, utility, etc.

In contrast to welfare economictheory and its focus on utility, the extra-welfarist approach asserts that the evaluation of welfare should focus on the characteristics of people, including and perhaps most importantly, non-utility characteristics. Two pivotal concepts that emerge from the characteristics of people approach are deprivation and need. Culyer argues that, "If the characteristics of people are a way of describing deprivation, desired states, or significant changes in people's characteristics, then commodities and their characteristics are what is often *needed* (emphasis in the original) to remove their deprivation..." (Culyer, 1990, p. 12). The most relevant characteristic in evaluating alternative policies in the health sector is health. Ill-health creates a need for health care, which restores a person's health (or forestalls a worsening of health).[6] If the relationship between specific health care services and changes in health status can be reasonably determined through clinical evaluation, analysts in the health sector can use the concept of need with more precision than in most other sectors. If a health care service does not improve health status, Culyer argues, it would not be judged to be needed, and indeed would not be wanted by most people aware of its ineffectiveness.

Though never stated unequivocally, Culyer's writings (1989, 1990), strongly imply that health should be *the* outcome of concern.[7] In the early articulations of

---

[5] Although the ethical problems associated with hypothetical compensation are recognized by many economists, the technical limitations of the PPI criterion are generally underappreciated. At the purely theoretical level, the PPI criterion does not produce unambiguous rankings because reversals are possible. And at a more practical level, the PPI criterion cannot serve as a conceptual foundation for using the net benefit criterion in cost-benefit analysis (Blackorby and Donaldson, 1990).

[6] Ill health does not, *per se*, create a need for health care. If there is no effective health care treatment for a condition, then there is no associated need for health care.

[7] He states that "In health economics, the extra-welfarist approach has taken "health" as the proximate maximand. This does not imply the complete ousting of "welfare" ..." (Culyer, 1989, p. 51). And again, "...extra-welfarism in health economics may be seen to take "health"output as the maximand.

his extra-welfarist framework, Culyer defined the objective of health care policy as maximizing population health. Adopting this "health-maximizing" stance did not, however, imply a lack of concern with equity. Rather, Culyer argued that equity and efficiency concerns could be reconciled within the extra-welfarist approach to maximizing health through a system of distributional weights based on the characteristics of people.[8] Culyer has since modified his views regarding equity in the health sector (Culyer and Wagstaff, 1993) in ways that make it less clear whether maximizing population health can be reconciled with achieving equity.

The extra-welfarist framework, therefore, is driven by the following analytic imperative: from the set of all characteristics of people, define the set of characteristics that are normatively relevant for evaluation in the health sector, measure the level of deprivation in these characteristics, assess the corresponding need for commodities (health care in particular) to address these deprivations, and determine alternative allocations of resources to reduce the deprivations.

At the conceptual level, therefore, the single most important break between the extra-welfarist approach and the welfare economic approach is the extra-welfarist's rejection of welfarism -- the principle that the goodness of any situation or allocation be judged solely in terms of the associated utilities achieved by individuals. Extra-welfarists argue that welfarism is inherently limited because "utility focuses too much on mental and emotional responses to commodities and characteristics of commodities and not enough on what they enable you to do" (Culyer, 1990, p. 15). A problem with focusing on such mental states, for example, is adaptation (Sen, 1987b; Elster, 1982; Kahneman and Varey, 1991). Those born in poverty with no hope of escaping often adjust expectations rather than suffer a life of constantly falling short of aspirations. Similarly, those suffering from disabilities often adjust and live lives full of satisfaction and meaning. That such individuals have high levels of "utility" (higher indeed than many wealthy or non-disabled) does not deny that they may have legitimate claims for special

---

The emphasis is in principle not exclusive..." (Culyer, 1989, p.55). But alongside these more qualified statements are numerous references that imply that health is the single outcome of interest. "There are also implications for rationing care (equalizing marginal products in terms of health per unit resource)" (Culyer, 1989; 51) and "optimal resource use is determined by equality of marginal health output per unit in various activities and across various groups" (Culyer, 1989, p.55).

[8] This is directly analogous to the system of weights that has been proposed to accommodate distributional concerns within cost-benefit analysis (*e.g.*, Weisbrod, 1968). Strictly speaking, however, such weights are not admissible in the welfarist framework because they constitute non-utility information.

considerations. An extra-welfarist approach, Culyer argues, can accommodate such concerns in a way that the welfarist approach cannot.

SHARED LIMITATIONS OF THE TWO FRAMEWORKS

The welfare economic and the extra-welfarist frameworks represent alternative, and in key respects, non-reconcilable frameworks for evaluating health policies and their attendant resource allocations. They derive from distinct conceptual foundations -- one utility-based, giving primacy to satisfying preferences, the other health-based. But perhaps what is more striking is the similarity of the two frameworks. Extra-welfarism has effectively substituted "healthism" for welfarism. This substitution has important implications, but the structural elements shared by the two frameworks, particularly restrictions on the types of information that can enter an evaluation and the way that information is used, means that both frameworks are subject to many of the same types of criticisms and limitations, criticisms that have grown more pronounced in recent years (Hausman and McPherson, 1993; Sen, 1979, 1987a). I focus on three shared problematic elements: consequentialism, monism (uni-dimensionality) with respect to outcomes, and the restricted range of equity concepts that can be accommodated within the frameworks.

CONSEQUENTIALISM

Both frameworks are strongly consequentialist. From this it follows that any aspect of the health care system, any policy or any action being evaluated can have only instrumental value for achieving a pre-determined outcome of concern. Strictly speaking, actions or processes can never be valued intrinsically. An emphasis on outcomes in evaluation is not unreasonable. After all, much human action and most policy making is purposeful (even if not maximizing) -- in general we try to accomplish things through our actions. But consequentialism, and the attendant focus on instrumental rationality, engenders an over-emphasis within these frameworks on efficiency compared to equity. Within the welfare economic framework, this tendency received further impetus from the fundamental theorems of welfare economics, which engendered a false dichotomy between efficiency and equity, with an undue emphasis on efficiency as a criterion of evaluation (Zajac, 1985; Reinhardt, 1992). This focus, and the extent to which it is at odds with deeply held values in society, was expressed nicely by Zajac, an economist with extensive experience in public utility regulation:

> Why do [public utility] regulators, and even the public generally, find it so hard to accept and apply the principles of economic efficiency - principles that are so obvious to trained economists? Is it simply that the public is economically illiterate? Or is it the economists who are out of step, insisting that everyone march to their drummer, when in fact they are deaf to a more fundamental beat that drives society? My continual immersion in public utility regulation has gradually led me away from "the public is illiterate" view and more toward the "economists are deaf" view (Zajac, 1985, p. 119).

Where equity considerations are included, they are nearly always restricted to distributional equity (i.e., the distribution of an outcome of interest).

Consequentialist reasoning is often contrasted with approaches that emphasize process over outcome, and which give virtually no weight to efficiency considerations. An outcome is fair and reasonable so long as it is generated by a fair and reasonable process. Such approaches often accord individual rights absolute status, so a policy or action is ethical only if it does not violate anyone's rights (*e.g.*, Nozick, 1974).[9]

By suitably defining the outcome to include process elements, consequentialist approaches can reflect at least some aspect of process concerns. Because utility functions can include nearly anything as arguments, the welfare economic approach is more malleable in this respect. The notion of "process utility" has developed to address some of these types of concerns (McGuire, Henderson, and Mooney, 1988). But even where this is possible, such concerns are captured only to the extent that they impinge on utility. The extra-welfarist framework, in which health is the outcome of concern, is severely restricted in its ability to accommodate process considerations.

In the end it appears that neither an exclusively consequentialist framework nor an exclusively process-oriented framework does justice to the range of concerns that deserve weight in an evaluative framework. Outcomes clearly matter, and indeed are often of primary importance, but one need not go to the extreme of violating basic rights to recognize that process considerations matter often in ways that are not well captured even by such measures as process utility. Concepts such as

---

[9] Within the health sector, for example, such reasoning underlies the prohibition against compelling a person to undergo a medical treatment, regardless of the consequent health benefits (except, perhaps, in extreme cases involving communicable diseases).

"duty," "fair," or "right" have value outside their utility effects. The challenge is to develop frameworks that can incorporate the full range of considerations in ways that reflect how they are valued.[10]

UNI-DIMENSIONAL OUTCOME SPACE

Monism, or uni-dimensionality in the outcome space, is one variant of consequentialism that restricts the consequences considered to a single outcome. In welfarism that single outcome is utility; in extra-welfarism it is health. Within economics, monism appears to be motivated in large part by its perceived pragmatic advantages in facilitating economic notions of rationality in decision making. Rationality entails ranking alternatives and then choosing consistently among them in accordance with the axioms of choice. If the measurement scale for the outcome is chosen suitably, monism can facilitate the process of ranking alternatives. The problems with it can be classified into three main areas.

First, focusing on only one consequence means that other consequences, some of which may be highly valued by individuals, often are excluded from an evaluation. In the case of extra-welfarism, no benefit other than health has a weight in the evaluation, a feature at odds with widely held views. For example, two consequences associated with universal, publicly funded health care insurance financed through a progressive tax system (such as in Canada) are risk spreading and a redistribution of income from the healthy wealthy to the sick poor. These non-health benefits do not fit easily into the extra-welfarist evaluative framework as it has developed in the health sector. Even in the evaluation of individual clinical services non-health benefits are often valued. In the evaluation of prenatal screening, for example, Mooney and Lange (1993) found important non-health, informational benefits for the women.

Because the utility functions of individuals can include a wide range of arguments, a welfarist approach is more amenable to at least reflecting a wider range of effects. But measuring all effects in the same, commensurate units creates its own problem, namely that of distortion. In the case of utility, the various effects can be viewed, and valued, only through the lens of utility. Many argue that the inherent diversity and incommensurability of different types of effects precludes meaningfully transforming each into a common metric (Taylor, 1982). This is

---

[10] Scheffler (1994), for instance, attempts to relax consequentialism to accommodate more easily rights and procedural concerns.

particularly a problem in applied work derived from these conceptual frameworks. In applied work derived from the welfare economic framework all effects are usually measured in dollars; in the extra-welfarist context all aspects of health must be reduced to a single-dimensional health measure such as a quality-adjusted life-year. In general then, monism may either seriously distort the measurement of benefits, or exclude consideration of certain types of benefits altogether.[11]

A second problem within monism is that less is gained by it than is commonly assumed (and asserted). In particular, uni-dimensionality in outcomes provides neither necessary nor sufficient conditions for generating complete rankings of alternative policies. The ability to evaluate and rank the alternatives depends also on the measurement properties of the outcome measure employed and the decision rule used. The critical importance of measurement properties is illustrated by using non-interpersonally comparable, ordinal utility as a measure of welfare. In such a context, one nearly always faces intractable aggregation problems, and one is left with decision rules such as the Pareto Principle, which produces incomplete rankings. Even if interpersonally comparable, cardinal utility is assumed, as long as the Paretian decision rule is retained, one cannot be sure of complete rankings because there may be multiple Pareto Optimal resource allocations, none of which can be compared against another. Within welfarism complete rankings can be generated only under the assumptions of cardinal, interpersonally comparable utility and a non-paretian decision rule, such as in classical utilitarianism (Boadway and Bruce, 1984). Analogous assumptions must be made within the extra-welfarist approach regarding measures of health and the decision rule employed.

If a uni-dimensional outcome space does not guarantee the ability to generate complete rankings, it is also important to note that multiple outcomes do not necessarily imply an inability to rank alternatives (though multiple outcomes obviously complicates matters). Nor do multiple outcomes necessarily generate inconsistency in choice (Sen and Williams, 1982b). In short, the links among uni-dimensionality, achieving a complete ranking of alternatives from best to worst, consistency in choice (rationality) is more complex than often supposed, and this complexity substantially undercuts the ultimate value of monism within evaluative frameworks.

The final consideration relates to the practical importance of achieving complete rankings within the economic analysis through a uni-dimensional outcome. When

---

[11] In many respects, this is an old, often-repeated criticism, but its age and familiarity do not lessen its veracity.

faced with the criticisms noted above regarding the inability of such approaches to include validly all relevant effects, economists often respond that the results of economic evaluations are only one piece of information intended to aid decision making and that other relevant considerations will enter via other avenues at the time a decision is taken. If true, then much of the force for monism and achieving complete rankings of alternatives evaporates. In such a decision-making process the information generated by the economic evaluation would ultimately have to be combined with other data measured in different units. If this is so, why should the entire structure of the economic evaluation be distorted so as to obtain a single number at the end of the analysis (the net benefit in welfarist based cost-benefit analysis, the cost-per-QALY in extra-welfarist cost-utility analyses)? Even from a strictly economic perspective, this single number is often inadequate for judging alternatives. Drummond, Torrance and Mason (1993), for instance, argue that the results of economic evaluations should be reported at a highly disaggregated level if they are to be useful and allow meaningful comparisons across programs. If true, it is not clear why an entire analysis should be structured to produce a single number, a number which, in the end, is of only limited value as an aid to decision making.

For both conceptual and practical reasons it would appear that monism may impose far greater restrictions on an evaluation than can be justified by the benefits it engenders.

EVALUATIVE ECONOMICS AND JUSTICE

Zajac's observation that individuals care deeply about issues of justice when evaluating economic policies falls squarely within a growing empirical literature documenting that justice and equity figure prominently in the allocation rules individuals adopt (Yaari and Bar-Hillel, 1985; Frohlich and Oppenheimer, 1992; Miller, 1992; Elster, 1991, 1992; Nord, *et al.*, 1995). Experiments have repeatedly demonstrated, for instance, that over quite a large range individuals are willing to trade-off efficiency (i.e., maximizing total output) for distributional equity, at times even to their own detriment. Therefore, on both empirical and philosophical grounds, there are compelling reasons for economists to take justice and equity more seriously in evaluative economic analysis. Yet, within both the welfare economic and the extra-welfarist frameworks, such considerations can enter in only limited ways, ways that cannot always accommodate factors consistently found to be important for assessing the equity of alternative policies and the resulting resource allocations.

Judgements of equity are complex, multi-factorial phenomena. Empirical investigations of such judgements indicate that universalistic theories of justice or equity often fail to reflect the contingent factors that make equity judgements context dependent (Walzer, 1983; Miller, 1992; Elster, 1992). Although such judgements are, indeed, context dependent, they are not necessarily *ad hoc*. Patterns and regularities have been identified, often relating to such factors as the nature of the resources in question, the purposes to which they will be put, the characteristics of the individuals affected, the relationships among them, etc. Such underlying principles, however, stop well short of a unified theory. In addition to this empirical literature, there is a growing recognition within philosophy that ethics should perhaps forego aspirations to develop an overarching, unified framework intended to be applied to all problems (MacIntyre, 1984, 1988; Taylor, 1989).

In the following section I discuss (non-exhaustively) some ways in which the welfare economic and extra-welfarist frameworks limit the range of equity concepts that can be incorporated into evaluative economic analyses.

DISTRIBUTIONAL EQUITY

The central concept of distributional equity underlying the welfare economic approach is that each member of society is weighted equally in an evaluation. According to the Paretian formulation, each person's preferences are accorded equal consideration -- in judging two resource allocations, a decrease in utility by any single individual is sufficient to block the judgement that one allocation is better than another. Within classical utilitarian formulation, each person's utility is weighted equally in the process of summing utility scores. However, strictly adhered to, each formulation cannot readily accommodate concerns relating to the distribution of utility among individuals. Within the Paretian framework, because interpersonal comparisons of utility are disallowed, distributional issues cannot be incorporated in any way. Hence, analytical welfare analyses generally assume either a single-person "society" with a representative consumer, or that all individuals in society have the same preferences. Within utilitarianism only the total utility matters; its distribution across individuals has no bearing.[12] Strictly

---

[12] Under the assumption that utility is interpersonally comparable it is possible to create a Bergson-Samuelson social welfare function (among others) that incorporates judgements of distributional equity (see, *e.g.*, Boadway and Bruce, 1984).

adhered to, the welfare framework is essentially mute with respect to assessing distributional issues.

The extra-welfarist framework is more accommodating to distributional issues, Culyer argues, because it can more naturally incorporate a system of differential weights based on equity -- relevant characteristics of individuals as discussed above.[13] The weights themselves could be based on any factor that affects how individuals value producing health for a person with the characteristic as opposed to a person without it (*e.g.*, age, social/occupational roles/family responsibilities, initial health status, etc.).

Distributional weights do offer scope for incorporating distributional concerns. It is vital, however, that in any such system the ethical basis for the weights be clear, as the identical system of weights may be motivated by very different ethical positions. Evidence suggests that in general people value differently the production of health among various sub-groups of the population (see, *e.g.*, Williams, 1988). This suggests a system of differential weights that is in accordance with the different values placed on producing health in the relevantly defined sub-groups. However, differential weights can also result from a fundamental desire to value health equally among individuals. Elster (1991) recounts the results of an experiment in which individuals were asked to allocate a fixed supply (48 pills per day) of pain relief medication between two individuals identical in all respects except their ability to metabolize the medication. Person A's metabolism is such that it takes three pills to provide one hour of relief, while B's is such that it takes only one pill to gain one hour of relief. In the experiment, more than three-quarters of respondents opted for an allocation that *equalized the pain experience by A and B*. Formally, this is equivalent to valuing the production of A's health three times more than in B's health. However, this interpretation misses a fundamental aspect of what is valued. A and B are valued equally and are equally deserving of being relieved of pain -- because they are equal, resources are allocated unequally to achieve equal outcome distributions. This type of result has been found in a number of different distributional contexts for a variety of goods (*e.g.*, Yaari and Bar-Hillel, 1985; Miller, 1992).

The Yaari and Bar Hillel (1985) work highlights the fact that choice problems that can be formally characterized identically (like the weights above) are nonetheless interpreted quite differently by individuals. It underlines in particular why pure preferences (and associated willingness-to-pay measures) are often an

---

[13] See note 8, above.

inadequate basis for making allocative decisions that reflect equity concerns.[14] Yaari and Bar-Hillel's investigations demonstrated that the reason why someone preferred a good was relevant -- was the good to be used to meet a health need or was it to be used to satisfy a taste? Other research demonstrates that individuals choose different allocation rules for formally identical problems depending on the relationships among the individuals involved (Miller, 1992; Mannix *et al.*, 1995). In settings where the relations are impersonal and possibly even competitive (*e.g.*, market contexts), priority is given to reward based on contribution or desert; in contexts where relations are more personal and/or cooperative, notion of equality and of responding to need are given priority. All of the above document how different allocation principles may be chosen for the same good depending on various aspects of context. Another line of investigation explored how the nature of the good being allocated affects the types allocation principles used (Walzer, 1983; Elster, 1992).

The importance of context is further reflected by the pervasive influence of reference states, particularly the *status quo*, on equity judgements. Judgements regarding the fairness of redistributions, for example, differ in important ways from judgements regarding the fairness of a final distribution. In Elster's pill experiment discussed above, if initially one pill provides one hour of relief for both A and B, so that each receives 24 pills daily and attains complete relief, followed several months later by a change in A's metabolism so that three pills are required per hour of relief while B's metabolism remains unchanged, only 50% endorse a redistribution to achieve an equal pain distribution. When the situation is reversed, however, so that, both A & B initially require three pills per hour of relief and B's metabolism subsequently changes to requiring only one pill per hour, 70% endorse a redistribution of pills to equalise pain relief. Asymmetric treatment of gains and losses is akin to what has been found in the more general decision making literature (*e.g.*, Tversky and Kahneman, 1981), and a significance attached to initial distributions of rights/claims pervades empirical research in this area.

BEYOND DISTRIBUTIVE JUSTICE

Both frameworks also exclude considerations of justice or equity beyond distributive justice. But again, research on beliefs about fairness demonstrates that

---

[14] Others have also questioned on conceptual grounds the place of pure preferences in ethical reasoning (Scanlon, 1975; Sagoff, 1994).

concepts of fairness extend to issues other than the distribution of rewards. Concepts of procedural justice play a prominent role in judging policies and their resulting resource allocations. Procedural justice focuses on process: How are decisions made? Who is involved in what ways? What factors are considered and what weight do they receive in the decision-making or the allocation process? Process considerations come to the fore in any context of explicit rationing of scarce resources, as for example, in the recent process used by Oregon to ration access to services within its Medicaid program. Among many observers and commentators, the process received more attention than the final decision as to what services would be eligible for funding. In such contexts, due process becomes a pivotal value. Rules used in areas where rationing has been practiced for a long time, such as allocating organs for transplant, reflect the importance for procedural concerns. Systems that are perceived as optimal are heavily influenced by procedural fairness and explicitly do not attempt to maximize the health produced by always giving the organ to the individual who has the highest-probability of successful transplant (Elster, 1991, 1992).

However, taking process concerns into account is not always straightforward. When good that is not infinitely divisible is in short supply, a lottery that gives each eligible individual an equal chance of receiving the good is often advocated on conceptual grounds as a fair process by which to allocate the good. Elster (1992) argues, however, that lotteries are seldom used, in part because, as a process, a lottery does not allow an individual's claims to be heard and taken account of in the allocation process. As noted above, to the extent that procedural concerns affect utility levels, the welfare economic framework can reflect them. But it can be questioned whether utility is the most appropriate metric in which to account for such effects. Measures of process utility may serve well when all that is at stake is choosing among processes to respond to "tastes," but when more fundamental issues of justice are at stake, utility may be less suitable.

WHERE DO WE GO FROM HERE?

This panoply of difficulties and limitations often engenders one of two polar reactions. One is to throw up one's hands and advocate abandoning structured economic evaluation altogether. However, this reaction is unhelpful, because, as economists and other analysts frequently point out, resource allocations and implicit evaluation will take place anyway. There are contexts in which implicit evaluation may be preferred to explicit evaluation (Elster, 1992), and indeed, we can never be sure that resource allocations based on implicit evaluations are inferior. However, as a society we have a responsibility to assess systematically the effects of policies in an attempt to ensure that they contribute toward social objectives in ways that reflect social values.

At the other extreme, many grow dogmatic, insisting on rigid adherence to "official," highly refined economic theory. Analyses that do not conform to the theory are simply labeled *ad hoc*.[15] This reaction overlooks a number of problems. First, as has been argued, it is not clear that the existing welfare and extra-welfarist frameworks accord well with social objectives and social values. Second, it is virtually impossible to conform with all aspects of the theory in practical policy analysis, and there is no evidence that violating only one precept necessarily gets one closer to the true answer (even in terms of the chosen framework) than violating two precepts.[16]

In closing I offer a few tentative suggestions for how we might proceed to develop evaluative frameworks with enough structure to be meaningful but enough flexibility to accommodate some of the complex, often conflicting, factors that are relevant to an evaluation. I do not offer an alternative framework; I try merely to point in what I believe are constructive directions.

A starting point is to think more carefully about the role of researchers and research evidence in addressing social issues. Many have argued that researchers ought to complement and support the policy making process by helping to identify relevant issues and provide information needed for deliberation over those issues (Lindblom and Cohen, 1979; Schmid, 1989). An important step in this direction is for economists (and other researchers) to be less ambitious with respect to the questions asked (though not in the policy issues addressed). Being more modest may have the paradoxical result of providing more useful information to decision makers. Both the welfarist and extra-welfarist frameworks emanate from a view that social problems can (should) be solved analytically, in wholly "rational" ways (i.e., as defined by the frameworks). The frameworks are structured to determine analytically which programs, interventions, or set of programs and interventions are best for society -- essentially trying to do a complete analysis for society.

In the face of rival conceptions of justice and equity, and the differing views

---

[15] See McCloskey (1985) for discussion of this practice in economics, which he labels the "Demarcation Problem."

[16] One is tempted here to make an analogy to the Theory of the Second Best.

held by members of society, to "close" such normative analyses economists have historically retreated to the Pareto Criterion -- a weak ethical position that would appear to be acceptable to everyone. The hope has been that it might still be possible to judge policies even with such an "innocuous" criterion. The result is a rather stilted framework, perhaps not surprising given the retreat to the lowest common denominator. But another type of retreat is possible in the face of this genuine and deep difficulty created by the diversity and complexity of ethical perspectives.

Analytical approaches are only one way to address social problems (Lindblom and Cohen, 1979; Frankford, 1994). It may be more fruitful for evaluators to provide the underlying information required for formulating an answer rather than to try to provide the answer itself. That is, perhaps we ought to refrain from determining definitively which policy is best for society (even if only from an economic perspective) and focus more on providing the "raw" information required to make such judgements. One of the purposes of many institutions in society, most obviously political ones, is to take information, evaluate trade-offs, and integrate varying perspectives and values to make decisions. Sometimes this is done analytically, but often it is not. Where such non-analytical processes are deemed most appropriate, the researcher should complement the process rather than try to replace it.

Such a retreat still leaves considerable scope for economists to utilize their specialized skills. In particular, economics still offers considerable insight into how various effects can be measured, the relation among important variables, and so on. Indeed, presumably much of the information currently collected in evaluations would be relevant. How it is assembled and presented, however, would be quite different. One immediate consequence of such an approach would be room for less rigid analytical frameworks. By forfeiting the need to produce an analytic solution, the imperative for certain features of the welfare economic and extra-welfarist frameworks recedes (*e.g.*, uni-dimensionality of outcomes; constraints imposed by need to aggregate explicitly all effects, etc.). A more pluralistic approach might also force researchers to think more carefully about taxonomic principles that can provide guidance in choosing methods and in determining which factors are most important in a given analysis.

It is clear, for example, that we care exclusively for neither utility nor health as an outcome. In some situations, non-health-related utility effects appear important; in others, we readily discount them (*e.g.*, extremely risk-averse individuals demanding high-cost tests for rare diseases). Similarly, one of the clear social objectives of health policy is to improve health -- it is not just one of many thousands of ways to increase utility in society -- health care has been singled out because the primary objective of health care is to produce health. In short, there are situations in which health effects appear to dominate, others where utility effects dominate, and others where other considerations altogether dominate.

The challenge is to develop defensible principles to guide analysts through such issues, a task that could have tremendous pay-off. The principles employed might reflect, for example, alternative levels of analysis (*e.g.*, system-wide issues, programmatic issues, interventions), the nature of the alternatives under examination (*e.g.*, clinical intervention; non-medical organizational issues); the nature of the groups affected by the policies under consideration, or the ultimate source of the benefit (*e.g.*, what underlies a utility benefit, satisfaction of some basic need or merely the satisfaction of some preference). The point is to let the question drive the analyses rather than simply imposing a pre-determined framework and making the question fit the framework in procrustean fashion.

The work of Leamer (1978) in econometrics may offer a useful analogy. The classical inferential statistics espoused in classrooms are regularly discarded in the computer room by those working with actual data. To conform to the strict standards of classical statistics would be nonsensical (don't look at the data ahead of time; only run the regression once; don't test alternative specifications, etc.). Applied statistical analysis is inherently judgement filled, and the gap between the theory and practical work leaves researchers in the lurch. In the absence of any real guide, researchers employ any number of purely *ad hoc* methods of specification testing. Leamer (1978) therefore set out to find the middle ground -- to systematically analyze alternative types of specification problems and how specification search strategies can be done legitimately (or at least understandably).

The hope is that within the area of normative analysis in health the taxonomic principles envisioned could offer both a middle ground for sound reasoning that reflects the real world of social values and the flexibility to respond to the particularities of different decision contexts while providing enough rigour to be meaningful.

Lastly, and perhaps most importantly, economists and others who conduct evaluative economic analyses must appreciate more deeply that such analyses are inherently exercises in social ethics. The developing methods for empirically investigating equity concepts, and the growing cross-fertilization between the empirical and conceptual equity literatures offer new possibilities for incorporating equity principles in ways congruent with social values. The development of methods for such evaluative economic analyses needs to occur in conversation with the broader literature on social ethics and moral philosophy.

REFERENCES

Blackorby, C. and Donaldson, D. (1990) The case against the use of the sum of compensating variations in cost-benefit analysis. *Canadian Journal of Economics* 23(3):471-494.

Bleichrodt, H. (1995) QALYs and HYES: Under what conditions are they equivalent? *Journal of Health Economics* 14:17-37.

Boadway, R. and Bruce, N. (1984) *Welfare Economics.* Oxford:Basil Blackwell.

Culyer, A.J. (1989) The normative economics of health care finance and provision. *Oxford Review of Economic Policy* 5(1):34-58.

Culyer, A.J. (1990) Commodities, characteristics of commodities, characteristics of people, utilities, and the quality of life. *In* S. Baldwin, Godfrey, C., and Propper,C., editors, *Quality of Life: Perspectives and Policies.* London: Routledge, pp. 9-27.

Culyer, A. and Wagstaff, A. (1993) Equity and equality in health and health care. *Journal of Health Economics* 12(4):431-458.

Drummond, M., Torrance, G., and Mason, J. (1993) Cost-effectiveness league tables: more harm than good? *Social Science and Medicine* 37(1):33-40.

Elster, J. (1982) Sour grapes and the genesis of wants. *In* Sen, A. and Williams, B., editors, *Utilitarianism and Beyond.* Cambridge: Cambridge University Press.

Elster, J. (1991) Local justice and interpersonal comparisons of utility. In Elster, J., and Roemer, J., editors, *Interpersonal Comparisons of Well-Being.* New York: Cambridge University Press, pp. 98-126.

Elster, J. (1992) *Local Justice.* New York: Russell Sage Foundation.

Evans, R. (1984) *Strained Mercy.* Toronto: Buttersworth.

Fox, D. (1990) Health policy and the politics of research in the U.S. *Journal of Health Politics and Law* 15(3):481-499.

Frankford, D. (1994) Scientism and economism in the regulation of health care. *Journal of Health Politics, Policy and Law.* 19(4):773-799.

Frolich, N. and Oppenheimer, J. (1992) *Choosing Justice: An Experimental Approach to Ethical Theory.* Los Angeles: University of California Press.

Gafni, A. (1989) The quality of QALYs: do QALYs measure what they at least intend to measure. *Health Policy* 13(1):81-83.

Gafni, A. and Birch, S. (1992) Equity considerations in utility-based measures of health outcomes in economic appraisals: an adjustment algorithm. *Journal of Health Economics* 10(3):329-342.

Hausman, D. and McPherson, J. (1993) Taking ethics seriously: economics and contemporary moral philosophy. *Journal of Economic Literature* 31(2): 671-731.

Johanesson, M. (1995) The ranking properties of health-years equivalent and quality-adjusted life-years under certainty and uncertainty. *International Journal of Technology Assessment* 11(1):40-48.

Johanesson, M., Plishkin, J., and Weinstein, M. (1993) Are healthy-years equivalent an improvement of quality-adjusted life years. *Medical Decision Making* 13(4): 281-286.

Kahneman, D. and Varey, C. (1991) Notes on the psychology of utility. In Elster, J. and Roemer, J., editors, *Interpersonal Comparisons of Well-Being*. New York: Cambridge University Press, pp. 127-163.

Leamer E. (1978) *Specification Searches: Ad Hoc Inference With Non-experimental Data*. New York: John Wiley.

Lindblom, C. and Cohen, D. (1979) *Usable Knowledge*. New Haven: Yale University Press.

MacIntyre, A. (1984) *After Virtue*. Second Edition. South Bend: University of Notre Dame Press.

MacIntyre, A. (1988) *Whose Justice? Which Rationality*. South Bend: University of Notre Dame Press.

Mannix, E., Neale M., and Northcraft, G. (1995) Equity, equality, or need? The effects of organizational culture on the allocation of benefits and burdens. *Organizational Behaviour and Human Decision Processes* 63(3):276-286.

McCloskey, D. (1985) *The Rhetoric of Economics*. Madison: University of Wisconsin Press.

McGuire, A., Henderson, J., and Mooney, G. (1988) *The Economics of Health Care*. London: Routledge and Keegan Paul.

Mehrez, A. and Gafni, A. (1989) Quality-adjusted life years, utility theory, and healthy years equivalent. *Medical Decision Making* 9(2):142-149.

Mehrez, A. and Gafni, A. (1993) HYE vs QALYs: in pursuit of progress. *Medical Decision Making* 13(1):142-149.

Miller, D. (1992) Distributive justice: what the people think. *Ethics* 102(3): 555-593.

Mooney, G. and Lange, M. (1993) Ante-natal screening: what constitutes a benefit? *Social Science and Medicine* 37(7):873-878.

Nord, E., Richardson, J., Street, A., *et al.* (1995) Who cares about cost? Does economic analysis impose or reflect social values? *Health Policy* 34(2):79-94.

Nozick, R. (1974) *Anarchy, State and Utopia.* New York: Basic Books.

Reinhardt, U. (1992) Reflections on the meaning of efficiency: can efficiency be separated from equity? *Yale Law and Policy Review* 10(302):302-315.

Sagoff, M. (1994) Should preferences count? *Land Economics* 70(2):127-144.

Scanlon, T. (1975) Preference and urgency. *Journal of Philosophy* 72(19): 655-669.

Scheffler, S. (1994) *The Rejection of Consequentialism.* Second Edition. Oxford: Clarendon Press.

Schmid, A. (1989) *Benefit-Cost Analysis: A Political Economy Approach.* Boulder: Westview Press.

Sen, A. (1979) Personal utilities and public judgements: or what's wrong with welfare economics. *Economic Journal* 89(September):537-558.

Sen, A. (1985) *Commodities and Capabilities.* Amsterdam: North Holland.

Sen, A. (1987a) *On Ethics and Economics.* Cambridge: Blackwell.

Sen, A. (1987b) *The Standard of Living.* New York: Cambridge University Press.

Sen, A. and Williams, B., editors. (1982a) *Utilitarianism and Beyond.* New York: Cambridge University Press.

Sen, A. and Williams, B. (1982b) Introduction. *In* Sen, A. and Williams, B., editors, *Utilitarianism and Beyond.* New York: Cambridge University Press, pp. 1-22.

Taylor, C. (1982) The diversity of goods. *In* Sen, A. and Williams, B., editors, *Utilitarianism and Beyond.* New York: Cambridge University Press, pp. 129-44.

Taylor, C. (1989) *Sources of the Self.* Cambridge: Harvard University Press.

Tversky, A. and Kahneman, D. (1981) The framing of decisions and the psychology of choice. *Science* 211:453-458.

Varian, H. (1978) *Microeconomic Analysis.* New York: W.W. Norton and Company.

Walzer, M. (1983) *Spheres of Justice.* New York: Basic Books.

Weisbrod, B. (1968) Income redistribution effects and benefit-cost analysis. *In* Chase, S.B., Jr., editor, *Problems in Public Expenditure Analysis.* Washington: Brookings Institute, pp. 395-428.

Williams, A. (1988) Ethics and efficiency in the provision of health care. *In*

Bell, M. and Mendus, S., editors, *Philosophy and Medical Welfare.* Cambridge: Cambridge University Press.

Yaari, M. and Bar-Hillel, M. (1985) On dividing justly. *Social Choice and Welfare* 1(1):1-19.

Zajac, E. (1985) Perceived economic justice: the example of public utility regulation. *In* Young, H.P., editor, *Cost Allocation: Methods, Principles, Applications.* New York: Elsevier Science Publishers, pp. 119-153.

17

Economics, Communitarianism, and Health Care

GAVIN MOONEY
Department of Public Health and Community Medicine
University of Sydney
New South Wales, Australia

ABSTRACT

This paper argues against the monopoly of the individualistic perspective in health economics. It proposes the need for a communitarian stance in examining issues in health economics. The particular focus of this paper is on the nature of the health care system as a community commodity. It is concluded that the preferences of citizens and not just patients are needed when evaluating health services, as otherwise health economists risk misspecifying the benefits of health care. There is a need to examine the community's "impersonal preferences" and to reflect more on what the community wants from its health care system.

Health, Health Care and Health Economics: Perspectives on Distribution
Edited by Morris L. Barer, Thomas E. Getzen, and Greg L. Stoddart
Copyright 1998 John Wiley & Sons, Ltd.

FOREWORD

This paper has emerged as a result of various thoughts and impetuses which I believe are important for the reader to appreciate in order to understand it. While working in Denmark from 1985 to 1990, I became acquainted with communitarianism through Uffe Juul Jensen, Professor of Philosophy at the University of Aarhus. Also, having moved there from the UK and then later to Australia, I could not help but notice the differences, not only in these societies' health care systems, but, more important in the context of this paper, the differences in attitudes of the peoples of these countries towards their health care systems. This was especially noteworthy in relation to equity. Without going into unnecessary detail, it seemed that Denmark had the "strongest" equity principle. The Danes were "proud" of that, yet seldom spoke about it. The UK had the next strongest commitment to equity and the British were particularly keen to talk about it, almost as if the country were unique or the world leader in this regard. The Australians, with what appear to be the weakest equity principles, seem best pleased with what they have. It may be significant that Australian Medicare is by far the "youngest" of these equity based systems. It is not as "embedded" in this society as in Denmark or the UK.

These observations may simply reflect the fact that different societies have different health services or that different societies have different objectives for their health services or that different societies have different cultural values which underlie their objectives and organisational arrangements. Yet the extent to which we, as health economists, account for any of these differences in our analyses is minimal. We seem not to see the health care **system** as contributing to the welfare of a society but concentrate much more on a micro-consequentialist view and value the outcomes (normally only the health outcomes) of the individual services that the system provides. The structural or organisational aspects of the commodity health care at the level of health care systems are seen as purely instrumental in health economics. There is no apparent interest or value in the social institution *per se*. I would hypothesise that this results in our missing out on certain key considerations in the economic analysis of health care. It is with respect to these that I want to mount an exploratory investigation in this paper.

INTRODUCTION

There is a need for health economists to think through just how best to represent the commodity of health care at two different levels. There is first the individual consumer level where the prime concern is with treatment for that individual. Some of this can be taken care of (as I have expressed elsewhere, see Mooney, 1992) by allowing a broader set of consequences than just health to enter the utility function. More can be taken care of by allowing process as well as outcomes to be utility bearing. Second, there is the community level where the concern is with the health care system as a social institution. There has been little interest in this community commodity among health economists.

While reference will be made in this paper to the first level of the commodity, the key focus is the latter, what I will describe as the "community commodity." It is here that we need to concentrate in any communitarian critique of health care economics. Looking at some more macro issues with respect to health care or more strictly speaking, with issues regarding social institutions, immediately lets us see that there is so much more to health care economics than we would be able to identify from the revealed preferences of our research in the last 20 years. The next section of this paper examines the issue of communitarianism *per se,* as well as related issues of preferences. Then health care is considered from a communitarian perspective before looking explicitly at the "community commodity" aspect of health care. Thereafter the paper examines whether it is necessary or desirable to abandon a utility framework before concluding that the ideas in this paper suggest that as health economists we need to research much more into health care systems *qua* systems than we have done to date.

COMMUNITARIANISM AND PREFERENCES

"Communitarianism is put forward in two spheres. One is methodological, the communitarians arguing that the premises of individualism such as the rational individual who chooses freely are wrong or false, and that the only way to understand human behaviour is to refer to individuals in their social, cultural, and historical contexts" (Aveniri and de-Shalit, 1992).

Additionally, in communitarianism there is a normative sphere that argues that individualism "gives rise to morally unsatisfactory consequences," among these being "the impossibility of achieving a genuine community, the neglect of some ideas of the good life that should be sustained by the state or others that should be dismissed, or...an unjust distribution of goods...the community is a good that people should seek for several reasons and should not be dismissed" (Aveniri and de-Shalit, 1992). Communitarians thus question the use of the preferences of individuals *qua* individuals rather than as members of a community.

Communitarians suggest that "to discuss individuals one must look first at their communities and their communal relationships" (Avineri and de-Shalit, 1992). These authors indicate that "the communitarians argue that active political participation is another good which is devalued by individualists, who at best regard it as an instrumental good." The consequentialism of classical utilitarianism misses out on issues of participation. Communitarianism can allow the incorporation of the value of participating in the community and of that feeling of identifying with the community. There is also emphasis on the values of individuals *qua* individuals rather than as members of a society or community who share mutual concerns. The community is not valued for itself.

Out of these statements on communitarianism a number of factors merit examination. There is the question of why individuals' preferences should count anyway; second is whether individually expressed preferences, which ignore others' preferences and others' actions, reflect or can be seen as reflecting the preferences of the community *qua* community rather than as being simply the aggregation of individuals' preferences (and on this see Shiell and Hawe, 1996 in the context of health promotion); and third, the issue of the value of the community *qua* community. Much of the rest of this paper will attempt to address these issues.

While there are many different interpretations of utility and welfare, it seems that what economists normally mean by any maximisation principle in this context is the maximisation of individuals' preferences. That raises an important question about preferences. As Sagoff (1986) states: "Is the satisfaction of preferences an intrinsic good, like pleasure or happiness, or is it good instrumentally because it leads to consequences that are good in themselves?"

Sagoff (1986) continues: "It cannot be argued that the satisfaction of preferences is a good thing in itself, for many preferences are sadistic, envious, racist, or unjust...It may be good in itself that certain preferences be satisfied, namely, preferences that are good in themselves." Sagoff also argues: "A contemporary utilitarian may reply that we should strive to satisfy preferences because this is what the people who have preferences prefer to want. If [this] means that a majority of citizens favor preference satisfaction as a national goal, it is plainly false" (and he cites evidence from the US Council on Environmental Quality [1980] to support this statement).

COMMUNITARIANISM AND HEALTH CARE

How can communitarianism be interpreted in the context of health care? One possibility is considered by Margolis (1982). He suggests that individuals have two sources of utility: first, the "normal" goods utility derived from "outcomes" and thus "consequentialist" in nature; and second, "participation" utility, which is derived from doing rather than getting and which may be seen as a form of "process" utility and is thus clearly not consequentialist (and possibly as a result not utility as a classical utilitarian would view it).

It is a short step from this (see Mooney, 1992) to the idea that, with respect to health services, individuals in a society may be prepared to pay **to make available** services for the population as a whole. It is not just that there is a fair society with respect to health care; it is also that the individual has done his/her bit to bring that fairness about. (It is to be noted that this does not rule out the prospect that the willingness to pay to make services available remains dependent on the effectiveness of the services made available.)

Before considering the extent to which this form of communitarianism and hence "participation utility" matter, let me examine a closely related issue raised by Sen (1992). With respect to linking Sen to Margolis's concept of participation and to communitarianism more generally, Sen's concept of agency seems particularly relevant. He writes: "A person's agency achievement refers to the realization of goals and values she has reasons to pursue whether or not they are connected with her own well-being....If a person aims at, say, the independence of her country, or the prosperity of her community, or some such general goal, her agency achievement would involve evaluation of states of affairs in the light of those objects, and not merely in the light of the extent to which those achievements would contribute to her own well-being."

Sen (1992) continues: "It is possible to make a...distinction between (1) the occurrence of such things that one values and one aims at achieving, and (2) the occurrence of such things brought about by one's **own** efforts (or, in the bringing about of which one has **oneself** played an active part)." He thus distinguishes between **realized** agency success" and "**instrumental** agency success." This seems a useful distinction. [Emphasis in original.]

At least two considerations are different between Sen and Margolis. First there is no parallel in Margolis to the agency goals that come about through no effort on the part of the individual. Clearly there is a simple solution to that particular issue and that is to build that element into Margolis' model. Second, however, and much more problematical, Sen is insistent (and there are echoes here of his concept of "commitment" in *Rational Fools* [Sen, 1977]) that this element can be independent of the individual's own well-being. In Margolis, of course, this is not the case as the individual does gain utility from participation-- from "doing his fair share." Thus, while Margolis can be accommodated within an extended utility framework, this is less feasible with Sen. (I will come back to this issue later.)

In one important respect, there is also a similarity between communitarianism and Tony Culyer's extra-welfarism. Culyer (1991) seems to exclude the possibility that individuals' diversities with respect to valuing health states should be allowed to count in extra-welfarism. This is the situation with QALYs where variations across individuals in their preferences for health are not allowed for. As Culyer states: "in extra-welfarism...the presumption is that external judgments may be imposed that replace or supplement the subjective utility numbers of principal or agent in the social welfare function." In a communitarian view of health care it might well be the case that a **community** would take the view -- make the "external judgment" -- to "replace or supplement the subjective utility numbers of principal or agent in the social welfare function." While of course the source of this "external judgment" could be other than the community, it is difficult to see what other more legitimate and acceptable source there might be.

The position taken by Sen (1992) is very much to favour allowing for such variations and indeed to frown upon ignoring or trying to bypass diversities across individuals in their valuations.

There are clear differences of opinion here between Culyer's extra-welfarism and with it the basis of QALYs where diversity of individual values is not to be allowed (because of some "external judgement" to the contrary) and Sen's view that such diversity is to be supported. My point is not to argue for or against either of these views. (Indeed it would be possible if not conventional to incorporate diversity of individual values into QALYs.) Rather I would propose that as economists we need to try to look at the communities in which health services are operating and ascertain what they want their health services to do when valuing health outcomes and whether the community believes that diversity of values across different individuals is to be allowed to count or not. (The related but separate issue of how a community might value differently health gains to different groups in the community (Williams, 1988) is discussed below.)

THE COMMUNITY COMMODITY HEALTH CARE

Let us then consider more explicitly the nature of the commodity health care. I do not want to disagree in terms of commission with the standard health economics treatment of the commodity health care. It is in omission that I see a problem. There is no allowance here for Sen's commitment. This phenomenon of commitment is in Sen's expression "counter-preferential." The inhibiting feature of any standard analysis here is not the concept of utility *per se* but the notion that each individual is maximising his or her **own** utility. It is thus in the assumed nature of the social welfare function and the form of aggregation from individuals' utility functions to the social welfare function that the problem lies. (It is, of course, possible to argue, as presumably utilitarians would, that it is not possible to act rationally **and** "counter-preferentially." It seems in large part because of this argument that Sen is critical of utilitarianism. It is also a major reason why we might have to consider abandoning the concept of utility in health economics as discussed in the next section.)

This problem can be overcome very simply. It would be possible to assume a social welfare function that is to be maximised independently of the maximisation of individuals' utility functions, **provided** the individuals involved are committed to that objective. The concepts of caring for and being cared about, for example (Wiseman, 1997), would then become easier to handle than in the standard "externalities" argument which does not allow (indeed cannot allow) for Sen's counter-preferential commitment. This form of maximand can include commitment in the sense that someone who cares for another can be committed to that other, be acting counter-preferentially at his/her own individual level but still be concerned about maximising the aggregate utility of the cared for and the carer, jointly.

It is this concept of "jointness" that seems to be missing from the analysis of health care as a commodity and I would suggest at two levels. The "caring externality," when it is conceived in terms of individuals' maximising utility, can handle Sen's sympathy (your pleasure is my pleasure), but it cannot handle Sen's commitment because, according to Sen, the commitment is counter-preferential **with respect to the individual**. It seems difficult to argue that it could be counter-preferential **for the society, group or community** to whom the individual is committed.

It is this sense of community, this context of caring in a **community**, that I think we have ignored in health economics. It is to these issues that I think we should devote more of our research efforts.

There are many issues that need to be considered with respect to the "communitarian commodity" health care. These might include the overall objectives of a health care system, what the equity objectives might be, who pays and how, etc. In examining these I am aware that some characteristics might be incorporated under other approaches and that consequently not all require a communitarian view. This is simply to recognise that most theories overlap with others. Nonetheless to see things in a communitarian light is, I believe, at least to allow the possibility that all of the relevant characteristics be viewed within a single coherent theory. In this paper I will consider the three areas in which some preliminary research has been done or where at least some work exists that might lead into grappling with these communitarian concerns. These are the objectives of health care systems generally (primarily related to health), the objectives related to equity, and the objectives of the doctor agent.

On health care objectives generally, the article by Culyer, Maynard and Williams (1981) on the ideological underpinnings of different health care systems lays out two possibilities that are at either end of the spectrum, one based largely on the standard reward system of the marketplace, the other on some social construct of need. Beyond this promising start, in the context of the arguments in this paper, what I am suggesting is required is some mechanism for asking communities to express their preferences between these possibilities.

In this context it is also useful to quote Tony Culyer (1988) when he suggests the following as possible objectives of health services: "to maximise freedom of choice in sickness, to maximise utility, to maximise consumers' sovereignty." He goes on to argue that there is an advantage "in choosing an objective that is...*likely* to command a consensus, which is not particularly quirky nor merely the idiosyncratic view of a particular pressure group or the tenet of a major but controversial political and social ideology." (Emphasis in original.) He proposes that the notion that "health services exist to promote health" is likely to "command a consensus."

He wants to pin this down further to suggest that there is a need for "something for which to strive and that can (at least in principle) yield indicators as to whether it is being attained." What he proposes is that: "given the resources available to the health services, the health of the community should be maximised."

My point in quoting Culyer at such length is neither to disagree nor to agree with him. Rather the point is that he has to conjecture what the objective of health services is because it is seldom the case that this is stated very precisely if at all and even less often have there been attempts to find out what the community view is as to the objective of its health service.

A view of what health services are about also emerges from the QALY literature. For example, Erik Nord and colleagues (1993) state that there is an ethical system underpinning the use of QALYs, which is that "social welfare is equal to a weighted average of individually determined utilities in which the weights ensure that each person's life-year is equally important, irrespective of the individual's personal characteristics or capacity to appreciate life-years." They continue: "The rule is almost certainly defective, as it ignores distributional considerations and issues of entitlement that are known to be important in decision making, especially in the health sector."

As mentioned above, Alan Williams (1988) has investigated a range of factors that he thought might have an influence on the weights that individuals might attach to health gains to different groups in the community. These included such considerations as age, having children, being a bread winner, etc. With colleagues I have attempted something similar, including existing health status, as a basis for discriminating in how health gains are to be distributed (Mooney et al., 1995).

Erik Nord, Jeff Richardson and others (1995), through a self-administered postal questionnaire surveying members of the Australian public, have examined the objective of health services being about "the maximisation of the QALYs gained, irrespective of how the gains are distributed." They found that there was little support for such a policy in a number of circumstances, for example "when health benefits to young people compete with health benefits to the elderly."

There is thus some limited work on this particular aspect of the community commodity health care, i.e., what the community sees as the objectives of the health care system. Given the potential importance of this issue, there is clearly a need for much more.

On specifically equity objectives there has been considerable debate in the literature. (See for example Culyer *et al.*, 1992 and 1992a; Mooney *et al.*, 1991 and 1992.) Certainly many countries do make explicit statements in policy documents about what the equity objectives are, at least in principle, that they want their health services to pursue. (See for example Donaldson and Gerard, 1993.) Little research, however, seems to have been undertaken to determine what citizens want from their health services in this respect.

The debate has proved somewhat sterile at least with respect to resolving what the appropriate dimension of equity is to be. This is because it has been conducted in a largely data free world. It has, however, stimulated Gunnar Rongen (1996) to try to examine empirically for local government areas in Norway which definition of equity -- equal health, equal use or equal access -- best seems to fit the data. Rongen found that individual variations in preferences with respect to equity do exist, especially between men and women. He went on to conclude that the results "indicate that individual preferences are important, and accordingly should be taken into account when equity is considered." While I would be very keen to agree with this (since it would support equality of access as the dimension of equity), it is not the case that because "individual preferences are important" it then necessarily follows that they should be taken into account. There remains a need to ask communities what they want with respect to an equity goal of their health care system and whether, if there are diversities in individuals' preferences, as Rongen's research suggests, these differences are to count or not.

There is thus some research on equity on which to build. It is small. Much more effort is needed here.

Turning to another key feature of health economics that would seem in need of consideration at a more communitarian level, the agency relationship between health care professional (usually doctor) and patient has been (surprisingly) little debated in the context of what the perfect agent is attempting to maximise. As I, together with Mandy Ryan, identified there is less than agreement in the literature as to what agency is about, i.e., what the agent is attempting to achieve (Mooney and Ryan, 1993). Possibilities here are: maximum health; information leading to better health; informed choice with respect to health; and maximising patient utility. There is also less than agreement as to who within the doctor patient relationship makes the decision under conditions of perfect agency and whether decision making in this context is potentially utility- or disutilitybearing for the patient.

Here again my intent is not to answer the questions underlying these issues but rather to point to the fact that health economists have done little to address them. "What do communities want from their doctors?" is not a question that has been on the lips of health economists of the last while. Currently the University of Sydney Medical Faculty is pushing through radical reforms to the training of doctors for the next century. If asked what health economists would want doctors of the next century to be trained for I suppose the best I could answer from the health economics community would be: "Doctors who produce health gains efficiently and possibly equitably." Further, given the baggage that we carry as health economists, there would seem little reason to suggest that perhaps we should go out and ask communities what they want from their doctors.

Why this rather bleak heritage? I think there are two prime reasons. First, health economists have concentrated on health to the exclusion of other arguments in the utility, interests, or welfare functions surrounding health care. We have tended to neglect those arguments at the level of the patient but even more so at the level of the citizen. Second we have not broken sufficiently from the neo-classical mould. Having rejected (largely) the invisible hand (Donaldson and Gerard, 1993), we have then neither recognised the need for it to be made visible nor accepted the need for health economists to be part of the process of making it visible.

UTILITY OR WHAT?

Returning to the comments above on Sen (1992), what are we to draw out of his ideas about agency and commitment, against the background of an extended concept of utility based in part on Margolis (1982)? One conclusion would be that if we extend the concept of utility enough, then we are bound to be able to incorporate anything we want to include. It might also be added that to do so might mean that utility would lose any meaning and all its substance.

If an individual wants only "states of the world" in the utility function or additionally wants actions or activities or giving or receiving or being loyal or having integrity or being honest or acting fairly or doing her fair share or having others acting in certain ways or having society taking a particular form or whatever, then it can be suggested that all of these are legitimate arguments in that individual's "utility function." Such a stance is also compatible with one that argues that man is a social animal, values that fact, and as a result values certain social institutions and social arrangements -- what amounts to a communitarian stance. (This does not mean that they are valued **irrespective** of what they produce but that they may be valued **additionally** to what they produce by way of intended outputs.)

In the foreword of his book on the economics of altruism, Collard (1978) addressed the issue of whether to work within a utility framework. His views seem highly relevant to this paper. He states: "It is true that the analysis is based on rational individualism into which altruism is permitted to enter only through the narrow gate of the utility function. Thus, it is said, an opportunity was missed to launch a more broadly based critique of orthodox economics." He argues for a retention of the utility function thereby "bringing altruism into the normal ambit of economic discourse: otherwise it will continue to be regarded as 'soft' rather than 'hard' and therefore not strictly part of economics. Mainstream economists could then regard it as part and parcel of some not yet accepted critique of orthodoxy or as belonging to one or more of the other social sciences. That would be a pity and, in itself, justifies some degree of intellectual conservatism."

Whether such "intellectual conservatism" is justified or not with respect to the ideas in this paper I am less sure. I am not loathe to give up utility or the utility function as long as somewhere we can retain a maximand. One way to move forward in relation to the ideas in this paper is to have what would amount to two functions. Let us call them "interests functions." One would be a patient's interests function and the other a citizen's interests function. The former would be concerned with what **patients** wanted from a health service; the latter with what **communities** wanted their health services to look like.

There is a need to find mechanisms and measurement instruments to get at these latter preferences, what Dworkin (1981) calls "impersonal preferences." These, according to Dworkin, are preferences that people have "about things other than their own or other people's lives or situations." Sagoff (1986) lists under these preferences such considerations as pollution control, wilderness preservation, and safety of workers. We could add health care systems. These are all aspects of social life which impinge on us, but often from afar, and which fall into the category of the nature of the society or the community that we as citizens want to have. It is possible to get some way down this road through option values *à la* Weisbrod (1964), but there he is concerned with options which may be consumed at some stage in the future. Here, while a close parallel, the issue is the community's concern to establish a good society.

One way we might get to a proxy for what we seek is to ask individuals to act in the role of community decision makers (somewhat along the lines adopted by Jan Abel Olsen [1993] in looking at time preferences). This gets closer to the "impersonal preferences" we want. That would still seem likely to lack the genuinely communitarian values that are sought. Interestingly, it seems that in some contingent valuation research such community preferences are being picked up anyway in the form of what Arrow *et al.* (1993) call "warm glows" which in one interpretation at least reflects the communitarian notion of individuals being "embedded" in a community. It may be that in allowing the values for "warm glows" to emerge, one route to getting at these communitarian values can be developed (instead of suggesting that these are in some sense not legitimate).

The prime difficulty and hence challenge here is to bring out that facet of communitarianism that makes it, as far as I can judge, uniquely communitarian, i.e., the notion that "it is morally good that the self is constituted by its communal ties" (Avineri and de-Shalit, 1992).

CONCLUSION

In communitarianism it is not just that we are interested in social values and aggregation of the preferences, interests, or whatever of individuals *qua* individuals but in these as part of a community or society where the community itself and its institutions (such as the health care system) are also valued.

While there is no totally agreed-upon view as to precisely what communitarianism is (is there with any school of philosophy?), Aveniri and de-Shalit (1992) suggest that what is common to all communitarians is that they advocate "involvement in public life." There is value *per se* in such involvement but, as discussed earlier, as in the case of preferences, such involvement is only good insofar as the institutions and communities are good. We cannot ignore this factor any more than we do when we judge that preferences based on envy, for example, are to be rejected. Thus, it is not just that there is a need to try to identify the values that might be used in health care in the various ways that I have suggested in this paper. Additionally what the communitarians would argue is that there is value in the very process of being active in such public decision making.

The challenge then is to elicit these communitarian values. I can see that by using conjoint analysis it is possible to get individuals to express preferences about the nature of the health care system they might wish. What equity principles should it embrace? What is the maximand? Should individual preferences for health be allowed to count and if so how? How should funding be arranged? What balance of care within and outside institutions is best? Who should be involved in decision making especially given the thrust for participation and the communitarian idea of there being value in public or community participation? (On this last issue see Julia Abelson and her colleagues, 1995.)

The further challenge, however, is to ensure that any expression of preferences includes "impersonal preferences" (*à la* Dworkin) as well. There is some limited evidence (see for example Abelson et al., 1995) that individuals respond differently to questions about preferences when this is done in groups as opposed to individually. More research on this front is needed, placing individuals into groups and/or making them play the role of representatives of their community.

The communitarian question -- in what sort of community would we prefer to live? -- is not one with which health economists have explicitly grappled. It can readily be argued that it is not our task to do so, that the responsibility for doing so lies elsewhere, for example with political scientists or philosophers. Certainly I would maintain that the task is a multidisciplinary one. Yet health care as a social institution is so important. For health economists not to get around to asking if not perhaps "in what sort of community would we prefer to live?" at least "what sort of health care system *qua* system do we as a community prefer?" would seem at best odd and at worst a dereliction of a responsible application of our analytical skills and talents.

In a recent guest editorial in *Health Economics*, Alan Williams (1993) indicated that he had no doubt "that the big issue for the 1990s is going to be outcome measurement" and he set out "important strategic research issues" for health economics. I would not want to remove any of the items from Alan's list. What I do note, however, is that, apart from the concerns with equity or more accurately its neglect by health economists, Williams' list is very much at the micro-individualistic end of the spectrum and the sorts of considerations that I am raising in this paper are ignored. In a more recent editorial, Charles Phelps (1995) does mention "increased attention to detailed institutional structures" but it is not the structures *per se* -- the main focus of this paper -- that he emphasises but "their effects on behaviour."

Yet, as I have tried to indicate in this paper, as health economists we have already begun to establish some of the agenda for considering "the community commodity" health care even if we have been very slow to recognise it as a research agenda that is ours to pursue. We have identified some of the issues but, for various reasons, some of which I have touched on in this paper, not picked them up. Perhaps things are changing however and will change still more in health economics in this respect in the next few years.

To try to sum up and exemplify what I have been trying to grapple with in this paper, it is relevant to quote from Nye Bevan, the founder of the British National Health Service: "Society becomes more wholesome, more serene, and spiritually healthier, if it knows that its citizens have at the back of their consciousness the knowledge that not only themselves but all their fellows, have access, when ill, to the best that medical skill can provide" (Foot, 1975).

As health economists are we not missing out on something when we turn our eyes away from valuing and measuring the impact of a health care system on a community's welfare and settle for looking only from the perspective of the patients?

ACKNOWLEDGMENTS

I am grateful for comments on an earlier draft of this paper to Steve Birch, Stephen Jan, Uffe Juul Jensen, and Alan Shiell. A version of this paper was presented at the International Health Economics Association Inaugural Conference, Vancouver, BC, Canada, May 1996 at which various helpful comments were received, in particular from Tony Culyer and Uwe Reinhardt. I am also grateful to NSW Health Department for financial support.

REFERENCES

Abelson, J., Lomas, J., Eyles, J., et al. (1995) Does the community want devolved authority? Results of deliberative polling in Ontario. *Canadian Medical Association Journal* 153(4):403-412.

Arrow, K., Solow, R., Portney, P.R., et al. (1993) Report of the NOAA panel on contingent valuation. *Federal Register* 58(10): 4601-4614.

Avineri, S. and de-Shalit, A. (1992) Introduction, In Avineri, S. and de-Shalit A., editors, *Communitarianism and Individualism*. Oxford: Oxford University Press.

Collard, D. (1978) *Altruism and Economy*. Oxford: Martin Robertson.

Culyer, A.J. (1988) Inequality of health services is, in general, desirable. In Green, D.G., editor, *Acceptable Inequalities*. London: IEA Health Unit.

Culyer, A.J. (1991) Equity in health care policy. Paper prepared for the Ontario Premier's Council on Health, Well-Being and Social Justice, Toronto: University of Toronto.

Culyer, A.J., van Doorslaer, E., and Wagstaff, A. (1992) Utilisation as a measure of equity by Mooney, Hall, Donaldson and Gerard. *Journal of Health Economics* 11:93-98.

Culyer, A.J., van Doorslaer, E., and Wagstaff, A. (1992a) Access, utilisation and equity: a further comment. *Journal of Health Economics* 11:207-210.

Culyer, A.J., Maynard, A.K., and Williams, A. (1981) Alternative systems of health care provision: an essay on motes and beams. In Olson, M., editor. *A New Approach to the Economics of Health Care*. Washington: American Enterprise Institute.

Donaldson, C. and Gerard, K. (1993) *Economics of Health Care Financing, The Visible Hand*. Basingstoke: Macmillan.

Dworkin, R. (1981) What is equality? Part I: Equality of welfare. *Philosophy and Public Affairs* 10:185-246.

Foot, M. (1975) *Aneurin Bevan*. London: Paladin.

Margolis, H. (1982) *Selfishness, Altruism And Rationality*. Cambridge: Cambridge University Press.

Mooney, G. (1992) *Economics Medicine and Health Care*. Hemel Hempstead: Harvester Wheatsheaf.

Mooney, G., Hall, J., Donaldson, C., and Gerard, K. (1991) Utilisation as a measure of equity: Weighing heat? *Journal of Health Economics* 10:475-480.

Mooney, G., Hall, J., Donaldson, C., and Gerard, K. (1992) Reweighing heat: Response to Culyer, van Doorslaer and Wagstaff. *Journal of Health Economics* 11:199-205.

Mooney, G. and Ryan, M. (1993) Agency in health care: getting beyond first principles. *Journal of Health Economics* 12:125-138.

Mooney, G., Jan, S., and Wiseman, V. (1995) Examining preferences for allocating health gains. *Health Care Analysis* 3:231-234.

Nord, E., Richardson, J., and Macarounas-Kirchmann, K. (1993) Social evaluation of health care versus personal evaluation of health states. *International Journal of Technology Assessment in Health Care* 9:4, 463-478.

Nord, E., Richardson, J., Street, A., et al. (1995) Maximising health benefits vs egalitarianism: an Australian survey. *Social Science and Medicine* 41:1429-1437.

Olsen, J.A. (1993) Time preferences for health gains: an empirical investigation. *Health Economics* 2:3, 257-266.

Phelps, C.E. (1995) Perspectives in health economics. *Health Economics* 4:335-353.

Rongen, G. (1996) *Equality, Choice and Local Preferences.* PhD Thesis. Oslo: University of Oslo.

Sagoff, M. (1986) Values and preferences. *Ethics* 301-316.

Sandel, M. (1984) The procedural republic and the unencumbered self. *Political Theory* 12:81-96.

Sen, A. (1977) Rational fools: a critique of the behavioural foundations of economic theory. *Philosophy and Public Affairs* 6:317-344.

Sen, A. (1992) *Inequality Re-examined.* Oxford: Clarendon Press.

Shiell, A. and Hawe, P. (1996) Health promotion community development and the tyranny of individualism. *Health Economics* 5:241-247.

US Council on Environmental Quality.(1980) *Public Opinion on Environmental Issues.* Washington DC: Government Printing Office.

Weisbrod, B.A. (1964) Collective-consumption services of individual consumption goods. *Quarterly Journal of Economics* 78:471-477.

Williams, A. (1988) Ethics and efficiency in the provision of health care. In Bell, J.M. and Mendus, S., editors, *Philosophy and Medical Care.* Cambridge: Cambridge University Press.

Williams, A. (1993) Priorities and research strategy in health economics for the 1990s. *Health Economics* 2:4, 295-302.

Wiseman, V. (1997) Caring: the neglected health outcome? or input? *Health Policy* 39(1): 43-53.

18

The Desirability of Market-Based Health Reforms: a Reconsideration of Economic Theory

THOMAS RICE

Department of Health Services
UCLA School of Public Health

ABSTRACT

This paper reconsiders the study of health economics by examining the foundations of competitive theory, and applying this to health care markets. It demonstrates that conclusions concerning the desirability of competitive markets are based on a number of assumptions — many of which have been largely ignored by the health economics profession — that are not met in the health care area. Market mechanisms are therefore shown to not necessarily provide the best means of enhancing social welfare. The paper then critiques key assumptions of the

Health, Health Care and Health Economics: Perspectives on Distribution
Edited by Morris L. Barer, Thomas E. Getzen, and Greg L. Stoddart
Copyright 1998 John Wiley & Sons, Ltd

conventional economic model, and then applies the arguments to health.

INTRODUCTION

In recent years there has been a surge of interest in reforming health care systems by replacing government regulation with a reliance on market forces. Although much of the impetus has come from the United States, the phenomenon is worldwide. Spurred by ever-increasing health care costs, many analysts and policy makers have embraced the competitive market as the method of choice for reforming health care. To a great extent, this belief stems from economic theory, which purports to show the superiority of markets over government regulation. This has led advocates to champion a number of policies, including:

> Providing low-income people with subsidies to allow them to purchase health insurance, rather than paying directly for the services they use

> Having people pay more money out-of-pocket in order to receive health care services -- especially for services with high demand elasticities

> Requiring that individuals pay more in premiums to obtain more extensive health insurance coverage

> Letting the market determine the number and distribution of hospitals and what services they provide, as well as the total number of physicians and their distribution among specialties

> Removing regulations that control the development and diffusion of medical technologies

> Eschewing government involvement in determining how much a country spends on health care services.

Through a reconsideration of economic theory, this paper examines the desirability of market-based health care reforms. It is my belief that health economists have been too quick to embrace conclusions about the superiority of market competition in health care, which are based on a large set of assumptions that are not, or cannot be, met in the health care sector. This is not to say that competitive approaches in health care are inappropriate; rather, their efficacy depends on the particular circumstances of the policy being considered and the environment in which it is to take place.

Much of the problem arises because health economists often tend to forget or ignore the many assumptions about markets upon which competitive prescriptions are based. This, in turn, leads many of them to believe — without resort to observation -- that competitive markets are the "correct" policy prescription for many ills facing our health care system. It also inclines health economists towards a number of more specific beliefs -- e.g., demand curves accurately reflect the marginal utility consumers obtain from health care services, comprehensive national health insurance is inefficient, patient cost sharing should be higher for more price-elastic services -- that also cannot be deduced through careful consideration of how economic theory applies to health. One should not put undue blame on health economists, however, because this problem pervades the entire economic discipline. In this regard, Thurow (1983) has written that, "Every economist knows the dozens of restrictive assumptions ... that are necessary to 'prove' that a free market is the best possible economic game, but they tend to be forgotten in the play of events" (p. 22).

It is not my view that relying on market forces in health care is always inappropriate. Rather, this paper attempts to demonstrate that such conclusions cannot be made by theory alone. Stated another way, theory is ambiguous on these and many other issues. It is only by conducting empirical studies that answers to these questions can be revealed.[1] But if this is the case, then it is essential that health economists approach such studies with an open mind.

The analysis contained in the paper is based on considering the lessons of the field of welfare economics. The literature contains many definitions of welfare economics; a representative one, by Henderson and Quandt (1971), states that, "The objective of welfare economics is the evaluation of the social desirability of

---

[1] This contention -- that we must seek all answers through empirical work -- is undeniable if one resorts to so-called "second-best" arguments (Thurow, 1983). The theory of the second best states that if there are multiple factors that cause a market to deviate from the assumptions of market competition, it is not necessarily appropriate to try to make the market more competitive in selected areas (Lipsey and Lancaster, 1956-57). Nevertheless, none of the arguments in this article rely on second-best considerations. For a review of how second-best issues apply to economic competition in the health care sector, see Fielding and Rice (1993).

alternative economic states" (p. 255). This encompasses many pressing economic and social issues, including how goods and services can be produced with the fewest inputs; how consumers can get the most utility from a limited budget; how to ensure that producers supply the things that consumers want the most; and how goods and services can be distributed in order to make society best off. One of the key issues in welfare economics is devising a way of weighing conflicting individual interests to derive a measure of aggregate or social welfare.

A not uncommon error is the belief that welfare economics provides objective or positive conclusions. In a recent debate, Pauly (1994), responding to an article by Labelle, Stoddart, and Rice (1994), stated that, "Using economic welfare, as it is customarily understood, rather than health status, allows one to avoid the murky area of 'societal decision making' " (p. 371). Culyer and Evans (1996), in their response to Pauly, cited Hume's Law[2] in contending that no such normative conclusions can be drawn from welfare economics. This point is consistent with a statement by Arrow (1973b): "The idea of a social welfare formulation is to make societal decisions in which there will be winners and losers" (p. 115), something which obviously cannot be done with value judgments.

Influential welfare economists of disparate political persuasions (e.g., Arrow, 1973a; Harberger, 1971; Little, 1957; Mishan, 1969a; Samuelson, 1947) would surely accept Nath's (1969) statement, that "value judgments are unavoidable in welfare economics" (p. 2) -- or perhaps even Sen's (1970) point, "that it must be regarded as somewhat of a mystery that so many notable economists have been involved in debating the prospects of finding value-free welfare economics" (p. 5). The real issue is, *what* assumptions are we willing to make in order to proceed? This article attempts to show that some rather heroic assumptions must be made in the health care area for one to conclude that reliance on market forces necessarily constitutes superior policy.

The stinginess of welfare economics with respect to what it can tell public policy is, of course, best known to its practitioners. To use Mishan's (1969a) words, "welfare economics is a meretricious[3] subject; it promises much, but yields little" (p. 33). Various tools have been used through the decades to try to make welfare economics "say something" that is useful for policy; perhaps the most

---

[2] Hume's Law, a label subsequently attributed to some of the writings of Scottish philosopher David Hume (1711-76), states that, "conclusions about what ought to be cannot be deduced from premises stating only what was, what is, or what will be" (*A Dictionary of Philosophy*, 1979).

[3] "of or relating to a prostitute" (Webster's Seventh New Collegiate Dictionary).

famous examples are the doctrine of utilitarianism[4] and the Kaldor-Hicks compensation criterion[5]. (Arrow's [1963a] Possibility Theorem does the opposite; it shows that any method of aggregating individual preferences into a social welfare function violates at least one reasonable and desirable ethical condition.)

Practitioners who have wished to have welfare economics say more have had to resort to certain assumptions. In his well-known "open letter to the profession," Harberger (1971) "plead[ed] that three basic postulates be accepted as providing a conventional framework for applied welfare economics:

"a) the competitive demand price for a given unit measures the value of that unit to the demander;

"b) the competitive supply price for a given unit measures the value of that unit to the supplier;

"c) when evaluating the net benefits or costs of a given action ... , the costs and benefits accruing to each member of the relevant group ... should normally be added without regard to the individual(s) to whom they accrue" (p. 785).

Much of this paper will be spent disputing postulate (a).[6]

Although these assumptions have been derided by some as evidencing a "*bravura* that is encountered rarely even within the Paretian camp" (Rowley and Peacock, 1975, p. 59), one can sympathize with Harberger and others who want to draw policy conclusions about the best way to maximize social welfare. At least Harberger admitted what his assumptions were. That does not mean, however, that

---

[4] Utilitarianism contended that society is at an optimum where the sum of individual utilities is greatest. Among the many criticisms of this doctrine are: the difficulty of attaching a cardinal number to a person's utility; the perhaps greater difficulty in summing these numbers across different persons; and the fact that utilitarianism can lead to the subjugation of a minority by a majority.

[5] The Kaldor-Hicks criterion states that an economic change is desirable if the "winners" can compensate the "losers" to get the latter to agree to the change -- but then they don't have to! (Reinhardt, 1992). The Kaldor-Hicks criterion has been much maligned in welfare economics because it is not necessarily welfare maximizing if no compensation is paid, but if compensation is paid then it is no different than the Pareto principle; and because it allows for economic changes that help the well-off at the expense of the poor.

[6] The author recently completed a monograph (Rice, 1998) that critiques the other two postulate as well.

we should accept these same premises when applying economic theory to health. But that is exactly what we do when we accept the "conventional wisdom" about the optimality of competitive equlilbria; when we accept that demand curves precisely show consumers' marginal utility; and when we employ any of several "tools of the trade" that are based on these premises.

It would appear that the traditional economic model of competition has a strong grip on health economists. This is supported by a 1989 survey of health economists in the United States and Canada (Feldman and Morrisey, 1990). One of the questions asked was whether the "competitive model cannot apply" to the health care system. Respondents were evenly divided on this question; half thought the model could apply, and half did not. More noteworthy, perhaps, were some of the response patterns to the question. Two-thirds of respondents who received their Ph.D.s from top economics departments thought that the competitive model could apply, versus 53 % with degrees from other economics departments. Few of those who received their training in non-economics departments believed that the competitive model could apply to the health care system. Other patterns showed that younger respondents were more likely to believe in the competitive model, as were U.S. (versus Canadian) respondents.

This paper is divided into two main sections. The first, on Market Competition, argues that one cannot conclude from theory that competitive markets are the best means of maximizing social welfare. The second, on Demand Theory, shows why demand curves do not necessarily represent either individual or societal benefits. Each of these two sections is divided into two parts: Problems with the Theory; and Implications for Health Policy.

MARKET COMPETITION

PROBLEMS WITH THE THEORY

This section considers three assumptions upon which conclusions about the superiority of market forces are based:

- The Pareto Principle is Desirable
- There are No Externalities in Consumption
- Consumer Tastes are Predetermined

The Pareto Principle

If certain assumptions are met, then allowing market competition to occur will result in Pareto optimality, where it is impossible to make someone better off without making someone else worse off. The premise is that making someone better off without making someone else worse off is a good thing; this premise has been called the Pareto principle. It is a value judgment. Some welfare economists find it to be a fairly mild one (e.g., Ng, 1979), while others, as we shall see, find it more problematic.[7]

Rarely do economists step back and consider whether Pareto optimality is indeed a desirable state of the world. But if the Pareto principle is thought to be problematic, then market competition -- which leads to Pareto optimality -- would not necessarily be the best way to bring about socially desirable outcomes. Rather, other policies, involving perhaps the regulation of certain industries and even restrictions on what consumers can purchase, could be superior.

It is not hard to see the appeal of the Pareto principle. Why not let people engage in trade until they are satisfied with their lot, and no longer wish to engage in further trades? Similarly, why not enact policies that convey benefits to some people and no cost to others? Wouldn't encouraging such trade, and enacting such policies, be in everyone's best interest?

The answer to this last question is, perhaps surprisingly, *"not necessarily."* Under standard economic theory consumers derive utility from the quantity of each of the alternative goods that they possess. It is important to think about what is *not* part of this conception of utility. There is no consideration given to how one's bundle of goods and services compares to, and affects or is affected by, that possessed by other people. Stated simply, only one's absolute amount of wealth matters; one's relative standing is irrelevant.

This has been pointed out a number of times in the mainstream literature but does not seem to have stuck. In his address to the American Economic Association in 1981, Robbins (1984), the leading exponent of the view that economics should confine itself to positive rather than normative issues, stated that Pareto optimality is "clearly a judgment of value," and that:

---

[7] Mishan (1969a) states that, "At first encounter, the Pareto improvement may appear a very modest value proposition, one that is readily acceptable. But ... when taken in conjunction with a distributional value judgment it can cause us a lot of trouble" (p. 26).

If the remaining groups regard their position relatively, they may well argue that the spectacle of such improvement elsewhere is a detriment to their satisfaction. This is not a niggling point: a relative improvement in the position of certain groups *pari passu* with an absolute improvement in the position of the rest of the community has often been a feature of economic history; and we know that has not been regarded by all as either ethically or politically desirable (pp. xxii-xxiii).

Similarly, Bator (1963), in his classic article on externalities, "The Anatomy of Market Failure," states that

market efficiency is neither sufficient nor necessary for market institutions to be the 'preferred' mode of social organization. ... If, e.g., people are sensitive not only to their own jobs but to other people's as well, or more generally, if such things as relative status, power, and the like, matter, the injunction to maximize output, to hug the production-possibility frontier, can hardly be assumed 'neutral,' and points on the utility frontier may associate with points inside the production frontier (p. 378).

We therefore need to ask, "Which conception of utility best represents people's actual behavior -- one in which only absolute wealth matters, or one where relative standing is important as well?" Intuition would tell us that the Pareto conception, in which only one's own possessions matter, is implausible if not downright wrong. It implies that people are indifferent about their rank or status in society. Rather, all that they care about is what they themselves have, irrespective of whether this is more or less, better or worse, than others with whom they have contact.[8]

In this regard, Pigou (1932), one of the founders of welfare economics, quotes and affirms John Stuart Mill's statement that, "Men do not desire to be *rich*, but to be richer than other men" (p. 90). In a lighter vein, Frank (1985) notes that, "H.L. Mencken once defined wealth as any income that is at least one hundred dollars more a year than the income of one's wife's sister's husband" (p. 5). Thurow (1980) has stated that once incomes exceed the subsistence level, "individual perceptions of the adequacy of their economic performance depend almost solely on relative as opposed to absolute position" (p. 18).

Is there any evidence to support the belief that people care about their relative standing in addition to their absolute level of wealth? One of the first to try to do so was Duesenberry (1952), who developed the relative income hypothesis. Under

---

[8] The interested reader may wish to peruse economist Robert Frank's (1985) book, *Choosing the Right Pond: Human Behavior and the Quest for Status*. Frank explains nearly all economic behavior on the basis of concern about one's relative position in society.

this hypothesis, people's drive for self-esteem makes them wish to emulate the consumption habits of those who are on a higher socioeconomic rung of the ladder; he states that "this drive operates through inferiority feelings aroused by unfavorable comparisons between living standards" and is heightened with more frequent contact between "the quality of the goods he uses with those used by others" (p. 31). The theory predicts that people with lower incomes will save a smaller proportion of their income because they will have more frequent contact with those in the economic class just above them, whose consumption patterns they will mimic. This prediction has been verified repeatedly through empirical studies.[9]

Further evidence is provided in Easterlin's study of human happiness in 14 countries and is particularly relevant here. He found that in a given country at a particular time, wealthier people tend to be happier than poorer people. Within a given country over time, however, happiness levels are surprisingly constant even in the wake of rising real incomes. Furthermore, average levels of happiness are fairly constant across countries; people in poor countries and wealthy countries claim to be about equally happy. The only way such findings can be reconciled is if both relative and absolute wealth matters. Easterlin (1974) concludes,

> there is a 'consumption norm' which exists in a given society at a given time, and which enters into the reference standard of virtually everyone. This provides a common point of reference in self-appraisals of well-being, leading those below the norm to feel less happy and those above the norm, more happy. Over time, this norm tends to rise with the general level of consumption ... (p. 112-13).

Suppose that one accepts the notion that people are concerned with how they compare with others. It could still be argued that even so, it is an irrational and/or flawed character trait that should not be respected by the analyst or policy-maker. However, this argument doesn't hold up for two reasons. First, traditional economic theory does not evaluate where preferences come from or whether they are good or bad. Instead, it views them as what has to be satisfied in order for an individual, and ultimately, a society to be in a best-off position. Second, concern about one's status, rather than being irrational or even undesirable, is an essential element of human nature allowing not only for individuals, but also a society, to

---

[9] In contrast, alternative theories such as the permanent income and life-cycle hypotheses do not correctly predict people's savings behavior in this regard (Frank, 1985).

prosper. In this regard, Scitovsky (1976) has written:

> The desire to 'live up to the Joneses' is often criticized and its rationality called into question. This is absurd and unfortunate. Status seeking, the wish to belong, the asserting and cementing of one's membership in the group is a deep-seated and very natural drive whose origin and universality go beyond man and are explained by that most basic of drives, the desire to survive (p. 115).

What others have can also be viewed as necessary information for a person in formulating his or her individual desires. It shows what can be had -- what is reasonable to expect.

Why is the Pareto principle so important to the belief that markets are superior? The answer is because markets are able to satisfy individuals only if people care about their absolute bundle of possessions rather than how they stand relative to others. Although health applications will be provided later, an example may help illustrate this. Suppose that an extremely expensive therapy is developed that can substantially reduce the chance of contracting a fatal disease, but only a few people can afford it. Under a market model, this therapy will be available only to those few. This will obviously increase their utility, but it would likely reduce the utility of a far greater group who would know that a life-saving technology were available -- but not to them. Relying on markets would therefore tend to reduce overall social welfare. To improve society's overall lot, it could be better if government intervened either to ensure equal access to the technology, or perhaps even to thwart its availability.

Externalities of Consumption

Economists are often concerned with the notion of "market failure," the circumstances under which a competitive market will not reach a Pareto optimum. The primary reason that a free market may fail is the presence of externalities. With externalities, the free market will not be Pareto optimal because too few goods and services with associated positive externalities will be produced and consumed, while too many of those with negative externalities are. Health economists are well aware of many of these externalities; commonly cited ones include smoking (a negative consumption externality), immunizations (a positive consumption externality), pollution (a negative production externality), and medical research (a positive production externality).

In this section we will deal with a consumption externality that has received far less consideration from economists: *concern about the well-being of others.* If we care about other people's needs as well as our own -- be they specific ones like food or medical care, or somewhat more vague concerns about how happy they think they are -- then there is a positive externality of consumption. Note that this does not contradict the previous discussion about people feeling envy or having concern about status. It is not unreasonable to believe that people would envy those who have more than they do, and have benevolence towards those who have less.

A few economists have recognized the importance of this assumption. Boulding (1969), in his Presidential address to the American Economic Association, remarked that:

> Many, if not most, economists accept the Paretian optimum as almost self-evident. Nevertheless, it rests on an extremely shaky foundation of ethical propositions. The more one examines it, for instance, the more clear it becomes that economists must be extraordinarily nice people even to have thought of such a thing, for it implies that there is no malevolence anywhere in the system. It implies, likewise, that there is no benevolence, the niceness of economists not quite extending as far as good will. It assumes selfishness, that is, the independence of individual preference function, such that it makes no difference to me whether I perceive you as either better off or worse off. Anything less descriptive of the human condition could hardly be imagined. The plain fact is that our lives are dominated by precisely this interdependence of utility function which the Paretian optimum denies. (pp. 5-6).

These considerations may be neglected precisely because of the damage their inclusion can do to the competitive model. In what must be considered one of the least sanguine statements ever written about the ability of economics to guide policy, J. de V. Graaff (1971), in his classic book, *Theoretical Welfare Economics,* writes:

> A theory which takes external effects in consumption into account seems to become so hopelessly complicated that any chance of ever applying it becomes exceedingly remote. Much of the appeal of what we might call *laissez-faire* welfare theory ... is undoubtedly due to its elegance and simplicity. Admit to the existence of external effects, and both disappear. Even under ideal circumstances, price no longer measures the marginal contribution a good makes to social welfare -- it measures the contribution it makes to private welfare, which may be something quite different. We have to retreat to banal statements about social rates of indifference, and can say virtually nothing that could ever have any bearing on problems of the day (pp. 1169-70).

Graaff believed that economics should focus on "*positive* studies -- through contributing to our understanding of how the economic system actually works in practice -- rather than through normative welfare theory (p. 170)," a conclusion, that, not surprisingly, did not go over too well with some other welfare economists.[10]

It is important to understand that this issue is not just about equity -- it concerns efficiency as well. Suppose for a moment that I care about poor people and want them to have more food and medical care. In order to increase my own utility, I would want to give some of my resources to the poor.

Why doesn't everyone just donate their optimal amount to charity, which should, in turn, maximize their personal utility? The problem is that many if not most people will attempt to become "free riders," recognizing that the poor will do about as well if everyone except themselves provide donations. This, in turn, will result in less redistribution than is economically efficient; people would feel better if there were a way to redistribute the optimal amount of resources rather than the lesser amount that occurs through the free market.

There is a standard "answer" to this problem in traditional economics. That is to rely on markets to efficiently allocate resources, and then to employ *lump-sum* taxes and subsidies to redistribute income. It is important to understand the nature of these lump-sum transfers. The idea is to come up with a way to tax, say, the wealthy, to subsidize, perhaps, the poor, without changing in any important way the efficiency-enhancing incentives of a competitive market.

The problem with this "lump-sum solution" is the virtual impossibility of establishing true lump-sum taxes and subsidies;[11] no such taxes exist which would also be politically acceptable.[12,13] The problem is nicely summarized by Nath (1969):

---

[10] Mishan (1969b) claims that, "Graaff's conclusions are too cavalier by far" (p. 80).

[11] For further discussion on problems in enacting such taxes and subsidies, see: Graaff (1971), pp. 77-82; and Samuelson (1947), pp. 247-249.

[12] There is, in theory, one sort of tax and subsidy that might work, but it has no practicality. This is a *poll tax* -- a tax that is levied irrespective of income.

[13] Another problem relates to the ability of the political system to approve of taxes of sufficient magnitudes. In this regard, Thurow (1980) has noted that government is much better at allocating gains or perks than at allocating losses. Similarly, Tullock (1979), one of the pioneers in the study of social decision-making, has written that: "So far as I know there is absolutely no reason to believe that majority voting or any of the variants of democratic government transfer an 'optimal' amount. Indeed, I would argue that they do very badly, since the bulk of the transfers they generate are transferred back and forth within the middle class; and, so far as I know, there are no arguments that would indicate that these transfers are desirable." (p. 172).

> If there is any kind of sales tax ... then the price paid by the consumers will be different than the price paid by the producer, and the Pareto optimality conditions will not be met. ... Only such taxes as do not produce a difference between the price of anything ... as received by the seller and as paid by the buyer are free from this shortcoming ... [I]f a tax is assessed on the basis of income ... -- as it must be if it is to bring about some desired change in the distribution of utility levels -- then the price received by the seller of the services ... is different from the price that the buyer pays for it ... (pp. 45-6).

However, if no such methods are feasible, then use of market competition becomes problematic when there are consumption externalities. If we do not redistribute income, the market is inefficient because people want the poor to be better off than they are. But if we do redistribute income -- say, by the traditional method, the income tax -- we damage the efficiency that the marketplace is designed to create.

Thus, in making policy, it is impossible to separate issues of resource allocation from issues of resource distribution. Rather, they both must be dealt with simultaneously. But this is not in keeping with the traditional method often preached by economists, in which markets are allowed to operate in an unfettered fashion and redistribution is only done afterwards -- usually through cash transfers rather than through the direct provision of goods and services.

This anomaly -- the impossibility of separating allocative and distributional activities of the economy -- has been raised, in a variety of contexts, by several writers, including Arrow (1963b), Mishan (1969b), Olsen (1969), Thurow (1983), Blackorby and Donaldson (1990), and Reinhardt (1992). In his famous article about the health care system, Arrow (1963b) states that,

> If ... the actual market differs significantly from the competitive model, or if the assumptions of the two optimality theorems are not fulfilled, the separation of allocative and distributional procedures becomes, in most cases, impossible (p.943).[14]

Mishan (1969b) writes,

> Far from an optimum allocation of resources representing some kind of an ideal output separable from and independent of interpersonal comparisons of welfare, a particular output retains its optimum characteristics only insofar as we commit ourselves to the particular welfare distribution uniquely associated with it (p. 133).

---

[14] The two optimality conditions referred to by Arrow are that (if certain assumptions are met): (1) a competitive equilibrium is Pareto optimal; and (2) any Pareto optimum can be reached by a competitive equilibrium corresponding to a particular initial distribution of resources.

Olsen (1969) notes that,

> In general, normative theories which separate equity and efficiency and use different principles
> to determine the optimal allocation of resources and distribution of welfare seem to yield
> solutions which are not Pareto optimal because of relevant disincentive effects (p. 41).

Blackorby and Donaldson (1990), perhaps more bluntly, remark that separating allocative and distributive decisions "require[s] a notion of efficiency that is independent of the distribution of income -- an idea that makes no sense in real-world economies" (p. 490).

The primary implication for policy makers is a crucially important one: allocative and distributive decisions by a society should be made in conjunction with each other, not separately. The belief that we should start with principles of fairness, and *then* proceed to considerations of efficiency, is embodied not only in much of contemporary moral philosophy (e.g., Rawls, 1971; Dworkin, 1981; Sen, 1992; Roemer, 1994), but it is also the foundation upon which most modern health care systems have been built (Wagstaff and van Doorslaer, 1992).

Thurow (1980) summarizes the issue in the following passage:

> Decisions about economic equity are the fundamental starting point for any market economy.
> Individual preferences determine market demands for goods and services, but these individual
> preferences are weighted by incomes before being communicated to the market. An individual
> with no income or wealth may have needs and desires, but he has no economic resources. To
> make his or her personal preferences felt, he must have these resources. If income and wealth
> are distributed in accordance with equity (whatever that may be), individual preferences are
> properly weighed, and the market can efficiently adjust to an equitable set of demands. If
> income and wealth are not distributed in accordance with equity, individual preferences are
> not properly weighted. The market efficiently adjusts, but to an inequitable set of demands
> ... One way or the other, we are forced to reveal our collective preferences about what
> constitutes a just distribution of economic resources (pp. 194-95).

Reinhardt (1992) has stated the same thing somewhat more succinctly:

> to begin an exploration of alternative proposals for the reform of our health system without
> first setting forth explicitly, and very clearly, the *social values* to which the reformed system
> is to adhere strikes at least this author as patently *inefficient*: it is a waste of time. Would it
> not be more *efficient* merely to explore the *relative efficiency* of alternative proposals that do
> conform to widely shared *social values*? (p. 315).

This concern would be eased if income were redistributed to the degree desired by members of society.[15] But if it is not, then other strategies are necessary to deal with both the inefficiencies and inequities that arise when there are positive externalities of consumption. One of the best ways to deal with Thurow's concern is to enact policies that ensure that those in need obtain goods and services even if they do not have the economic resources to purchase them in the marketplace. Programs like Medicare and Medicaid -- which are not in keeping with some economists' recommendations to rely on competition and then redistribute resources through cash subsidies -- offer good examples of how society grapples with problems like these.

Consumer Tastes are Predetermined

Of all of the assumptions in the traditional economic model, perhaps the one that is most often forgotten is that consumers' tastes are already established when they enter the marketplace. This turns out to be very important; this section will attempt to show that it is not realistic, and that when it is dropped, the competitive model loses many of its advantages.

One facet of other social sciences is that, in general, they seek to determine how people and groups *actually* behave, not how they *ought to* be behaving. In contrast, Thurow (1983) contends, "while the reverse is true in the other social sciences that study real human behavior...prescription dominates description in economics" (p. 216). In this regard, in economics one commonly sees the word "ought" (e.g., people ought to maximize their utility, or otherwise they are being "irrational"; to maximize social welfare a society "ought" to depend on a competitive marketplace).

In economic theory, individual tastes and preferences "simply exist -- fully developed and immutable" (Thurow, 1983, p. 219). This is what Boulding (1969) has referred to as the "Immaculate Conception of the Indifference Curve," because "tastes are simply given, and ... we cannot inquire into the process by which they are formed" (p. 1). Milton Friedman (1962) provides one explanation for this:

---

[15] See Tullock's quotation in footnote 13.

economic theory proceeds largely to take wants as fixed ... primarily [as] a case of division of labor. The economist has little to say about the formation of wants; this is the province of the psychologist. The economist's task is to trace the consequences of any given set of wants (p. 13).[16]

The overriding issue concerning the formation of tastes is whether they are *endogenous* -- that is, a product of the economic system or even the society in which they exist. Although not a central focus by any means, the issue has received some attention from mainstream journals such as the *American Economic Review* and the *Journal of Economic Theory*. In one of these articles, Pollak (1978) succinctly demonstrates the gravity of the issue:

Taste formation and change pose more difficult problems for welfare analysis. Variable tastes undermine the normative significance of the fundamental theorem of welfare economics which asserts ... that in competitive equilibrium everyone gets what he wants ... However, if tastes are sufficiently malleable, then this may be no more than a corollary of the more general proposition that *people come to want what they get* (p. 374, emphasis added).

Similarly, von Weiszacker (1971) notes that taking endogenous tastes as predetermined leads to a situation where "the *status quo* is not Pareto optimal even though none of the usual kinds of externalities are present" (361). He further states that:

One of the reasons why economists [do] not very deeply discuss this question may be that their present concepts of Pareto optimality and efficiency possibly are not flexible enough to cope with endogenously changing tastes. It may become necessary to change the conceptual framework of our theory; we may be forced to ask almost philosophical questions about the concepts we use. In every discipline, there is always a reluctance to engage in this kind of activity (p. 346).

The unrealistic nature of the assumption of exogenously determined tastes is easy to see. Consider the case of advertising. The reader, who is likely well-versed in the tactics of the media, probably will admit that most advertising is not aimed at providing objective information so that consumers can obtain the best value. Rather, it is designed to: (a) *minimize* the consumer search process, and more

---

[16] Gary Becker (1979) provides another reason: The assumption of stable preferences provides a stable foundation for generating predictions about responses to various changes, and prevents the analyst from succumbing to the temptation of simply postulating the required shift in preferences to 'explain' all apparent contradictions to his predictions (p. 9).

generally, (b) change consumer tastes, in part by exerting social pressure. It is hard to claim that the tastes people come to have, as the result of exposure to this sort of advertising, are sacrosanct. In fact, people often make "bad" or non-maximizing decisions by acting on the message -- the hallmark of a successful advertising campaign!

Why, then, does economics consider tastes predetermined rather than subject to the forces of change? Most economists believe that the consumer is the best judge of what will maximize his or her utility. Consequently, to maximize overall social welfare, we should set up an economic system that is best at allowing consumer choices to be satisfied. Where these choices come from, as Friedman said, is beside the point.

In contrast, it might be true that your current tastes are determined not on the basis of preferences that are endemic to you so much as on what you consumed in the past. This implies a strong advantage for whatever is the status quo; familiarity breeds preference (as opposed to breeding contempt), so what exists now will be demanded in the future. But if that is the case, it could be argued that in demanding goods and services in the marketplace, you are *wanting what you got* rather than getting what you want (Pollak, 1978).

If what you want depends on what you had in the past, or on the influence of advertisers, then it is not clear that a competitive marketplace is the best way to make people better off. In the paragraphs below, three examples are provided in which people's market behaviors are not predetermined but rather are a result of their past or present environments. In each case, it is not clear that fulfillment of their personal choices would make them best off.

The first example, and perhaps the least important of the three given, concerns addiction. Suppose that, while growing up, you are in a peer group that smokes cigarettes, and you become addicted. Once you leave that peer group, you will still have a "taste" for cigarettes and are more likely to demand them than someone who is not addicted. Can we really say, in such an instance, that satisfying this "taste" through the marketplace is efficient from a societal standpoint -- in the same way as satisfying the demand for bread or literature? Might not you be better off if cigarettes are taxed so prohibitively (or even banned) by the government to make you stop smoking?[17]

---

[17] Note that this argument for government intervention does not rely at all on any externalities associated with cigarette smoking.

A second and much more general application is habit formed by past consumption patterns.[18] Suppose you live in a community that has not discovered the joys of music. A resident of such a place will therefore have not developed a taste for music. But, as Marshall (1920), one of the fathers of modern economics, once noted, "the more good music a man hears, the stronger is his taste for it likely to become" (p. 94). The aforementioned resident might likely be better off with music than without, but he or she has not been sufficiently "educated" to know this. Government intervention, in the form, perhaps, of funding for culture in the arts, could make people better off than pure reliance on the marketplace.

The third example concerns occupational choices. In the traditional economic model, it is assumed that people make occupational choices based on weighing all alternatives; factors considered would include how much satisfaction they obtain from the work and the wages that it offers. Whatever choice is made in a competitive labor market is assumed to be utility-maximizing. But this might not be the case if tastes are a product of one's environment. Suppose, for example, that a person grows up in a factory town and later decides to work in the factory. This might not necessarily be utility maximizing; it is possibly a poor choice for some such people, which was made because of their limited opportunities. As another example, imagine that one person works to perform house cleaning services for another. This may not reflect the personal preferences as much as lack of good alternatives (Buchanan, 1977). In this regard, Roemer states that:

> people learn to live with what they are accustomed to or what is available to them. ... Thus the slave may have adapted to like slavery; welfare judgments based on individual preferences are clearly impugned in such situations (p. 120).

Again, we see that the status quo would be favored by competitive markets, even though people might be better off if society, in some way, intervened in these choices. A public job training program would be an example of the type of intervention that could be beneficial to society.

If this is true and people's tastes are indeed the product of their environment, why is this an indictment of market forces? It is because people's demand for goods and services might not reflect the things that would make them best off.[19] In health care, for example, people may not demand certain preventive services that

---

[18] For a good discussion of these issues, see Hahnel and Albert (1990).
[19] This line of reasoning is pursued in the next section, which concerns demand for health care.

would make them better off in part because they grew up in an environment in which more high-tech medical interventions were stressed. In such an instance, having the government provide or subsidize such services would then be superior to relying on the market, where they are not purchased in sufficient quantity. But if consumer tastes are viewed as predetermined, as they are in the market model, people become "stuck" with whatever they demand because they are assumed to always know best.

IMPLICATIONS FOR HEALTH POLICY

The previous discussion attempted to show that, despite popular belief to the contrary, economic theory does not provide a strong justification for the superiority of market competition in the health care area because the competitive model is based on certain assumptions that do not appear to be met. This section provides some implications of these conclusions for health care policy.

Equalizing Access to Health Care Services

The Pareto principle states that if society can make someone better off without making someone else worse off, it should do so. At first glance, it might appear that most developed countries do believe in the Pareto principle when it comes to health policy. After all, almost all countries, even those with comprehensive universal health insurance programs, allow their citizens to spend their own money on additional health care services if they wish to go outside of the government-sanctioned program.

However, upon closer examination, it can be demonstrated that health care policy has, and continues to be, conducted on principles quite contrary to the Pareto principle. This is even true in the United States, where, it will be argued, society has not tended to tolerate large differences in access to care.

Evidence supporting this belief dates back many years. Beginning with the post-World War II period, public funding for building and expanding hospitals under the Hill-Burton Act directly reflected a belief that poorer, rural areas of the United States should not be disadvantaged *relative to* wealthier, urban areas of the country. By defining the need for hospitals based on the per capita availability of beds, the philosophy behind Hill-Burton was that no areas of the country should be given greater access than others to hospital care.

More recent evidence is provided by state mandates concerning the content of health insurance coverage. If the Pareto principle were viewed as desirable, insurance companies would be allowed to provide whatever health insurance coverage they wished. In fact, this is not the case; states, which have almost all regulatory authority over the sale of insurance, have enacted numerous "mandates" concerning the eligibility for, and content of, health insurance policies. One study found that by 1988, there were more than 730 mandates across the different states (Gabel and Jensen, 1989). It reported, for example, that 37 states require insurers to cover alcohol treatment, 28 require that mental health care be covered, and 18, maternity care. It is true that special interest groups provide much of the support for these mandates; nevertheless, consumer groups, and particularly people who need certain services (or know someone who does) also strongly support them.

Similar evidence can be seen by examining the political fallout that arose from the Oregon proposal for Medicaid reform, which was dubbed as requiring "rationing" of services. Early versions of the proposal engendered a great deal of opposition, mainly because program beneficiaries would not be able to receive coverage for the same services as the rest of the population. Rather, what services would be paid for would depend on how much money was available. Less cost-effective services would not be covered if program money was exhausted after paying for more cost-effective services. This prompted Vladeck (1990), who later became director of the federal government's Health Care Financing Administration, to write,

> this will be the first system in memory to explicitly plan that poor people with treatable illnesses will die if Medicaid runs out of money or does not budget correctly, and providers will be excused from liability for failing to treat them. The Oregonians argue that it is healthier for society to make such choices explicitly, but it is hardly healthy to establish rules of the game that require such choices (p. 3).

In fact, the proposal was cleared by federal officials only after methodology was revised to ensure that disabled individuals would not face discrimination in coverage (Fox and Leichter, 1993) and after the state made it clear that all essential services would be provided.

A final, and probably the most compelling example of how health policy operates in conflict of the Pareto principle, concerns coverage for new health care technologies. Traditionally, when new and potentially effective technologies become available, they are viewed as experimental until their safety and efficacy are established. But once established, insurers almost always cover them; failure to do so first results in strong pressure from policyholders, and eventually lawsuits that the insurer is withholding necessary medical care. Having these technologies covered by public and private insurance ensures that their access is available to the large majority of the population that possesses health insurance. In this regard, Reinhardt (1992) writes:

> Suppose [that a] new, high-tech medical intervention [is available] and that more of it could be produced without causing reductions in the output of any other commodity. Suppose next, however, that the associated rearrangement of the economy has been such that only well-to-do patients will have access to the new medical procedure. On these assumptions, can we be sure that [this] would enhance overall *social welfare*? Would we not have to assume the absence of social envy among the poor and of guilt among the well-to-do? Are these reasonable assumptions? Or should civilized policy analysts refuse to pay heed to base human motives such as envy, prevalent though it may be in any normal society? (p. 311).

If public policy were based on the Pareto principle, then we would see a market-driven gap between the services that are available to the wealthy and those available to the rest of the population. This would likely result in reduced social welfare, as noted by Reinhardt. But we do not see such a gap -- once a procedure is found to be safe and effective, everyone with private health insurance is potentially eligible to receive it. And, if insurers are not sufficiently quick enough to adopt new procedures, states can and do mandate their provision.[20]

What Comes First: Allocation or Distribution?

In the traditional economic paradigm, a competitive market ensures that resources are allocated efficiently. However, if there are positive externalities of consumption -- for example, society wants poorer people to have more resources -- then the "free-rider effect" will prevent a competitive economy from achieving allocative efficiency. The traditional economic solution to this problem is to institute lump-sum taxes and subsidies because they do not distort incentives and reduce efficiency, but in practice, no such mechanisms are available.

Rather than relying on this economic paradigm, what all developed countries

---

[20] States cannot currently mandate provision of services under employer sponsored health plans that fall under the jurisdiction of the Employee Retirement Income and Security Act (ERISA). Although this has effectively reduced the strength of state mandates, there is little doubt that such mandates would still exist if ERISA were repealed.

do instead is confront allocative and distributive issues concurrently. In the U.S., public programs like Medicare and Medicaid were established outside of the competitive marketplace in order to ensure that our priority -- access to medical care services for the elderly and the poor -- was met. There is now much discussion about introducing more competition into both programs, and perhaps that will occur. Nevertheless, such proposals have engendered a tremendous amount of opposition because it is contended that the introduction of more competition will jeopardize the principles that formed the basis of these programs in the first place.

The belief that we should start with principles of fairness, and then proceed to considerations of efficiency, is also the foundation upon which most other health care systems have been built. In their comprehensive study of health care financing and equity in nine European countries and the United States, Wagstaff and van Doorslaer (1992) found that:

> There appears to be broad agreement ... among policy-makers in at least eight of the nine European countries ... that payments towards health care should be related to ability to pay rather than to use of medical facilities. Policymakers in all nine European countries also appear to be committed to the notion that all citizens should have access to health care. In many countries this is taken further, it being made clear that access to and receipt of health care should depend on need, rather than on ability to pay (p. 363).

No countries have adopted the economic approach of starting with a market system and then engaging in redistribution policies so that the poor can afford to purchase privately-provided care. There are many good reasons for this. The key one, however, is that it would provide no assurance that people who find themselves without insurance would purchase it. This, in turn, would lower the welfare of a society where people feel better in knowing that the poor can receive health care services.

Should Cost Control Be a Public Policy?

A larger issue that arises if consumer tastes are pliable concerns cost control. Health economists often point out that we cannot say that a country spends too much of its national income on health care. Who is to say that 14% or even 25% is "too much"? It is contended that there is nothing necessarily wrong if a society wants to spend more of its money on, say, expensive technologies. But this viewpoint is harder to justify if one views consumer tastes not as predetermined but rather as the product of previous experiences.

Take the example of medical technology. People are likely to demand the fruits of new technologies in part because they come to expect them. Rublee (1994) has provided data on the relative availability of six selected medical technologies in Canada, Germany, and the United States. For all six technologies shown, the number of units per million persons is far higher in the United States than in Canada and Germany. With regard to open heart surgery, the figures are almost three times as high in the United States as in Canada, and nearly five times as great as in Germany. For magnetic resonance imaging, availability in the United States is ten times as great as Canada and three times as great as Germany. Because of this, the U.S. public -- and perhaps more importantly, their physicians -- are likely to have developed greater expectations of such technologies. Some analysts argue that it is the growth of these technologies -- or, as Joseph Newhouse (1993) termed it, "the enhanced capabilities of medicine" (p. 162) -- that is primarily responsible for rising health care costs in the United States.

The point -- that perhaps people would be equally well-off without so many expensive (not to say duplicative) life-saving interventions -- is made only tentatively. One would not want to claim that people want to live longer because they are inculcated into believing that is desirable. Clearly, though, quality-of-life issues become relevant to such a discussion, as does the fact that the United States ranks near the top of the world in only one major vital statistic category -- life expectancy after reaching age 80.[21] One must take pause when considering Easterlin's results presented earlier -- that people in poor countries seem to be equally happy as those in wealthier ones -- or perhaps more relevant to health care, the fact that citizens of other countries, which spend far less money on medical care, tend to be much happier with their health care systems. This latter point is supported by Blendon (1993) and his colleagues in writing on the satisfaction that citizens in ten developed countries have in their health care systems. Only Italians show as low satisfaction levels as do Americans. Ten percent of Americans thought that only minor changes were needed in their health care system, compared to 56% of Canadians, 41% of Germans, 32% of Swedes, and 27% of British. Thus, more spending on technologies does not seem to be increasing utility levels

---

[21] Data from 24 developed countries show that female life expectancy in the United States at age 80 is rivaled only by Canada, and male life expectancy at that age, only by Canada and Iceland. In contrast 15 countries exceed the United States in female life expectancy at birth, and 17 in male life expectancy. See Schieber and Poullier, 1992.

very much.

As was argued above, if tastes are based on past consumption, then perhaps in demanding things like more medical technology, patients and their physicians are, in part, wanting what they got rather than getting what they want. It follows that greater medical spending to support more of these technologies might not enhance social welfare so much as it represents the fulfillment of expectations that were built on the availability of such technologies in the past. Having said this, one must be very careful because in the case of health care, people's utility would appear to depend a great deal on absolutes rather than relatives. (If you feel pain, it is little consolation if your neighbor does too.) Nevertheless, the belief that more and more spending on technologies may not increase utility levels very much -- because it raises people's expectations to unrealistic levels -- is consistent with a rather sober quotation from Mishan (1969b):

> As I see it, the main task today of the economist at all concerned with the course of human welfare is that of weaning the public from its post-war fixation on economic growth; of inculcating an awareness of the errors and misconceptions that abound in popular appraisals of the benefits of industrial development; and also, perhaps of voicing an occasional doubt whether the persistent pursuit of material ends, borne onwards today by a tidal wave of unrealisable expectations, can do more eventually than to agitate the current restlessness, and to add to the frustrations and disillusion of ordinary mortals (p. 81).

DEMAND THEORY

PROBLEMS WITH THE THEORY

In *Candide*, the philosopher Dr. Pangloss attempts to prove that the obviously flawed state of nature and society is, nevertheless, the best of all possible worlds. Voltaire (1759) quotes his character as stating:

> It is demonstrated that things cannot be otherwise: for, since everything was made for a purpose, everything is necessarily for the best purpose. Note that noses were made to wear spectacles; we therefore have spectacles. Legs were clearly devised to wear breeches, and we have breeches. ... And since pigs were made to be eaten, we have pork all year round. Therefore, those who have maintained that all is well have been talking nonsense: they should have maintained that all is for the best (p. 18).

Although perhaps not recognized by most economists, the theory of revealed preference in particular, and consumer theory in general, bears a striking resemblance to Pangloss' philosophy. By choosing a particular bundle of goods, people demonstrate that they prefer it to all others; consequently, it is best for them. And, if all people are in their best position, then society -- which is simply the aggregation of all people -- is also in its best position. Therefore, allowing people to choose in the marketplace results in the best of all possible economic worlds.

This section questions this line of reasoning because it is based on assumptions that are difficult to support, particularly in the health area. In doing so, it questions the conventional meaning of the demand curve -- that it represents the marginal utility obtained by consumers through the purchase of alternative quantities of a good. If one accepts the arguments presented here, there are profound implications for the field of health economics.

An economic system that allows for consumer choice will, subject to some caveats (mainly that externalities are unimportant or corrected for by policy) result in Pareto optimality. Then, if society can reach some agreement on the distribution of wealth, social welfare can be maximized. Here, we will make the assumption that an acceptable redistribution does take place. By doing so, we can focus on the resulting implication about competitive markets under economic theory -- that reaching Pareto optimality through market competition will ultimately lead to the maximization of social welfare.

With this assumption about redistribution in hand, we can form the following syllogism:

If:

A: Social welfare is maximized when individual utilities are maximized, and

B: Individual utilities are maximized when people are allowed to choose, then:

C: Social welfare is maximized when people are allowed to choose.

This is obviously a strong conclusion because it implies that the type of consumer choice brought about by market competition will result, as Dr. Pangloss would say, in the best of all possible worlds. In the health care field, it would provide strong ammunition for the superiority of competitive approaches. But if either propositions A or B do not hold, then such a conclusion about the superiority of competition is not warranted. The following two sections will attempt to cast doubt first on B, and then A.

Are Individual Utilities Maximized when People are Allowed to Choose?

One of the basic tenets of market competition is that people are most satisfied when they are allowed to make their own choices. If, instead, some entity such as government makes the choices for them, it would be extremely unlikely that consumers would fare as well; each person is different, and it would seem to be impossible for an outsider to appreciate an individual's exact desires. Although this is a persuasive argument, this section will attempt to demonstrate that, at least in the health care field, allowing people to make their own choices does not necessarily make them best off.

The belief that consumers will find themselves in a best-off position when they have sovereignty over their market choices is based on several assumptions in the competitive economic model:

-- People know what's best for themselves

-- People have ability to make choices that are in their best interest:
  ● there is sufficient information available
  ● they have the internal wherewithal to do so

-- The resulting choices indeed reveal their preferences.

Each of these will be considered in turn.

Do People Know What's Best for Themselves?

The first question that needs to be addressed when considering if sovereignty is best for consumers is whether they know what is best for themselves. In many instances they unquestionably do, but this may not always be the case. If, in some instances, consumers are not the best judge of what is in their interest, then such choices might be better handled through public intervention.

There is no way to test the proposition directly. Thus, we consider how society goes about making allocation decisions about particular goods and services. In many instances, societies set rules that are explicitly designed to thwart the sanctity of individual choice.

Some of the activities that a libertarian -- that is, a person who believes in the sanctity of individual sovereignty -- would likely believe should be left to individual choice rather than be proscribed by society, include personal use of narcotic drugs, gambling, prostitution, riding a motorcycle without a helmet, selling one's own organs, and suicide. This list was chosen specifically because these are all decisions that mainly affect the individual in question rather than others.

Why would society act in a way to abridge individual choice when consumer theory indicates that people can and do make welfare maximizing choices themselves? Frank (1985) suggests an interesting possibility: people are overly concerned with their status and will make the wrong economic, social, and/or moral decisions in order to enhance this status. But this does not seem to fully account for such laws. There is nothing status-raising about going to Mexico to purchase a supposed cure for cancer. Thus, another reason for paternalistic laws that limit individual choice is that some types of spending decisions are simply a waste of money or an unnecessary danger; society is protecting people against their own foolishness. A final reason, and the one that is usually raised in this regard, is that in health care there are often "experts" who know much more than individual consumers. This would also help account for the laws against the sales of remedies that have not been approved of by the governmental authorities.

Do People Have the Ability to Make Choices that are in Their Best Interest?

Even if people know what is in their best interest, they may not have the ability to make choices that are in their best interest. There are both external and internal reasons for this. On the external side, they may not have sufficient information or might be unable to adequately process the information that is available. With respect to their internal resources, they may not behave in a rational manner. Each will be considered in turn.

Beginning with the information issue, the first question is whether people have enough information available to make the health care choices that are best for them. This obviously depends on the type of health service being considered, and unfortunately, there is, as of yet, very little research available upon which we rely. Some empirical research has been conducted on how consumers go about trying to collect information on the alternatives they face in the health care market. A number of fairly old studies have found relatively little evidence of "consumerism" in health care, with one physician observer sardonically noting that consumers "devote more effort selecting their Halloween pumpkin than they do choosing their physician."[22] A more recent study, by Hoerger and Howard (1995), examined how pregnant women search for a prenatal care provider. The sample included women from Florida who gave birth in 1987. Women who believed that they had a choice of prenatal providers were asked, "Before you selected your actual prenatal care provider, did you seriously consider using another prenatal care provider?" If they answered that in the affirmative, they were further queried, "Did you actually speak with or have an appointment with another prenatal care provider?" Curiously, only 24% of respondents seriously considered using another provider, and only 14% actually had contact with another provider. The authors conclude,

> This amount of search is surprisingly low, given the importance of childbirth, the ample opportunity for choice, and the relative surplus of information about prenatal care providers compared to providers of other physician services. Recall that we expected the choice of prenatal care providers to establish a benchmark or *upper bound* on the extent of search for other physician services (italics added) (p. 341).[23]

A related issue is whether consumers are able to successfully use information that *is* made available to them. Hibbard and Weeks (1989a, 1989b) conducted studies of how being given information about physician fees affects consumer knowledge levels and their use of services. They found little if any resulting change in behavior, as measured by asking about the costs of visits, procedures, tests, or medications; or changing physicians or insurance plans. They also found that receipt of the information had no effect on costs per physician visit, the number of visits, or on annual health care expenditures.

One important, relatively new area in which consumers will need to be skilled at using information, is for health care "report cards." Currently there is not any one standard report card format, and it is not clear how well data items on early versions of these report cards can be used. Examples include utilization rates for alternative services, or the relative importance of survival rates from high versus low incidence procedures.

Relevant here is a study on the type of information consumers look for on report cards, which was conducted by Hibbard and Jewett (1996). The authors

---

[22] This quote, from Dr. Harvey Mandell, is from Hoerger and Howard (1995), which contains a good review of the literature on consumer search for physicians.

[23] Interestingly, experience from previous births did not explain the results. For most women the birth examined was the first child, and furthermore, women with previous births were more likely to search for a provider than those who were having their first child.

found that most consumers indicate that the key type of information for them in choosing a health plan are so-called "desirable events," such as utilization rates for mammograms, cholesterol screening, and pediatric immunizations. Less important to them were "undesirable events" such as hospital death rates from heart attacks, rates of low birth weights, and hospital acquired infections. Curiously, then, when given report cards on two alterative health plans -- one with a better record on desirable events and the other with a better record on undesirable events -- consumers overwhelmingly chose the latter. Although far more research is needed in this area, this sort of inconsistent behavior casts doubt on how well consumers can use report card information to make the best choices for themselves. The mere existence and dissemination of information, even if objective and complete, does not guarantee that it will be used properly by an individual.

A final informational concern is whether consumers can predict the results of their choices. If they cannot, then another entity might be better able to make some choices for them. This issue is best understood by considering something known as the "counterfactual"[24]; counterfactual questions can never be answered with certainty.

Health care poses many counterfactual questions. Suppose a person seeks health care from a primary care physician, and tries to determine what he or she learned from the experience. It turns out to be very difficult for the person to determine whether they made the right decision in seeking care from that provider, because to do so would involve answers to several counterfactual questions, such as: "Would the problem have gone away if I had left it untreated?" or "What would have happened if I had sought the care of a specialist instead of a primary care physician?" or "Would the result have been different if I had seen a different primary care physician than the one I sought?"

In this regard, Weisbrod (1978) has written that,

> For ordinary goods, the buyer has little difficulty in evaluating the counterfactual -- that is, what the situation will be if the good is not obtained. Not so for the bulk of health care . . . Because the human physiological system is itself an adaptive system, it is likely to correct itself and deal effectively with an ailment, even without any medical care services. Thus, a consumer of such services who gets better after the purchase does not know whether the improvement was because of, or even in spite of, the "care" that was received. Or if no health care services are purchased and the individual's problem becomes worse, he is generally not

---

[24] Counterfactual questions are those that are hypothetical in a special way: they concern what would have happened if history had been different.

in a strong position to determine whether the results would have been different, and better, if he had purchased certain health care. And the consumer, not being a medical expert, may learn little from experience or from friends' experience . . . because of the difficulty of determining whether the counterfactual to a particular type of health care today is the same as it was the previous time the consumer, or a friend, had "similar" symptoms. The noteworthy point is not simply that it is difficult for the consumer to judge quality before the purchase . . ., but that it is difficult even after the purchase (p. 52).

Moving on to internal or cognitive reasons that individuals may be unable to make choices in their best interest, we consider the issue of consumer rationality. Here, rationality is seen as indicating *reasonable* behavior.[25] For example, if an adult in the United States smokes cigarettes, we would not necessarily regard this as irrational. This is because there are several potentially reasonable bases for some people to smoke: pleasure, vanity, or addiction. Thus, smoking can be a reasonable decision if these benefits outweigh the various costs. Now suppose that such a person also claims that smoking does nothing to harm health. If the person is even minimally educated, that sort of behavior should be viewed as irrational because it is not based on reason. To deny that cigarette smoking can harm one's health simply does not make sense.

Economists, in contrast to social scientists in other disciplines, sometimes suppose that consumers must be rational and must therefore act to maximize their utility. But that supposition would seem to be false. In this regard, Leibenstein (1976) has noted that, "the idea of utility maximization must contain the possibility of choice under which utility is not maximized" (p. 8). Similarly, Thurow (1983) writes,

Revealed preferences ... is just a fancy way of saying that individuals do whatever individuals do, and whatever they do, economists will call it "utility maximization." Whether individuals buy good A or good Y they are still rational individual utility maximizers. By definition, there is no such thing as an individual who does not maximize utility. But if a theory can never be wrong, it has no content. It is merely a tautology (pp. 217-18).

Obviously, the topic of whether consumers are rational or not is a broad one. To confine the issue a bit, we will discuss only one such issue here because it has been well-researched in the field of social psychology but only touched upon by economists -- cognitive dissonance.

---

[25] Economists often use a more technical definition, in which choices are consistent and transitive. See Mishan (1982).

The theory of cognitive dissonance concerns a central aspect of human behavior -- self-justification or rationalization. As explained by Aronson (1972),

> Basically, cognitive dissonance is a state of tension that occurs when an individual simultaneously holds two cognitions (ideas, attitudes, beliefs, opinions) that are psychologically inconsistent ... Because [its] occurrence ... is unpleasant, people are motivated to reduce it ... (pp. 92-93).

Whether people act in a way that we might define as rational or irrational depends on how difficult it is to change the behavior in question versus the cognition. Smoking offers one of the best examples. Suppose that a person smokes but knows that it is very dangerous to health. This causes cognitive dissonance; how can you continue to do something that is so self-destructive? If the person is not addicted or has particularly strong will, he or she may quit. But an addict or weaker person will typically find it easier to change the cognition rather than the behavior, by either attributing more pleasure to smoking than is truly obtained, or by denying that it is dangerous (Aronson, 1972). Although this latter type of behavior has been repeatedly confirmed and is certainly understandable, it would seem to be a violation of the English language to deem it as "rational."

Akerlof and Dickens (1992) have used cognitive dissonance to explain various economic behaviors. Examples include explaining the choice of risky jobs, technological development, advertising, social insurance, and crime. Regarding social insurance, they write:

> If there are some persons who would simply prefer not to contemplate a time when their earning power is diminished, and if the very fact of saving for old age forces persons into such contemplations, there is an argument for compulsory old age insurance. ... [They] may find it uncomfortable to contemplate their old age. For that reason they may make the wrong tradeoff, *given their own preferences*, between current consumption and savings for retirement (italics added) (p.317).

Note that saving is what would make the person best off in his or her own eyes, but the person fails to do it anyway. Hence, society makes the decision to override individual choice by establishing social insurance programs -- like Social Security and Medicare. In summary, when cognitive dissonance is important, there is little reason to suppose that people will act in a rational manner -- that is, make decisions that maximize their utility.

Do Individuals Reveal their Preferences through their Actions?

The final aspect of whether market choices are best left to the individual concerns a perhaps more abstract issue: whether people's actions really reflect their preferences. Demand theory assumes that what people choose to buy or do reflects their preferences. This might not be the case.

Sen (1982, 1987, 1992) has written several persuasive essays and books on this issue. The basic problem concerns an issue addressed earlier -- interdependencies in people's utility functions. If people make their choices based not only on their own preferences but those of others as well, then these choices will not necessarily reflect their own preferences. This becomes important because it casts doubt on the conventional meaning of demand curves, which purport to show the marginal utility that people obtain from additional units of consumption.

One argument that Sen makes is that much human behavior flies in the face of the notion that your actions indicate your personal preferences. He does this by distinguishing two concepts, sympathy and commitment. A person who acts on feelings of sympathy is indeed showing his personal preferences through his actions; you feel better if you help. Commitment, however, is different; you would rather do something else but you don't because you are committed to a particular cause. Sen uses recycling as an example. He argues that people don't recycle because they enjoy it or because they think that their own actions will convince anyone else to do it. In spite of that, they do it anyway because of their commitment to a cleaner environment. Sen (1982) summarizes this point, noting that:

> One way of defining commitment is in terms of a person choosing an act that he believes will yield a lower level of personal welfare to him than an alternative that is also available to him. (p. 92)

and that this concept:

> drives a wedge between personal choice and personal welfare, and much of traditional economic theory relies on the identity of the two (p. 94).

People's actions therefore seem to be motivated by things other than selfishness, and thus, the choices one observes do not necessarily indicate the level of welfare derived by the individual or by society. [In this regard, Sen (1982) writes, "The *purely* economic man is indeed close to being a social moron."(p. 99)]

But the results of this behavior can go in either direction: either choosing something that enhances social but not personal welfare (e.g., commitment); or choosing not to help others when it would be personally beneficial to do so. Nath (1969) provides a useful example of the latter behavior.

Suppose we observe a person *not* giving to a charity aimed at improving the health of the poor. Using revealed preference, one would conclude that the person would rather have something else -- the good or service purchased with the money that could have been spent on the charity. This might not be the case, however. It may be that the person would benefit from providing such a donation because his utility function contains an element encompassing the health of the poor. But he may believe that his contribution will not be of much help because others are not compelled to follow suit. Thus, the person would like the poor to have better access to health care, but this is not evident by examining his or her market behavior. Nath (1969) states that there is a "fallacy in the assumption that an individual's welfare function coincides with his utility function as revealed by his market choices. This is a very common fallacy in economic writings." (p. 141).

In summary, what we have tried to show is that proposition B in the syllogism presented above -- that individual utilities are maximized when people are allowed to choose -- very well may not be met in the health care area. The next section examines the validity of the other proposition that must be met in order for consumer choice to necessarily result in what is best for society.

Is Social Welfare Maximized When Individual Utilities are Maximized?

This section examines the proposition A of the syllogism presented earlier, that social welfare is maximized when individuals maximize their own utility.[26] Although the proposition that social welfare is based solely on individuals' welfare is a philosophical issue and cannot be proven true or false, there are two reasons to question its validity. The first of these arguments is also from Sen (1982, 1987, 1992), who disputes this notion that individual welfare is the only legitimate component of social welfare. He calls such a philosophy "welfarism," which "is

---

[26] Recall that we are making the assumption that society can and does redistribute income so that any Pareto optimum that is reached through a competitive marketplace will result in maximum social welfare. This allows us to explicitly examine the advantages of allowing for consumer choice in the health care market without worrying about issues of equity.

the view that the only things of intrinsic value for ethical calculation and evaluation of states of affairs are individual utilities." His arguments, which span several books, are too lengthy to be properly summarized here. One of the reasons that Sen rejects the welfarist approach is that it does not allow us to distinguish between different *qualities* of utility. An example he gives is that if you get pleasure from my unhappiness, that counts as much under the welfarist approach as anything else. Alternatively, one might believe that a society should devote its resources to meeting somewhat more lofty desires. Another reason is that the concept of individual welfare does not seem to be well captured simply by the goods you have; other aspects of life, such as freedom, would also seem to be important. In this regard, Hahnel and Albert (1990) point out that conventional theory would make you equally well off if you are *assigned* a bundle of goods, versus a situation in which you *choose* the bundle. It does not take much introspection to realize that the latter may indeed result in higher utility.

A second and more fundamental reason to doubt that social welfare is the sum of individual welfare is brought up by Frank (1985), who notes that much of what individuals seek out is status or rank. But these are relative things; if my status goes up, yours goes down by definition. This leads to a situation where people engage in consumption that does not add to the social welfare. For example, if I buy a fancy car, I get utility both from the various characteristics of the car, as well as from the fact that I have distinguished myself from you. Once you (and others like us) buy the car, the latter part of my utility is canceled out. Total utility (or social welfare) is thus lower than the sum of our individual utilities.

IMPLICATIONS FOR HEALTH POLICY

The previous section has attempted to show that there are various problems with inferring that the goods and services people demand in a competitive marketplace will necessarily make them best off. This section provides a number of implications concerning the tools used, and the issues studied, by health economists.

Is Comprehensive National Health Insurance Necessarily Inefficient?[27]

Health economists have long contended that people in the United States and other developed countries are "overinsured." This is because when people are fully insured, they may demand services that only provide a small amount of benefit. But these services are likely to cost just as much as any other services. Thus, the benefits people derive from the purchase of these "marginal" services might be swamped by their cost, which in turn means that social welfare is lower.

This has made many economists conclude that there is a societal "welfare loss" associated with the ownership of too much health insurance -- one recent set of estimates puts this loss somewhere between $33 and $109 billion (1984 dollars), representing between 9 and 28% of U.S. health care spending (Feldman and Dowd, 1991). In this regard, in a survey of U.S. and Canadian health economists conducted in 1989, 63% strongly or mildly agreed with the statement that health insurance causes societal welfare loss (Feldman and Morrisey, 1990).

The argument supporting the notion of welfare loss from full health insurance, and estimates of its magnitude, are based on the assumption that the demand curve shows the marginal utility a person derives from an additional service. Consumers determine exactly how much an additional service is worth to them, and then compare this to its price to determine if it is worth their while to purchase the service. In the previous section we questioned whether consumers can and do behave in such a manner.

There is a method of testing whether in fact consumers do exhibit such behavior. It will be recalled that welfare loss occurs because consumers with health insurance have an incentive to purchase additional services that provide little benefit to them. We can therefore examine whether this occurs by observing the kinds of services that consumers forgo when they are provided with less comprehensive insurance coverage. The results from the RAND Health Insurance Study and other research show that utilization will go down in the presence of co-insurance (Newhouse *et al.*, 1993; Feldstein, 1988; Phelps, 1992). Welfare loss theory tells us the types of services which ought to be forgone: those that provide relatively little utility.

The nature of this test is clarified in Figure 1, which is taken from an earlier work of the present author's (Rice, 1992). The horizontal line indicates the

---

[27] For a more detailed discussion of this issue, see Rice (1992).

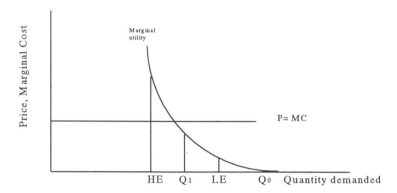

Figure 1: Change in demand for services of differing effectiveness

marginal cost of producing a service, which can be viewed as the cost to society -- that is, the resources that have to be expended in providing a service. The curved line, which is a demand curve, shows the marginal utility of each additional service. At a zero price -- that is, with comprehensive insurance -- the consumer will demand Q_0 services; the last such service provides very little utility.

Now suppose that there are two types of services -- those that are highly effective (HE) and those that are less effective (LE). Further suppose that the person no longer has health insurance, and his demand for care declines from Q_0 to Q_1. It is clear from Figure 1 that the person would be expected to forgo the low-effectiveness service, LE, because its benefits are now outweighed by its costs. But service HE would still be purchased because its benefits exceed costs, even in the absence of insurance coverage. If people actually behave as predicted, then we would have some confidence that the demand curve for medical care really shows the marginal utility consumers obtain from additional services. This, in turn, would provide support for the welfare loss estimates discussed above.

The problem with operationalizing this test is coming up with a way of determining the marginal utility consumers receive from a service. The proxy used here is a measure of the medical effectiveness of a service -- as judged by medical experts. Although consumers and experts may differ in what they think is important, it seems logical that consumers would prefer those services that are thought to be the most effective.

As part of the RAND study, Lohr (1986) and her colleagues grouped services into several categories based on their expected medical effectiveness and found that,

> [C]ost sharing was generally just as likely to lower use when care is thought to be highly effective as when it is thought to be only rarely effective (p. S32)

and that it

> did not seem to have a selective effect in prompting people to forego care only or mainly in circumstances when such care probably would be of relatively little value (p. S36).[28]

What does all this mean for the theory of welfare loss from excess health insurance? That consumers do not seem to be able to evaluate the usefulness of medical services and to make the types of decisions that economic theory calls for. This view -- that patient demand curves show how much consumers buy at different prices, but not necessarily the utility they derive from such services -- runs very much against the grain of conventional economic theory. It is not, however, unique among economists. One noteworthy example is from an article by Ellis and McGuire (1993), who write:

> we are skeptical that the observed demand can be interpreted as reflecting 'socially efficient' consumption, [so] we interpret the demand curve in a more limited way, as an empirical relationship between the degree of cost sharing and quantity of use demanded by the patient (p. 142).

If one is skeptical that there is such a large welfare loss from excess health insurance, a related issue naturally arises: Are there other substantial sources of waste in the provision of medical care services? Over the years health services researchers have shown strong agreement that many of the services provided are not medically necessary -- estimates go as high as 30% (Leape, 1989). Indeed, probably the major research effort being conducted by the health services research community today is determining what services are and are not medically effective.

Under the traditional theory, the source of the waste is clear: patients demand too many services when they have complete or nearly complete insurance coverage. The alternative being presented here is that most of the waste is in the provision of

---

[28] Another component of the RAND study (Siu *et al.*, 1986) reached a similar conclusion regarding the impact of co-insurance on appropriate vs. inappropriate hospitalization.

services that do little or no good to improve the patients' health.[29] The policy implications of the two approaches are very different. If one believes the conventional theory, policies should be enacted that make the user of services more sensitive to price. In contrast, if the problem is provision of services that are not useful, one would target the provider of services.

It is noteworthy that many analysts -- economists as well as practitioners of other disciplines -- believe that managed care strategies that are based on capitating health plans offer the best hope for improving efficiency and controlling U.S. health care costs. These strategies are aimed almost entirely at changing what services are provided by providers, rather than changing the demand by consumers. In fact, what is perhaps most noteworthy about the HMO approach to cost containment is that copayments are *lower* than in fee-for-service medicine. If these strategies are designed to reduce waste, it would seem clear that the waste is thought to be generated through the provision of unnecessary services far more so than through excess demand by patients. And if this is true in the United States, it must be even more true in other developed countries, where, with very few exceptions, there are very few patient copayments, with almost all cost-control activities being focused on the providers of care.

Indeed, most policies aimed at controlling health care costs not only in the United States, but in the rest of the developed world, are aimed at the supply rather than demand side. By focusing on the supply side, other countries find themselves able to provide the population with comprehensive national health insurance. This can improve equity, and, if supply-side measures are more effective than demand-side ones in bringing about other policy goals, can enhance the efficiency of their health care systems as well.

Should Patient Cost-Sharing be Encouraged, or Should We Use Other Policies?

As indicated above, the thrust of the "welfare loss" literature is that more patient cost sharing will be beneficial to society. There is a danger in this sort of analysis which has been noted by Evans (1984): "the welfare burden is minimized when there is no insurance at all" (p. 49). If one takes this reasoning very far, it becomes apparent that the conventional analysis will always find that the country with higher

---

[29] Other writers have also advocated calculating welfare losses based on the provision of unnecessary services. See Phelps and Parente, 1990; Phelps and Mooney, 1992; Dranove, 1995; and Phelps, 1995.

patient cost-sharing requirements will have the more efficient health care system (Reinhardt, 1992). Thus, the U.S. system would be deemed most efficient in the world not because of a comparison of outcomes to costs, but rather simply from the fact that the U.S. imposes patient copayments, which in turn reduces utilization.

Non-U.S. health economists have been more amenable to the idea that a fee-for-service system could be efficient in the absence of patient cost sharing. Evans and his colleagues (1993) argue that the case for patient cost sharing is difficult to make if four questions can be answered in the affirmative: (1) is the service really health care?; (2) does the service work?; (3) is the service medically necessary?; and (4) is there no better alternative? If a service passes all of these tests, "the standard argument against user charges, that they tax the sick, seems wholly justified" (p. 26).

There are two broad arguments that can be made against relying on patient cost sharing to control health care costs. First, of course, is the issue of equity. It is frequently argued that cost sharing is more burdensome on people with lower incomes. In this regard, one of the key findings of the RAND Health Insurance Experiment was that the sick and the poor had the most adverse health consequences as a result of cost sharing.[30]

The other issue concerns efficiency -- specifically, are there alternative ways of encouraging efficiency and containing health care costs besides cost sharing? We mentioned various supply-side policies above. Here, we mention a *demand side* lever that is not concerned with price -- influencing behavior. Although estimates about the cost of so-called "bad behaviors" -- smoking, alcohol consumption, drug abuse -- abound, economists rarely consider these to be social welfare losses in the sense that too much health insurance is considered to be. This is particularly curious given the estimated sizes of these losses -- in the United States alone, an estimated $67 billion annually for drug abuse, $99 billion for alcohol abuse, and $91 billion for smoking (Robert Wood Johnson Foundation, 1994). These figures far exceed all estimates of the welfare losses from health insurance.

Sociologists and psychologists have been concerned about the factors that influence behavior, and ways in which it can be altered. (In contrast, economic theory views behavior as either immutable or something which should *not* be

---

[30] Newhouse *et al.*, 1983. For a summary of literature on the impact of cost sharing, see Rice and Morrison, 1994.

altered as it reflects individual choices.) The field of health education focuses, to a large degree, on how behaviors can be changed. David Mechanic (1979) has stated that,

> Reducing needs involves the prevention of illness or diminishing patients' psychological dependence on the medical encounter for social support or other secondary advantages. Reducing desire for services requires changing people's views of the value of different types of medical care, making them more aware of the real costs of service in relation to the benefits received, and legitimizing alternatives for dealing with many problems (p. 11).

The task of changing behavior is not easy, however. In this regard, he writes:

> it is prudent to recognize the difficulty of the task, the forces working against change, and the depths of ignorance concerning the origins of these behaviors and the ways in which they can best be modified (p. 12).

The point is not that health economists need to be conducting this research. Rather, it is that policy levers like these need to be recognized by policy makers even if they are not derived from traditional economic analyses.

Should People Pay More for Price-Elastic Services?

Another common economic conclusion is that the magnitude of patient coinsurance rates should be directly related to the price elasticity of demand. More specifically, services for which consumers show a high demand elasticity should have higher cost sharing requirements than services for which consumers are less price-sensitive (Ellis and McGuire, 1993).[31]

What services are the most price elastic and therefore should, according to theory, have the highest patient cost sharing requirements? The major source of data to answer this question is the RAND Health Insurance Experiment. Its results in this regard are somewhat ambiguous because the calculated elasticities vary

---

[31] This is because if the possession of insurance leads to a large increase in utilization, then welfare loss will be larger because more services will be purchased where the marginal costs exceed marginal benefits. Thus, one would improve social welfare by assessing higher patient coinsurance rates for such services, thereby reducing usage. In contrast, if utilization rates are not very sensitive to the possession of insurance, then there is little welfare loss, and less need to charge high coinsurance rates.

depending on the level of coinsurance.[32]

These elasticities, shown in Table 1, do not vary a great deal by type of service. One noteworthy exception is that so-called "well-care services," while showing a comparable elasticity to other outpatient services (acute and chronic) in the 0-25% range, had a much larger one in the 25-95% range. Dental services also showed a relatively high elasticity in the 25-95% range. The well-care services considered in the study would include preventive care, but other services as well. This, unfortunately, is most of what is currently known about the elasticity of demand for preventive services.

Table 1 Arc Price Elasticities of Medical Spending in the RAND Health Insurance Experiment*

Range	Dental	Acute	Chronic	Well	Total Out-Patients	Total Hospital	Medical
0-25	-0.16	-0.20	-0.14	-0.17	-0.17	-0.17	-0.12
25-95	-0.32	-0.23	-0.43	-0.31	-0.14	-0.22	-0.39

*Source: Newhouse, J.P., *et al.* (1993) Free for all?: lessons from the RAND health insurance experiment. Cambridge, MA: Harvard University Press, p. 121

The implications of the standard economic model are nevertheless clear: If preventive are the most price responsive, they should have the highest patient coinsurance rates, which in turn will discourage their usage. This would be true even if it were shown that some of these services were particularly effective in improving health and/or well-being.

There are, of course, alternative criteria that one could use in determining patient copayment levels that are in the best interest of society. One model, popular in a number of recent proposals for U.S. health reform, would have made preventive services free of any copayments -- the *opposite* of what the economic model would recommend.

------

[32] In the study, patients were assessed 0% or 25% or 95% of the total charge. Some patients were charged 50% coinsurance rates, but they were not used in the demand elasticities presented by authors of the study.

There are several possible justifications for basing copayment rates on factors other than price elasticities, all of which have been discussed in other contexts, above. First is the issue of whether consumers have sufficient information. If they do not, then they may underestimate the value of investing in preventive services. Second, even if the appropriate information is available, people may not use it correctly. As noted, it is difficult for people to make "counterfactual" choices. Furthermore, because of people's tendency towards cognitive dissonance, they may avoid seeking some types of services that are of value to them. Third, medical experts may be better aware of the benefits of certain services than are individuals -- and these experts routinely recommend more preventive services than people are obtaining. Fourth, people might be short-sighted in their views, particularly when they are young. Finally, there is a public good aspect of preventive care. If it makes you healthy, I want you to have it, but the free-rider effect will prevent me from subsidizing you. Subsidized, low-copayments for preventive care therefore could improve social welfare.

CONCLUSION

This is a long paper -- no effort will be made to summarize its content. Although its major theme may be viewed as somewhat "downbeat," it will end on a somewhat positive note.

If one accepts the viewpoint that economic theory does not demonstrate the superiority of market forces in health, the obvious corollary is that all important questions must be answered empirically. And, to a large extent, that is exactly what most health economists and health services researchers are trying to do. I have few reservations about the kinds research studies that are being conducted; they address many key issues. I am, however, very concerned that the work will suffer if researchers come in with preconceived notions of what the results *ought* to be.

Economists often take the viewpoint that the way to test a theory -- such as the purported advantages of market competition -- is to see how well it predicts. This may work well when we are evaluating so-called *positive* issues -- say, the impact of a change in patient copayments on service utilization -- but it is less helpful in evaluating *normative* issues -- those that involve the word "should."

Welfare economics deals in the latter -- e.g., *should* we rely on competitive policies in health care? In such instances, it does little good to assess how well the theory predicts because different analysts will disagree about which alternative state of the world is at a higher level of welfare. For example, if the United States adopted a Canadian-style health care system, there would likely be little agreement among health economists whether the population is better off under the new system or the old one.

In this regard, Graaff (1971) has written:

> welfare ... is not an observable quantity like a market price or an item of personal consumption [so] it is exceedingly difficult to test a welfare proposition. ... The consequence is that, whereas the normal way of testing a theory in positive economics is to test its conclusions, the normal way of testing a welfare proposition is to test its assumptions ... The result is that our assumptions must be scrutinized with care and thoroughness. Each must stand on its own two feet. We cannot afford to simplify much (pp. 2-3).

The primary purpose of this paper has been to engage in this activity and to speculate about the implications that arise when many important assumptions that underlie the advantages of competition are not met in health care.

In conclusion, I believe very strongly that it is important that we get our theory right. If analysts misinterpret economic theory as applied to health, then they will blind themselves to policy options that might actually be best at enhancing social welfare, many of which simply do not fall out of the conventional, demand-driven economic model. It is my belief that market forces have a place in health care organization and delivery; what I have tried to convey in this paper is that economic theory does not show them to *necessarily* be a superior approach to health care policy.

ACKNOWLEDGMENT

I would like to thank a number of people for providing comments on the research that resulted in this article: Ronald Andersen, William Comanor, Katherine Desmond, Robert Evans, Rashi Fein, Paul Feldstein, Susan Haber, Diana Hilberman, Donald Light, Harold Luft, David Mechanic, Glenn Melnick, Joseph Newhouse, Mark Peterson, Uwe Reinhardt, John Roemer, Sally Stearns, Greg Stoddart, Deborah Stone, Pete Welch, and Joseph White. All conclusions and any errors are entirely my own.

Another version of this research appears in a paper published in the Spring 1997 issue of the *Journal of Health Politics, Policy, and Law*. Both works are part of a larger inquiry, a book entitled, *The Economics of Health Reconsidered*, to be published by Health Administration Press in 1998.

REFERENCES

Akerlof, G.A. and Dickens, W.T. (1992) The economic consequences of cognitive dissonance. *American Economic Review* 72:307-319.

Aronson, E. (1972) *The Social Animal.* San Francisco: W.H. Freeman & Co.

Arrow, K.J. (1963a) *Social Choice and Individual Values.* New York City: John Wiley.

Arrow, K.J. (1963b) Uncertainty and the welfare economics of medical care. *American Economic Review* 53:940-973.

Arrow, K.J. (1973a) Some ordinalist-utilitarian notes on Rawls's theory of justice. *Journal of Philosophy* 70:245-263.

Arrow, K.J. (1973b) Formal theories of social welfare. In Wiener, P.P., editor, *Dictionary of the History of Ideas*, Vol. 4. New York: Scribner.

Bator, F.M. (1963) The anatomy of market failure. *Quarterly Journal of Economics* 53:351-379.

Becker, G.S. (1979) Economic analysis and human behavior. In Levy-Garboua, L. editor, *Sociological Economics.* Beverly Hills, CA:Sage.

Blackorby, C. and Donaldson, D. (1990) A review article: The case against the use of the sum of compensating variations in cost-benefit analysis. *Canadian Journal of Economics* 23:471-94.

Blendon, R.J. *et al.* (1993) Satisfaction with health systems in ten nations. *Health Affairs* 9:185-192.

Blendon, R.J., Leitman, R., Morrison, I., and Donelan, K. (1990) Satisfaction with health systems in ten nations. *Health Affairs* 9(2):185-92.

Boulding, K.E. (1969) Economics as a moral science. *American Economic Review* 59:1-12.

Buchanan, J.M. (1977) Political equality and private property: The distributional paradox. In Dworkin, G., Bermant, G., and Brow, P.G. editors, *Markets and Morals.* Washington, D.C.: Hemisphere Publishing Corp.

Culyer, A.J. and Evans, R.G. (1996) Mark Pauly on welfare economics: normative rabbits from positive hats. *Journal of Health Economics* 15:243-251.

Dictionary of Philosophy (1979) London: Pan Books.

Dranove, D. (1995) A problem with consumer surplus measures of the cost of practice variations. *Journal of Health Economics* 14:243-251.

Dworkin, R. (1981) What is equality? *Philosophy & Public Affairs* 10:185-246 & 283-345.

Duesenberry, J.S. (1952) *Income, Saving and the Theory of Consumer Behavior* Cambridge, MA: Harvard Univ. Press.

Easterlin, R. (1974) Nations and households in economic growth: Essays in honor of Moses Abramovitz. David, P.A. and Reder, M.W. editors. New York City: Academic Press.

Ellis, R.P. and McGuire, T.G. (1993) Supply-side and demand-side cost sharing in health care. *Journal of Economic Perspectives* 7:135-151.

Enthoven, A.C. (1993) The history and principles of managed competition. *Health Affairs* 10 (Supplement):24-48.

Enthoven, A.C. and Kronick, R. (1989) A consumer-choice health plan for the 1990s. *New England Journal of Medicine* 320:29-37.

Evans, R.G. (1984) *Strained Mercy.* Toronto: Butterworth.

Evans, R.G., Barer, M.L., Stoddart, G.L., and Bhatia, V. (1993) *It's not the money, it's the principle: Why user charges for some services and not others?* Vancouver: University of British Columbia.

Feldman, R. and Dowd, B. (1991) A new estimate of the welfare loss of excess health insurance. *American Economic Review* 81:297-301.

Feldman, R. and Morrisey, M.A. (1990) Health economics: a report on the field. *Journal of Health Politics, Policy, and Law* 15:627-46.

Feldstein, P.J. (1988) *Health Care Economics.* New York City: John Wiley.

Fielding. J.E. and Rice, T. (1993) Can managed competition solve the problems of market failure? *Health Affairs* 216-228.

Fox, D.M. and Leichter, H.M. (1993) The ups and downs of Oregon's rationing plan. *Health Affairs* 12:66-70.

Frank, R.H. (1985) *Choosing the Right Pond: Human Behavior and the Quest for Status.* New York City: Oxford Univ. Press.

Friedman, M. (1962) *Price Theory.* Chicago: Aldine Press.

Gabel, J.R. and Jensen, G.A. (1989) The price of state mandated benefits. *Inquiry* 26:419-431.

Graaff, J. de V. (1971) *Theoretical Welfare Economics.* London: Cambridge University Press.

Hahnel, R. and Albert, M. (1990) *Quiet Revolution in Welfare Economics.* Princeton, NJ: Princeton University Press.

Harberger, A.C. (1971) Three basic postulates for applied welfare economics: an interpretive essay. *Journal of Economic Literature* 9:785-797.

Henderson, J.M. and Quandt, R.E. (1971) *Microeconomic Theory,* Second Edition. New York: McGraw-Hill.

Hibbard, J.H. and Weeks, E.C. (1989a) Does the dissemination of comparative data on physician fees affect consumer use of services? *Medical Care* 27:1167-1174.

Hibbard, J.H. and Weeks, E.C. (1989b) Does the dissemination of comparative data on physician fees affect consumer use of services? *Medical Care* 27:1167-1174.

Hibbard, J.H. and Jewett, J.J (1996) What type of quality information do consumers want in a health care report card. *Medical Care Research and Review* 53:28-47.

Hicks, J.R. (1941) The rehabilitation of consumers' surplus. *Review of Economic Studies* 9:108-116.

Hoerger, T.J. and Howard, L.Z. (1995) Search behavior and choice of physician in the market for prenatal care. *Medical Care* 33:332-349.

Labelle, R., Stoddart, G., and Rice, T. (1994) A re-examination of the meaning and importance of supplier-induced demand. *Journal of Health Economics* 13:347-368.

Leape, L. (1989) Unnecessary surgery. *Health Services Research* 24:351-407.

Leibenstein, H. (1976) *Beyond Economic Man.* Cambridge, MA: Harvard University Press.

Light, D.W. (1995) *Homo Economicus:* escaping the traps of managed competition. *European Journal of Public Health* 5:145-154.

Lipsey, R.G. and Lancaster, K. (1956-7) The general theory of the second best. *Review of Economic Studies* 11:32.

Little, I.M.D. (1957) *A Critique of Welfare Economics,* Second Edition. London: Oxford University Press.

Lohr, K.N., Brook, R.H., Camberg, C.J., *et al.* Effect of cost-sharing on use of medically effective and less effective care. *Medical Care* 24(Supplement):S32-S38.

Luft, H.S. (1980) Trends in medical care costs: Do HMOs lower the rate of growth? *Medical Care* 18:1-16.

Marshall, J. (1920) *Principles of Economics.* London: MacMillan and Co.

Mechanic, D. (1979) *Future Issues in Health Care.* New York: The Free Press, MacMillan and Co.

Mishan, E.J. (1969a) *Welfare Economics: An Assessment.* Amsterdam: North-Holland.

Mishan, E.J. (1969b) *Welfare Economics: Ten Introductory Essays.* New York City: Random House.

Mishan, E.J. (1982) *What Is Political Economy All About?* Cambridge, England: Cambridge University Press.

Nath, S.K. (1969) *A Reappraisal of Welfare Economics.* London: Routledge & Kegan Paul.

Newhouse, J.P. (1993) An iconoclastic view of health cost containment. *Health Affairs* 10 (Supplement):152-171.

Newhouse, J.P. *et al.* (1985) Are fee-for-service costs increasing faster than HMO costs? *Medical Care* 23:960-966.

Newhouse, J.P. *et al.* (1993) *Free for All? Lessons From the RAND Health Insurance Experiment.* Cambridge, MA: Harvard University Press.

Ng, Y-K. (1979) *Welfare Economics.* London MacMillan and Co.

Olsen, E.O. (1969) A normative theory of transfers. *Public Choices* 6:39-58.

Pauly, M.V. (1994) Editorial: A re-examination of the meaning and importance of supplier-induced demand. *Journal of Health Economics* 13:369-72.

Phelps, C.E. (1992) *Health Economics.* New York City: Harper Collins.

Phelps, C.E. (1995) Welfare loss from variations: Further considerations. *Journal of Health Economics* 14:253-60.

Phelps, C.E. and Parente, S.T. (1990) Priority setting in medical technology and medical practice assessment. *Medicare Care* 29:703-723.

Phelps, C.E. and Mooney, C. (1992) Correction and update on priority setting in medical technology assessment in medical care. *Medicare Care* 31:744-751.

Pigou, A.C. (1932) *The Economics of Welfare*, 4th Edition..London: Macmillan and Co.

Pollak, R.A. (1978) Endogenous tastes in demand and welfare analysis. *American Economic Review* 68:374-9.

Rawls, J. (1971) *A Theory of Justice.* Cambridge, MA: The Belknap Press of Harvard University.

Reinhardt, U.E. (1992) Refections on the meaning of efficiency: can efficiency be separated from equity? *Yale Law & Policy Review* 10:302-315.

Rice, T. (1992) An alternative framework for evaluating welfare losses in the health care market. *Journal of Health Economics* 11:88-92.

Rice, T. (1998) *The Economics of Health Reconsidered.* Chicago, IL: Health Administration Press.

Rice, T., Brown, E.R., and Wyn, R. (1993) Holes in the Jackson Hole approach to health care reform. *Journal of the American Medical Association* 270:1357-1362.

Rice, T. and Morrison, K.R. (1994) Patient cost sharing for medical services: a review of the literature and implications for health care reform. *Medical Care Research and Review* 51:235-287.

Robert Wood Johnson Foundation (1994) *Annual Report: Cost Containment.* Princeton, NJ: Robert Wood Johnson Foundation.

Robbins, Lord (Lionel) (1984) Politics and political economy. In, *An Essay on the Nature and Significance of Economic Science*, Third Edition. London: MacMillan Press.

Robinson, J.C. and Luft, H.S. (1987) Competition and the cost of hospital care, 1972 to 1982. *Journal of the American Medical Association* 257:3241-3245.

Roemer, J.E. (1994) *Egalitarian Perspectives.* Cambridge, MA: Cambridge University Press.

Rowley, C.K. and Peacock, A.T. (1975) *Welfare Economics: A Liberal Restatement.* New York: John Wiley.

Rublee, D.A. Medical technology in Canada, Germany, and the United States: an update. *Health Affairs* 13:113-117.

Samuelson, P.A. (1938) A note on the pure theory of consumer's behavior. *Economica* 5:61-71.

Samuelson, P.A. (1947; republished in 1976) Foundations of Economic Analysis. New York: Atheneum.

Scitovsky, T. (1976) *The Joyless Economy.* New York: Oxford University Press.

Sen, A.K. (1970) *Collective Choice and Social Welfare.* San Francisco: Holden-Day.

Sen, A. (1982) *Choice, Welfare and Measurement.* London: Basil Blackwell.

Sen, A. (1987) *On Ethics and Economics.* Oxford, England: Basil Blackwell.

Sen, A. (1992) *Inequality Revisited.* Cambridge, MA: Harvard University Press.

Sui, A.L., Sonnenberg, F.A., Manning, W.G., *et al.* (1986) Inappropriate use of hospitals in a randomized trial of health insurance plans. *New England Journal of Medicine* 315:1259-66.

Thurow, L.C. (1980) *The Zero-Sum Society.* New York: Penguin Books.

Thurow, L.C. (1983) *Dangerous Currents: The State of Economics.* New York City: Random House.

Tullock, G. (1979) *Objectives of Income Redistribution. In, Levy-Garboua, L., editor, Sociological Economics.* Beverly Hill, CA: Sage.

Vladeck, B.C. (1990) *Simple, Elegant, and Wrong.* New York City: United Hospital Fund.

Voltaire (1759) *Candide*, translated by L. Bair (1981). New York City: Bantam Books.

von Weiszacker, C.C. (1971) Notes on endogenous change of tastes. *Journal of Economic Theory* 3:345-372.

Wagstaff, A. and van Doorslaer, E. (1992) Equity in the finance of health care: Some international comparisons. *Journal of Health Economics* 11:361-387.

Weisbrod, B.A. (1978) Competition in the health care sector: Past, present, and future, edited by Greenberg, W. Washington, DC Bureau of Economics, Federal Trade Commission.

19

Toward a Healthier Economics
Reflections on Ken Bassett's Problem

ROBERT G. EVANS
Centre for Health Services and Policy Research and Department of Economics
University of British Columbia
Vancouver, Canada

From 1978 to 1990 Dr. Ken Bassett practised as a family physician in Invermere, a small town in southeastern British Columbia. As part of that practice, he and his colleagues cared for a number of obstetrical patients. And in managing the delivery process, they would commonly use an electronic foetal monitor (EFM) to check on the condition of the foetus. In this their behaviour was no different from that of most other physicians, in North America at least. But they may have been somewhat unusual in reflecting upon and being troubled by their own behaviour. As they were well aware, there is an extensive research literature on the effectiveness of electronic foetal monitoring that stretches back about twenty years. Over time, the early enthusiasm for this diagnostic tool has given way to the now predominant view that, on balance, EFM provides no benefits for normal deliveries. Yet it continues to be used routinely. And it continued to be used routinely in Invermere, by family practitioners who *knew* that their practice had no scientific basis. Unlike most practitioners (and most other

Health, Health Care and Health Economics: Perspectives on Distribution
Edited by Morris L. Barer, Thomas E. Getzen, and Greg L. Stoddart
Copyright 1998 John Wiley & Sons, Ltd

people) they found this discrepancy troubling and tried to understand it.

Dr. Bassett went further, however, and in 1985 began to study for a doctorate in medical anthropology during winter sessions at McGill University. Not surprisingly, intensive further analysis of EFM from an alternative disciplinary perspective has shown that the application of a particular medical intervention is the result of a wide and quite complex array of interrelated factors (Bassett, 1996). The balance of findings from randomized trials and other forms of "scientific" evaluation of effectiveness is only one of these factors, and is rarely decisive in itself.

Of particular interest was the role of EFM in supporting first an increase and then a decrease in rates of use of "augmentation" (acceleration) of labour through the administration of oxytocin to the mother. This is a highly controversial procedure with some risk to both mother and child. The "objective" data provided by the EFM, available for interpretation by anyone, supported a corresponding sense of a "normal" birth process that could be defined objectively and represented by mathematical models.

Departures from the model, usually taking the form of "prolonged" labour, were then "abnormal," and the intervention was indicated. The EFM could then be applied to ensure that the foetus was not getting into trouble, becoming hypoxic, during the procedure. The technology thus enabled clinicians to act with greater confidence in augmenting more patients.

But when, for a variety of reasons, including the sheer unpleasantness of the procedure and its dubious value, augmentation fell from favour, *the same* "objective" EFM data (which were, in any case, usually rather ambiguous) could be read to show that the foetus was not in trouble during an extended birth, and that no augmentation was necessary. Rates fell. "Only years later did ... local doctors come to see augmentations as almost irresistible opportunities to behave badly, to be impatient, to project their fears onto patients, or to take out their general job frustrations on a particular individual." (Bassett, 1996, p. 291).

Dr. Bassett now works with the B.C. Office of Health Technology Assessment at the University of British Columbia, where a range of disciplinary perspectives are brought to bear to try to understand *why* particular technologies are adopted, and how to influence the process. Improving these decisions requires far more than simply presenting the findings of research, however relevant or competent.

The processes by which particular technologies come to be employed (or not) in medical practice are of obvious interest to economists, simply because of the impact these decisions have on patterns and levels of resource utilization -- costs and outcomes. But that is not the focus of this paper. Much more fundamental, as the Invermere physicians well understood, is the issue raised by the observation of informed practitioners knowingly (and in this case unhappily) applying an intervention that they knew to be inappropriate. I believe that this phenomenon generalizes, and not just among physicians; and I suggest the following label.

Ken Bassett's Problem:

"Why would intelligent and competent professionals routinely behave in ways that they know to be illogical and scientifically unsound?"[1]

My focus will of course be on economics and economists, particularly on economists studying the health care sector. This paper thus complements that by Uwe Reinhardt (this volume), in which he documents quite specifically such behaviour within our own "profession." Like him, I feel best equipped to talk about the inadequacies of the field I know best.

Ken Bassett's Problem, however, refers to a more general process, even if we ourselves have a narrower focus. And while in economics (as in medicine) this behaviour is revealed in the work of particular individuals, we are not or should not be engaged simply in finger-pointing. A systematic pattern of behaviour is unlikely to be explained solely by the lapses and inadequacies of particular individuals; at least this is not the first hypothesis upon which we ought to seize.[2]

Also at the outset we should set to one side, or at least hold in check, a hypothesis that may come most easily to the minds of economists. Ken Bassett and his colleagues were not paid more when EFM was used. The equipment was owned by the hospital, not the physicians, and the hospital was reimbursed on a global budget. They did not do it for the money. We economists are trained and habituated to reach first for economic incentives in explaining human behaviour,

---

[1] One has to be a bit careful with language like "illogical." As Dr. Bassett's subsequent anthropological research made clear, there *were* reasons for the pattern of behaviour that he and his colleagues observed and participated in. In Marmor's paraphrase of Hegel, "Nothing that is regular, is stupid." The reasons were not to be found, however, in the overt objectives of the physicians themselves; these did not in general include providing their patients with ineffective care.

[2] That would be akin to attributing unhealthy lifestyles such as smoking to the moral inadequacies (or the "tastes"!) of smokers. In fact, we know that smoking is a physiological addiction, taken up in childhood, in response to marketing carefully targeted at children. The presence of a sharp social gradient in this and other "unhealthy lifestyles" reflects more fundamental social processes influencing individual behaviour. Ken Bassett's Problem is similarly indicative of broader social forces at work.

and of course such motivations *are* both powerful and widespread. As Morone (1986) has pointed out, however, while incentives are powerful, economists are not very good at predicting their effects.[3] There is usually much more going on than simple financial gain (Giacomini *et al.*, 1996). And indeed (and quite inconsistently) we are much less ready to adopt economic explanations for *our own* behaviour.

In addressing Ken Bassett's Problem in the context of health economics, I am not proposing to argue for the *existence* of this form of professional behaviour in our field. Such behaviour is described elsewhere in this volume, not only by Reinhardt, but also by Hurley and Rice, among others. Nor are they the first to point it out; much of what they say is old news -- and yet the patterns they describe persist. Observing this persistence, in economics as in medicine, I am arguing that this behaviour is a systematic phenomenon to be described and understood, not merely an aberration to be deplored. I will also indicate what seems to me to be a relatively effective corrective strategy.

It may, however, be helpful to start by illustrating what I regard as persistent illogical and unsound analysis by competent professionals. Consider the classic summary of welfare economics by Bator (1957). As Reinhardt reminds us, in this volume and elsewhere (Reinhardt, 1992), that paper makes crystal clear a point that every professional economist knows: to rank social outcomes, you need a ranking rule, a social welfare function, embodying a set of values, that cannot be derived from economics itself. If you want to generate recommendations, normative conclusions that state A is better than state B, using economic analysis, then you must introduce those values first, explicitly or more often implicitly.

The Pareto criterion is one such externally imposed ranking rule; it imports a particular set of values into the analysis from outside. The justification may be that these are widely held, "sort of universal" values -- surely no one could object to changes that make some better off without making anyone else worse off? Indeed, they could object -- the Pareto criterion actually does impose restrictions on individual utility functions (non-malevolence, for one). But maybe in practice

---

[3] "[Law] 4. Beware of Incentives. Economists and other rationalists restlessly tinker with peoples' incentives. This is a dangerous game. Although incentives are important for understanding problems and fashioning solutions, they are also tricky devils, always veering off in unanticipated ways.....People are complicated, social systems almost infinitely so. A great many uninvited incentives lurk in each policy change" (Morone, 1986, p. 818).

they don't? (And anyway maybe malevolent people's values "shouldn't" count?).

As it happens, however, there may be a much more fundamental flaw in the Pareto criterion as a representation of our values. And it is a flaw that health economists, in particular, need to be aware of if they are serious about their subject matter. Consider a pattern of economic growth in which all the gains go to a very small group of people at the top percentile of the income distribution, and everyone else's income is held constant (in real terms). This is not merely a hypothetical case; Krugman (1992), for example, argues that this pattern characterizes growth in the United States over the last two decades.[4] By the Pareto criterion, such growth unambiguously improves overall well-being. But do we approve this trend? Do we think our neighbours would (Rice, this volume)?[5]

More than mere envy is at stake. As van Doorslaer and Wagstaff (this volume) show, inequalities in health status are correlated, across countries, with inequalities in income. If this relationship is causal, then the "Pareto-improvement" above may actually increase the dispersion of health outcomes -- life expectancy, disability, morbidity. Do we still approve *this*?

Well we might, if health is related to absolute income. Income gainers become healthier, on average, but non-gainers do not become less so -- though it is not so clear that most of us would in fact view with approval a widening gap in *e.g.* life expectancies. But evidence is now accumulating of a relationship between health and *relative* income status (Wilkinson, 1994; Kaplan *et al.*, 1996; Kennedy *et al.*, 1996). "...these associations...seem to show that inequality *per se* is bad for national health, whatever the absolute material standards of living." (Davey Smith, 1996). The evidence for this "big idea" (Editor's choice, 1996) is still controversial (Judge, 1995) for a variety of reasons, but it is growing steadily stronger.[6]

---

[4] In the 1980s, people in the lowest quintile actually became poorer, on average (Krugman, 1992); such a change could not be a Pareto-improvement.

[5] And if we think our neighbours *would* approve, why would the editors of the *Wall Street Journal*, among others, argue so strenuously, "display[ing a]...combination of mendacity and sheer incompetence" (Krugman, 1992, p.19), that this "Pareto-improvement" is not in fact occurring?

[6] Data on both health status and income distribution, in every country, are not nearly as good as one would like, though they are rapidly improving (Smeeding and Gottschalk, 1995). The pathways through which a relationship between inequality and ill-health might operate, involving "social and cognitive processes, rather than...[material] effects" (Wilkinson, 1994), have been somewhat obscure, although recent work in neuro-biology is rapidly generating candidate possibilities (Evans *et al.*, 1994; Evans, 1996b). The principal reason for the controversy, however, and especially for its intensity, is probably the obvious ideological and political challenge implied by such findings. The interpretation

If the overall health status of a community *is* in fact lower, *cet. par.*, when inequality is greater, that would mean that the "Pareto-improvement" of more for the wealthiest was actually making people, on average, sicker. Do we approve this? If so, would you like to explain to your neighbours, just *why*?[7]

The criterion of Pareto-optimality may thus turn out to be a good deal more ethically troubling than we economists have previously assumed. In any case it does not actually rank very much. Not only does it not permit points on the utility-possibility frontier to be ranked relative to each other; it does not *in general* permit them to be ranked relative to points inside that frontier. Only points northeast (southwest) of a given point in n-dimensional utility space can be declared superior (inferior) to that point.

In the Paretian context words like "optimal" or "efficient" have very specific technical meanings that are different from, and much more limited than, their meanings in general English usage. Accordingly, as Reinhardt (1992) has pointed out, if economists use such words in their technical sense when communicating with non-technical audiences, they are likely to mislead (whether or not deliberately).

In particular we talk of, and encourage others to believe in, the possibility of an "equity-efficiency trade-off" when in fact no such trade-off exists *when efficiency is used in its Paretian sense*. Nothing is given up -- "traded off" -- by a move from a Pareto-efficient point in utility possibility space to a non-efficient point, if the latter ranks more highly on the relevant social welfare function. There is an unambiguous welfare gain; that's all.

A trade-off may exist when "efficiency" is used in its more everyday, non-technical sense, as an engineer or a clinician might -- trading off total QALYs against their distribution, for example, as Williams describes in this volume. Perfectly legitimate; but quite different from the meaning of "efficiency" when the word is applied to a general discussion of the institutions governing resource allocation -- markets and all that. Encouraging others in confusing the two

---

of research, positively or negatively, becomes entangled with advocacy and with well-defined political agendas.

[7] A quick answer might be that the Pareto criterion refers to making one or more people better off while making no one else worse off, and if inequality breeds illness, clearly the criterion has not been met. Others *are* worse off. That's true, but it is not what we do. In fact we apply the criterion to models in which individual utility depends only upon commodity (or commodity/leisure) bundles, or indirect functions of incomes and prices. So we *do* use (real) income to stand for well-being.

meanings is not honest.[8]

Being well aware of the limits of Pareto, economists have historically tried to extend the range of their analysis by proposing the "compensation tests" associated with the names of Kaldor, Scitovsky, and Hicks. If the gainers from a given policy could compensate the losers, and/or the losers could not bribe the gainers to abandon it, then the policy is "good" *even if no compensation is actually paid*.

This illustrates the point of this paper. How could competent economists, among the most eminent in the profession, imagine that such a test made sense *as economic analysis*? Reinhardt (1992) has skewered the idea memorably as the "unrequited-punch-in-the-nose test"; other economists have, over the years, been equally if less entertainingly scathing. Why should the *losers* find such tests convincing?

The compensation tests embody interpersonal comparisons, value judgements as to whose interests should be sacrificed to whose gain. These are made constantly in the real world of politics and policy; the compensation test is simply one way of making a political choice, suggested by certain citizens with an interest in the political process.

But suppose a majority of economists -- or even all of us except Reinhardt -- found such compensation tests plausible as a basis for making normative policy recommendations. *So what*? Economists are not priests. Our normative judgements, our political preferences, have no claim to special weight relative to those of our fellow-citizens. The relevant question in a democracy (as different from a theocracy) is whether such value judgements are acceptable to the man on the Clapham omnibus, or T.C. Pits, or the median voter. Economists are entitled

---

[8] The "equity-efficiency trade-off" is often presented as a claim that egalitarian redistributive social policies may have a cost in total social *output* -- the GDP will be lower, for example. That may or may not be so; but it is a statement about *product* space, not *utility* space. The Pareto criterion does not apply to commodities *per se*, only to the utilities presumed to be derived from them. And again, all professional economists know this.

The persistence of the fallacy is probably rooted in conflicts over the social welfare function itself. Those who would lose from redistribution can be expected to resist with any argument that comes to hand. "We'll all be worse off, if I have to give up anything!" And of course there may be circumstances in which this is true. But a move toward greater equality in utility space, *even if* it involved falling inside the utility-possibility frontier (say, because GDP is lower), might still increase the value of the SWF. It depends on the shape of that function. To assert a *necessary* trade-off is simple political deception, and economists know it.

to one vote each.[9]

Yet the urge to derive normative conclusions from positive propositions, to offer purely objective, scientific recommendations on issues of public policy, remains fully alive and very strong. Just because it is impossible -- "No ethics in, no ethics out" in Archibald's paraphrase of Hume -- does not stop us from trying *even though we know it is impossible!*[10]

Harberger (1971), for example, states quite explicitly that economists have no special competence in making value judgements or interpersonal comparisons, and then in the same breath proceeds to do precisely that. "...costs and benefits...*should* (my emphasis) normally be added up without regard to the individual(s) to whom they accrue." (p.785) *i.e.*, each individual should be given equal weight. How could an intelligent person and eminent economist miss the obvious fact that equal weighting is one particular form of interpersonal comparison?

Coming down to the present, Mark Pauly (1994a,b; 1996) writes that welfare economics *given its assumptions* permits normative policy conclusions to be drawn. But to support normative conclusions, these assumptions must themselves be normative. So *whose* assumptions are they? *People* have values, and make normative assumptions; but a body of analysis, such as welfare economics, cannot. A body of thought that includes normative assumptions is a religion, not an academic discipline, much less a science (Culyer and Evans, 1996).

When Pauly (1994b) says "Improved health status that results from demand distorted by incorrect information...*cannot generally be endorsed by welfare economics*." (my emphasis), he is formally correct, because analytic frameworks are not in the business of handing out endorsements of anything. Only people can do that. Pauly is simply attaching the label of "welfare economics" to his personal

---

[9] But do any of us believe otherwise? No, or at least I have never heard any economist openly claim special normative insight. So why do we make policy recommendations, *qua* economists, that implicitly embody just such a claim?

[10] We appear to follow Tertullian, the early father of the Church (and later heresiarch) who formulated the "Credo quia impossible!" But are we all so knowledgeable? Styles change in the teaching of economic theory; Reinhardt, in his opening address to the 1996 inaugural iHEA Conference, suggested that a professional economist trained in the major graduate schools of today can no longer be assumed to be familiar with the fundamental theorems of welfare economics. The currently dominant American political ideology, with its emphasis on "markets *über alles*," has sunk so deeply into what is taught as "economic theory" that some in the younger generation *may* in fact simply be ignorant. If he is right, then Ken Bassett's Problem is a question for their instructors.

ideology, no more. He may share that ideology with some other economists, and even some non-economists; but that does not make his values part of "welfare economics."

A critical normative assumption for Pauly (1996) is that the distribution of income is "accepted as ethically correct." This permits one to avoid distributional issues and interpersonal comparisons. But accepted *by whom*? The most that one could ever say, on the basis of economic analysis alone, would be that if *you* believe that the distribution of income (and any health implications associated with it -- recall the discussion above) is ethically acceptable, then for you policy A is better than policy B. But if not, not.

In fact matters are a bit more complex than that. Pauly (1996) refers to *the* distribution of income, but particular policies raise distributional questions precisely because they are expected to *change* that distribution in a material way. Otherwise we *could* legitimately abstract from distributional questions (but we might not find many such policies to analyze).

Thus one would have to say that the distribution of income was ethically acceptable *both before and after* the implementation of a policy, suggesting that one were pretty neutral about distribution anyhow, at least over the relevant range. It does not matter if some gain and some lose, or how the gainers and losers are situated. One doubts that many people would share this ethical position with Pauly; and if most people do not accept a particular ethical assumption, what does it mean to say that "welfare economics" does? We're back to religion again.

But is any of this news? A quarter century ago, Arrow (1973) introduced a mathematical analysis of the welfare effects of coinsurance charges for health care by "....ignor[ing] distributional considerations and *assum[ing] a single person in the economy* (my emphasis)." Without that assumption no welfare conclusions could be drawn *a priori*. One would have to introduce explicit value judgements about interpersonal deservingness -- and of course identify interpersonal effects.

And indeed Pauly (1996) in replying to Culyer and Evans (1996) asks what all their fuss is about? Surely all economists know this? Pauly (1997) and Gaynor and Vogt (1997) take the same approach in critiquing Rice (1997a). Why reiterate the obvious as if it were new learning?[11]

Because we know it, and ignore it. At the time Arrow wrote, and ever since, eminent (and less eminent) health economists have been drawing *a priori*

---

[11] Similar comments were made from the floor about Uwe Reinhardt's presentation at the 1996 iHEA conference.

conclusions about the welfare effects of coinsurance charges (*e.g.*, M. Feldstein, 1973; Manning *et al.*, 1987). Never do they mention that these depend upon specific distributional value judgements, let alone identify and justify the ones that they make implicitly.

More generally, the academic literature contains numerous papers by health economists that draw normative conclusions about "efficiency" and "optimality," and approve or reject public policies, without a second thought about the normative content of their work. They assume a spurious objectivity without even bothering to claim it, purporting to be doing economic "science." Yet they are neither stupid, nor ignorant, nor malicious.[12]

This discrepancy between knowledge and practice was one of the most consistent themes of plenary and other sessions at the inaugural iHEA conference. A common response to this criticism of so much of contemporary economic practice was to mutter about "market-bashing," or simply to ignore the issue and continue with business as usual. Interestingly, these are also the common responses of physicians confronted with questions -- however solidly based in scientific research -- about the appropriateness of *their* practices. What else is there to do? -- the charges are true. So they cannot be answered -- but neither are they heeded.

So why do economists knowingly misrepresent the scope of economic analysis, by pretending to draw normative conclusions from positive propositions, and in the process mislead the public, other economists, and themselves?

The news is not all bad, however, in economics any more than in medicine, and I am not trying to be the Ivan Illich of health economics. There are, in fact, some very positive features of health economics in particular, that can be strengthened

---

[12] But see Note 10 supra. There may be more ignorance around than we think. In this context it is worth reflecting upon a comment by Gaynor and Vogt (1997), highlighted by Rice (1997b), "It is not clear to us in what way an economist saying `trade barriers make everyone worse off than...' is any more or less normative than an engineer saying `bridges made out of cardboard will fall down more frequently than...'"

Nor are they alone. Fuchs' (1996) questionnaire identifies the statement "Third-party payment results in patients using services whose costs exceed their benefits..." as a *positive* statement! Costs and benefits can be defined, indeed *evalu*ated, without introducing any value judgements...(we're just doing economic science). And almost all of his respondents dutifully agreed.

and built upon. In important ways we are in better shape than some other branches of economics. We are healthier, and we should strive to stay that way.

From that perspective, one could have chosen two alternative titles for this paper:

"What Do They Know of Economics, Who Only Economics Know?"

and

"Two Cheers for Health Economics."

The first title emerges from the observation that economics *per se* has remarkably little specific content. One is tempted to say, none at all. Harberger's argument for "equal weighting" was that without some sort of value judgements as to interpersonal weightings, we as economists can make few, if any, recommendations on policy. Arrow had the same reason for abstracting from distributional considerations, as did the proposers of compensation tests. But the problem runs deeper; on the basis of economic analysis *alone* we cannot say very much of anything.

That, I think, is why we find a definition of economics so elusive. The common ones are vague and over-general -- "the study of people in the ordinary business of life," "optimization under constraint," "the study of the allocation of scarce resources among competing wants...etc." -- or trivial -- "what economists do."[13] We tend to fall back on references to a way of thinking, or a particular perspective on social phenomena, that leads one to ask certain characteristic sorts of questions and to try to organize the description and prediction of human behaviour in particular ways. But there is in fact no distinct body of *knowledge*, settled or unsettled, that we can point to and say, even provisionally, "That is economics."[14]

---

[13] Jacob Viner's definition is, however, far from trivial in its potential consequences. If economics is "what economists do," then an obvious inference (though not a logical implication) is that "what non-economists do" is, whatever its content and findings, "not economics." The field becomes defined not by its substantive content, but by the identity of its practitioners. If these form a self-identifying club, then economists can achieve something of the monopolistic privileges that other professions have gained through regulation.

[14] There is however a body of "tools and techniques" that tends to be the characteristic possession of economists. To the extent that these are exclusive to economists, then defining the field in terms of those tools and techniques leads back to Jacob Viner's definition -- see the previous Note.

The standard jokes about looking for a one-armed economist, or "no matter how many economists one lines up end-to-end, they never reach a conclusion," have point. Judicial comments on the testimony of economic experts -- not "hired guns" but leaders of the profession -- have been more brutal, and equally justified. Reputable and defensible economic opinion can be found on every side of almost every public issue, or at least every one that comes to prominence. Nor are disagreements and disputes confined to the leading edges or the fringes of the discipline, where matters might be expected to be unsettled. They persist across the whole range of questions with which economists have concerned themselves. Even when consensus appears to be established for a time, old ideas and controversies break out again in new language. Nothing ever seems permanently settled.[15]

This indeterminacy does not, I think, arise because economists are more confused or more attracted to controversy than practitioners of other disciplines.[16] Insofar as they aspire to "scientific" status, economists seek to generate their own body of positive, "if...then" statements, that have been consistently confirmed by various forms of empirical analysis. These would therefore command general assent among not only economists but anyone else familiar with "scientific" modes of demonstration.

Armed with such convincingly demonstrable propositions, as well as with a professional consensus as to their validity, economists could then make unambiguous positive statements to their fellow citizens. We could, in Wildavsky's phrase, "speak truth to power," not in the normative form of, "You should do A and not B," but "if you do A, C will follow."

A generation ago this was the great hope. "Give us the data, and we will finish the job!," as the members of the graduate Economic History Seminar proclaimed at Harvard in the 1960s. With new and more powerful mathematical and statistical techniques, new and massive sources of data, and, of course, explosive progress in computing capacity, a rapid increase in the supply of confirmed positive propositions seemed guaranteed -- just over the next hill. And these in turn would

---

[15] Particular *theoretical* propositions that can be given formal mathematical representation are settled, once they are proved or refuted. Thus there is a steady accumulation of information about the properties of such mathematical relationships. But there is no necessary connection between this form of "progress," and our understanding of the behaviour of actual human beings, either individually or in (small or large) groups.

[16] They may in fact be either, or both, but I do not think that that is the whole explanation.

permit economists to make unambiguous and more or less consensual statements about the impact of different public policies -- predictions, not recommendations.[17] Has it come to pass?

Clearly not. Despite the accumulation of empirical studies -- particularly multivariate statistical analyses -- over the last three decades, it has turned out to be remarkably difficult to confirm or refute hypotheses in a way that is generally recognized as decisive.

What we neglected, is that all positive statements have a "third component." Fully specified, they take the form: "If... [and...] then...." The contents of the [and...] term are absolutely critical; like the gate in a triode or a transistor they amplify or suppress (or reverse) the connection between intervention and response. Under what circumstances does a relationship hold?[18]

But the range of potentially relevant circumstances is exceedingly diverse, and open to all sorts of interpretation and disagreement as to what should be included. Without some sort of restriction, anything can happen. And conclusions of the form "If A,...then anything" are a weak intellectual basis for a science. (They may not elicit much respect or financial support from the rest of society, either.)

There are two ways of dealing with the contents of the [and...] term:

- Go and find out; and
- Make them up.

The predominant response among economists has been the latter.

We impose radical simplifications on the contents of the [and...] term, by making substantive assumptions about the circumstances we are studying. (Sometimes we are conscious of this process, and of its significance, but repetition

---

[17] Friedman (1953) not only laid out this objective, but advocated a particular methodology for reaching it which appeared to liberate economists from the need for any substantive information about the processes they were studying. That "bootstrap" methodology was flawed at its core, and has had no shortage of critics. But it retains a superficial attractiveness, perhaps because it is easy to understand, and offers the illusion of general insights without the effort of acquiring specific knowledge. ("Ignorance is Strength.") Indeed Friedman's proposed methodology may have contributed to Ken Bassett's Problem, in suggesting that it doesn't matter if analysis is based on false assumptions. Go ahead and do things you know are wrong; empirical testing of consequences will sort things out. Well, *that* prediction was thumpingly falsified!

[18] This is not quite the same as the traditional *ceteris paribus* assumption. "If A, then B" requires that C, D, etc. not be changing at the same time; *ceteris paribus* isolates the change in a single variable A to focus on its effects alone. But the point here is that the effects of A will depend on the specific pattern of other circumstances, even when these are held constant. And in the real world, these patterns are typically very complex.

forms habits that economize on scarce cognitive resources.) The resulting "If...then" propositions refer to abstract transacting entities -- "consumers," "firms" -- with highly stylized properties, interacting in very specific circumstances. Their relationship to entities in the world of observation and experience is always problematic.

Through this process we are enabled to make certain definite predictions, although the range of unambiguous predictions that can be supported in this way is much more limited than its practitioners -- present company not excepted -- typically admit. ("Demand (supply) curves always slope downward to the right (left), except when they don't.") And even such limited results are bought at a very steep price. The substantive assumptions "made up" in traditional economic theory are at best based on radically impoverished and obsolete theories of human behaviour, long abandoned by students of the relevant disciplines. At worst they are in flat contradiction with "reality" as understood by those professionally concerned with such matters.

For example, we can set up an analytic framework postulating that consumer behaviour can be represented as the outcome of maximizing some objective function, but this framework tells us nothing at all about the arguments of that objective function. When we specify them *a priori*, we are acting as amateur psychologists -- and often rather poor ones. Likewise, when we not only hypothesize the existence of the relationships we call "production functions," but try to specify their arguments and functional forms, we are acting as (typically very bad) engineers, or in health economics, epidemiologists or clinicians.

But these specifications matter -- minor changes in either the arguments or the functional forms that we use can lead to radically different predictions. (See, for example, Frank, 1985; Frank and Cook, 1995.)

The point is definitely *not* that one should not "build models," in the sense of consciously or unconsciously introducing simplifying assumptions about the processes that we are trying to describe and understand. That would be silly; we cannot *not* do so if we are to think at all, or even to perceive. The full range of possibly relevant impressions is far beyond the capacity of our senses to record, let alone of our brains to manipulate.

The art of simplifying is that of excluding the differences that do not make a difference, of capturing the essence of a process and ignoring the unimportant. Some do and some do not; there are good and bad models. If essential features of the underlying reality are left out of the [and ...] term, the resulting model becomes at best useless, and quite often actively deceptive and mischievous.

But *as economists*, we have no advantage, comparative or otherwise, in choosing the appropriate simplifications. To do that, you actually have to know something about the processes, activities, institutions, people, that you are trying to analyse. Left to his/her own devices, the economist without content knowledge tends to select the simplifications that yield analytic tractability (and follow convention). And if one does not know any better, why not?

More reliable results, however, emerge from the more interesting and productive alternative -- to go and find out. This can be done by immersing oneself in the relevant literature from other disciplines, and building their observations and conclusions into economic analyses in a fundamental way. One may also engage in direct observation "on the shop floor."

But the most efficient approach, entailing less effort and greater reliability, is to seek out and work with specialists in other disciplines.[19] Find out what are the relevant "other circumstances" in a particular situation, from those who know. Working closely with people from other disciplines protects economists from a good deal of sin and error, by forcing them to justify their intellectual behaviour to other informed and intelligent analysts. Such people are unlikely to accept, as support for an otherwise implausible assumption, the explanation that many economists have made it before. (That may be why economists, in general, tend to hold themselves and their work apart from other disciplines -- arrogance rooted in a deep and justifiable sense of vulnerability.)

Health economists *do* have, I think, an unusual proclivity for following the second route. Many of us work closely with clinicians, epidemiologists, and "social scientists" of various persuasions, on a long-term basis. We are thus more willing -- we have no choice! -- to modify or abandon, when they do not fit, the traditional assumptions that have been "made up" in formulating the corpus of general economic theory. We also have unusual opportunities to become informed about the technological relationships underlying the production of both health care and health.

But we deserve only two cheers. Not all of us have had that good fortune, or been able to profit from it through a genuine melding of perspectives. More fundamentally, we have come at best only part way in the reconstruction of our theoretical frameworks to accommodate what we have learned from our colleagues in other disciplines. Cross-disciplinary work is not just intellectual "parallel play";

---

[19] Few of us are likely to have the opportunity to take Ken Bassett's route, and to *become* a specialist in another discipline. And in any case, even two disciplines *is* only a beginning.

the (relevant) understandings of one field must actually change the content of another. To the extent that this does not happen, we find ourselves working with theoretical frameworks based on the traditional "made up" contents for the [and...] terms, while trying to grasp the realities of the health care field as we now understand them. Ken Bassett's Problem emerges.

It emerges in a number of specific contexts across the whole field of health economics. I will focus only on a few leading examples that particularly interest me. In each case, we find important discrepancies between what health economists know, and what they assume in much of their theoretical structures -- discrepancies that have material consequences for the outcome of their analyses.

But in each area we also find important examples of health economists having learned from other disciplines in ways that significantly improve the quality of our analysis. And as it happens, under each head we can find a nugget or two of illustrative information from Fuchs' (1996) informal survey of economists and physicians, reported in his presidential address to the American Economic Association.

INDIVIDUAL TASTES

"Standard" economic theory postulates that individual consumer behaviour can be analyzed and predicted on the assumption that only commodities (or commodities and leisure) contribute to well-being. If other state variables matter -- individual health status, for example -- they do not interact with commodities and so can be held in the pound of *ceteris paribus*. They are not in the [and...] term.

On the other hand it is pretty obvious that the value of the commodity "health care" to a user depends critically on whether s/he is ill or injured, or more generally whether s/he has reason to believe that the care will improve his/her health status. Perceived effectiveness of care is central to the user's decision (when s/he is in a position to decide) to use care.

No one challenges this overtly, at least not in ordinary language.[20] Yet one finds a radical split among health economists as to how or whether this obvious fact should be built into their analyses. On one side of the Atlantic, for example, the centrality of health status is so generally accepted that the consideration of

---

[20] Mathematical formulations, on the other hand, permit one to say things that would be pretty dubious, if not simply silly, in other languages.

direct utility effects constitutes an extension to the research program. Certain forms of health care, in particular circumstances, may have a value to the user independent of their effects on health status. Health is not *all* that matters.

On the other side, we occasionally find explicit arguments that health effects are, or should be (the normative economist again), irrelevant to the evaluation of resource allocation. The decisions of the (fully informed) consumer, facing prices that reflect opportunity costs, within an ethically acceptable income distribution, are the only relevant criteria (Pauly, 1994a,b).[21] If a particular form of care contributes to such a consumer's well-being, its effect on health is irrelevant; if it does not, *ditto*. Any health effects are subsumed into the (informed) consumer's evaluation.[22] More typically we find this assumption being built into analysis without supporting comment. Health care is treated as just another commodity, a "widget"; health as such is implicitly irrelevant.[23]

Whether or not health status *per se* is inserted in the utility function for analytic purposes is not, however, simply an academic point. It matters a great deal for the normative evaluation of particular health services, and of the institutions and systems that produce and deliver them. Are they to be judged by their ability to contribute to health, or by their response to the preferences -- as expressed, for

---

[21] Does such a consumer exist, has s/he ever existed, *could* s/he exist? Or rather, does this "transacting entity," endowed by assumption with certain properties, and operating in a hypothetical informational and institutional environment, bear a sufficiently close relationship to any human person or family to be of any relevance to the analysis of health care systems in the world around us?

If the answer were "yes," the judgements of such a hypothetical "consumer" might be an ethically plausible guide to resource allocation. Of course there is no way of knowing whether our fellow citizens would agree; and remember, we economists are neither legislators nor priests. But the answer is in fact "no"; and the hypothetical situation serves primarily as a distraction from attempts to understand health care systems in the real world.

[22] The legendary Muslim (substitute preferred faith) read only the Koran because other books would either confirm its truth, and be superfluous, or deny it, and be blasphemous.

[23] There is a dodge that can be added to this, but it *is* only a dodge. To avoid the obvious absurdity of the insertion of health *care* in the individual utility function -- *i.e.*, that people will want care regardless of their health state ("Take two appendectomies, they're free!"), one can postulate that individuals are indeed concerned not about health care but about their health state. But the latter is then modelled as a "capital stock" in which people "invest" by, *inter alia*, purchasing and consuming health care. This formulation has problems of its own, but it is then augmented by the assumptions that (a) individuals are fully informed about the relation between health care and their "health capital," and (b) more health care always produces more health. Both of these are clearly counter-factual; they serve in effect to reinsert health care into the utility function while camouflaging the absurdity. Health status is introduced into the analysis, but then finessed out again.

example, in willingness to pay -- of "consumers"?[24]

Research on what people actually want indicates (not surprisingly) that more is not better, that people do *not*, in general, want ineffective or minimally effective care, especially when it is inconvenient, unpleasant, or dangerous. Moreover their judgements as to the effects that matter, and the risks that are and are not worth taking, will often differ from the views of practitioners. The only way to discover these preferences, is to go and look for them. Inference from observed utilization is notoriously deceptive.

In any case, people are often not in a position to make their wishes effective, because of either lack of knowledge or lack of effective control. Lack of knowledge is pervasive; loss of physical control typically occurs in extreme situations and not in the general run of patient contacts with the health care system. But a large proportion of health care resources are used up, and costs generated, in just such extreme situations.

When people have been given either greater information or greater control (*e.g.*, Wennberg, 1992; Molloy and Guyatt, 1991), it has been found in certain important cases that they want *less* care, not more. But it is apparently much more difficult than one might think to achieve this; the resistance and simple inertia are substantial (*e.g.*, SUPPORT, 1995). For our purposes, however, there is direct evidence (apart from introspection!) that health care *per se* -- most of it, anyway -- is not a direct (positive) argument in the utility function of the normal consumer.[25]

But the role of (perceived) health status is also central to the endless debate among health economists about the role of physicians and other professionals in generating the demand for their own services. (Other students of, and policy makers in, the health care systems of the world have settled this debate long ago. *Of course,* capacity generates use, that is why capacity control -- hospital beds, physician supply -- is always among the first steps taken in strategies for cost control.) The relationship between health care and health status is a technical "production" relationship about which professional providers are (perceived to be)

---

[24] Implicit in this distinction is the assumption that users of care, though they may know the value of health to themselves, will not, in general, be knowledgeable about how health status is produced from health care. The whole apparatus of professional regulation is built around just this assumption; and if/when an economist assumes perfectly informed "consumers," s/he is very much in the minority. One might speculate about the personal care-seeking behaviour of such economists.

[25] A form of mental illness, Münchausen's Syndrome, is characterized by seeking out care services, and counterfeiting illnesses in order to undergo various diagnostic and therapeutic interventions. Such people apparently *do* derive direct utility from using health services.

more knowledgeable than patients. So, their advice -- recommendations, or still more revealingly "doctor's orders" -- powerfully affects use, independent of price.

If these recommendations are themselves endogenous, varying according to the economic circumstances of the provider (workload, income, prices/fees received), then the "demand curve" disappears, or at least becomes endogenous to supplier behaviour. (And it is hard to imagine any sensible economic model of provider behaviour in which their recommendations would *not* be endogenous.) Thus the inclusion of health status in the individual utility function provides the channel through which "supplier-induced demand" operates.

But as we know, this relationship cuts to the positive foundations of standard economic theory, as well as the normative significance typically adjoined to it. It is therefore not surprising that many economists have resisted it, particularly but not exclusively in the United States. What is remarkable is Fuchs' (1996) finding that an overwhelming majority of the economists, as well as the physicians, that he surveyed agreed that *doctors can and do shift the demand curve for their own services,* and are more likely to do so when demand is low. Yet an overwhelming majority of the formal analyses carried out by American economists in particular, and of the normative interpretations given to them, suppress this reality (without comment).

When pressed, analysts in the exogenous demand tradition tend not to deny the existence of such shifting, but to emphasize the empirical difficulties in establishing its existence beyond all doubt, and especially in measuring its extent. Both concerns are valid; they also apply to virtually every (perhaps every) other behavioural relationship that economists study and build into their theories. In this case, however, incomplete information is translated for analytic purposes into a specific assumption -- zero effect. This is the Harberger manoeuvre.

Intriguingly, while two-thirds of both health economists and physicians believed that such shifting occurs. among general economic theorists, the proportion was over three quarters. One is tempted to infer that this reflects the views of the general public, as economic theorists not elsewhere classified have no specific interest in this area. Health economists will be more aware of the extent of the analytic modifications required by such an effect; and physicians may realize -- as the leaders of professional associations certainly do -- its potentially awkward political implications.

But that is all speculative, and the sample is small. The key point is that -- unless Fuchs found a very unrepresentative sample of American health economists -- knowledge (or at least belief) and practice appear to diverge at a point fundamental to virtually all of health economics.

But whatever the role of health status in the individual utility function, we cannot legitimately define that function only over arguments pertaining to a single individual. As is well-known, there are "external effects," interactive relationships among people, both in the form of contagion and at more general levels of benevolence. What one assumes about these -- including ignoring them -- will significantly influence the results of any formal analysis.[26]

Nothing here is new; the theoretical terrain has been mapped for years. Moreover it is now understood that simply inserting interpersonal terms in the individual utility functions leaves us with a "welfarist" social welfare function (Culyer, 1991) that is still quite restrictive.[27] What is new and interesting is the sort of work that Williams (this volume) is doing, in exploring the more detailed structure of these interpersonal concerns in a way that can link them to policy decisions. Rather than simply assuming them away, or assuming that they exist and then weighting each individual, or individual life-year, or QALY, equally on *a priori* grounds, he has gone to find out.

But the more general question of whether such concerns exist, is easy. People, even Americans, *tell* you when questioned, that other peoples' health matters to them, that people should get the care they need, whether or not they can pay for it, financed through government. And (outside the United States) they vote that way.

Fuchs' (1996) respondents are about two-thirds in favour of a universal health insurance plan for the United States, and well over half of them think it should be tax-based. They are about 85% (physicians and health economists) against charging higher private insurance premiums to people born with costly genetic defects, though much more dubious about requiring general community rating by private insurers. (Physicians are over two-thirds for it, theorists over two-thirds

---

[26] Economists can be appallingly stupid about personal interactions. We routinely illustrate the importance of prices by telling the little homily of the group of diners who go out to lunch together and agree to split the cheque equally. Each of them, acting as an independent utility maximizer, eats more than s/he would if s/he had to pay the full cost of his/her meal. All end up eating, and spending, too much relative to what they really wanted. See how bad socialism is, and how much better are private markets? But why did this group decide to eat together (and split the cheque) in the first place? People who act like individual utility maximizers in such settings, very soon find themselves dining alone.

[27] Archibald characterized this class of models as "dog-and-master" models. The well-being of the dog takes on broader social significance only insofar as the master cares about it. There is no general community concern for equity that might serve as a basis for entitlements for dogs (including stray dogs).

against, health economists split down the middle.) But that could simply reflect the economists' greater understanding of the dynamics of private insurance markets.

Yet those same economists, in their professional lives, will work quite happily with theoretical structures in which "consumers" are completely selfish, and in which tax-based universal (thus, in effect, compulsory) insurance coverage can easily be demonstrated (provided all consumers are identical in all relevant respects) to create a large "welfare burden" for society as a whole.[28] The potential losers from such a policy could easily compensate the potential gainers for abandoning the idea -- though they won't, and should not have to.

And what about uncertainty? Do people react to incomplete information by trying to maximize their expected utilities, or do they employ other strategies and heuristics? The answer is known; the psychologists can demonstrate the latter quite conclusively. The departures from E(U) maximization are large and the circumstances under which they occur are to some extent predictable. (The insurance salesman's maxim is that insurance is sold, not bought.) Yet many economists continue to assume the former.[29] The "efficiency" of markets for risk, where they exist, does rather depend upon how people behave under uncertainty!

The overall point of the above discussion is not that *I* know how individuals' utility functions should be structured in setting up formal models, but that this knowledge:

a) matters a lot for the outcome of the analysis; and
b) is not and cannot be derived from economics *per se*; but
c) is commonly assumed in economic analysis, often in defiance of evidence generated by non-economist experts,
d) despite the fact that most, if not all, health economists know better.

It might be a better idea to go and find out.

---

[28] Or alternatively provided that a strict interpersonal comparative rule is in effect that "a buck is a buck is a buck" (*pace* Kenneth LeM. Carter) regardless of who gets it -- the Harberger SWF.

[29] Moreover the economic theorists have shown that expected utility maximization by each individual (argument) in a given "welfarist" SWF will not, except in very special cases, yield the maximum expected value of the SWF itself (Hammond, 1982, 1983). But health economists interested in private insurance markets seem to have ignored this result.

TECHNOLOGY

The same four points can be illustrated by the ways in which we understand and model "technology." And here Fuchs' results suggest that health economists well deserve their two cheers. 83% of economic theorists believe that widespread screening and early diagnosis could cut health care costs significantly. And that's a pretty reasonable view -- for the 1950s. Ninety percent of health economists, however, (and even most physicians) knew that the evidence is in and that this is a false hope. And indeed economists, working with epidemiologists and clinical specialists, have helped to produce that evidence. *A priori* reasoning provides no substitute.

Another cheer: *no* health economists identified differential access to health care as the *primary* reason for health status differences across socioeconomic groups. Most of the other economists also understood that (at least on the present evidence) the principal determinants of health lie elsewhere. One does get a little twitchy, however, in recognizing that this is an *American* sample. Class differences in access to (effective) care are especially marked in that country, and *do* appear to contribute to differences in health outcomes. It would be ironic if the health economists' responses were correct for all developed countries *except* their own. But the word "primary" is key.

But then we, or at least Fuchs' sample, go and blow it. Eighty-one percent of the health economists believed that "technological change" is the primary reason for the increasing share of GDP devoted to health care over the last 30 years! Only 37% of the economic theorists fell for that. The health economists should each be required to write out, one thousand times: "The technology does *not* dictate its own range of application." And that, of course, is why American health care costs have travelled such a different path from those in other countries.

Causality is always problematic; but it is pretty obvious that all the health care systems of the developed world have had access to the same technologies. Indeed, several of the most prominent technological innovations were first developed outside the United States. How extensively those technologies have been used, however, and whether or not they have been translated into escalating costs, has depended upon the ways in which health care has been organized, delivered, and funded in different countries.

Twenty, or even fifteen years ago one could perhaps claim that, on average, health expenditures were rising as fast (relative to GDP) outside the United States as in it. (There were significant exceptions, like Canada and the United Kingdom.)

But that ceased to be true in the mid- to late 1970s, and since then the United States has been on a trajectory all its own. As an international common factor, technological change cannot "explain" patterns that show so much cross-national variation.

Again, we all know that. So why would we find not only Fuchs' sample, but also eminent members of the profession, resorting to this "technology" story and presenting something that cannot be true as if it were established fact? Well, it could be that "technology" is short-hand for a more value-laden story. Improved technology has led to more and better care, and people want this new care and are willing to pay for it, individually and/or collectively. Thus use and costs go up, as they should when new and better products meet consumer needs/tastes.

But why, then, is this escalation so much more rapid in the United States? When costs were escalating at similar rates in most countries one might have argued that some aggregate analogy to an income effect was at work. It could then be claimed that costs were higher in the United States because Americans were wealthier, but that rising incomes were pushing up costs everywhere. Other countries, when they were as rich as the United States, would have similar spending patterns. (They're just a bit backward, that's all.)

But that argument ceased to hold water long ago. As noted above, the gap in health spending between the United States and the rest of the developed world has actually been widening since the late 1970s. And there is no corresponding income gap opening up in Americans' favour; on the contrary, incomes in other countries have, on average, pulled closer to the U.S. level.[30] Now, presumably, one would have to claim that costs do not go up, or not as fast, in other countries because care is being "rationed"; other people are being denied things that they value and would be willing to pay for. So, they are made worse off as a result. The United States does not spend too much; everyone else spends too little.[31]

---

[30] The OECD Health Data 96 database (OECD, 1996) assembles a wide range of health-relevant data for these countries from 1960 to 1994. Over the first half of this period, prior to 1977, the U.S. share of GDP spent on health care was rising in parallel with the (unweighted) average of OECD countries, though at the top of the pack. After 1977, however, the average for OECD countries has grown much less rapidly and the United States has pulled away. The share of health spending in GDP in the United States is now about 50% larger than that in any other OECD country. Over this same period, 1977-94, the (unweighted) average of GDP per capita, measured in purchasing power parities, rose from 71% to 76% of the U.S. level (in the nineteen OECD countries for which data are available since 1960).

[31] Indeed this is precisely the conclusion reached by "National Economic Research Associates" (NERA) in an international study of health care spending (Hoffmeyer and McCarthy, 1994), with an interesting qualification. "Needs/demands" for health spending were allegedly met (in 1990) in *two*

If this *is* the underlying story, it neatly inverts the evaluation implicit in Abel-Smith's (1985) description of the United States as the "Odd Man Out," or White's (1995) identification of an "international standard" in health care organization and finance from which only the United States departs. It also requires that one bypass the evidence that *prices* for health care are much higher, in relative terms, in the United States (Gerdtham and Jönsson, 1991; see also Fuchs and Hahn, 1990; Nair *et al.*, 1992; Redelmeier and Fuchs, 1993), implying that Americans do not in fact get much more care but just pay more for it.[32]

In effect, everyone is out of step but Uncle Sam. But Americans are not healthier than people in other developed countries, so the "rationing" that is presumably being practised wherever costs are lower (everywhere else) does not appear to have the health-damaging effects routinely alleged by medical alarmists. It must then be "tastes" for care that are being suppressed by rationing -- which brings us back to the questions of the arguments of the individual utility function and, since almost all care is collectively financed anyway, the nature of the

---

countries -- the United States and Switzerland. These two countries spent vastly different shares of their national incomes: 12.4% of GDP in the United States; only 7.8% in Switzerland. Yet both are alleged to have been spending the "right" amount, while all the countries *between* these rates were spending far too little. The United States and Switzerland were the only countries in the OECD (except for Turkey) with a high proportion of private funding, suggesting that NERA's criteria for "meeting needs" depended much less on how much was spent than on how it was spent -- and raised.

But even the United States, they claim, should spend a much larger share of its national income on health care by the year 2000, and this will not be politically acceptable. The study then proposes a new international "prototype" model of health care organization and finance (replacing White's (1995) "international standard"). In effect, this would ensure that health care costs were once again out of control, so as to escalate as "needed/demanded" by the various national populations. (The percent of GDP spend on health has escalated significantly since 1990 in both the United States and Switzerland.)

The study is critiqued in Towse, ed. (1995): NERA were commissioned by Pharmaceutical Partners for Better Health Care, a lobby group for the international pharmaceutical industry.

[32] One might then argue that if care is higher priced, it must be higher "quality" -- a "quality" reflected not in better health outcomes, but, in the minds of the recipients, in greater satisfaction. It must be so, or else higher prices would not be paid.... But higher American prices are to a large extent caused by the extraordinarily high costs of administering the *payment system*, not of providing better care (Woolhandler and Himmelstein, 1991). Well, that provides greater "choice," not of care but of mode of reimbursement. Do Americans want that? They must, or they would not pay for it.... And so it goes. There is in fact counter-evidence that might bear on each of these points; but the *a priori* argument forever slides away into circularity.

interpersonal relationships across utility functions.[33]

But this is all a bit speculative. The positive point is that on substantive issues of the relationship between health care and health outcomes, health economists have learned from their other professional colleagues, and get the answer right. Only when we get into "technology" in the abstract, are we vulnerable to confusions that may have a political dimension.

The political significance of technological assumptions, however, has deeper roots in economic theory. In micro-economic theory we impose certain substantive assumptions on the shape of the production function, at least in the short run. The average and marginal cost curves had better turn up, beyond some level of output, or else not only is the firm "size" (equilibrium output level) indeterminate in a competitive environment, but marginal cost pricing is impossible. And the normative significance that we attach to markets, and the prices they generate, depends critically upon those prices reflecting opportunity costs.[34]

We all know why we need to specify the technology, the shape of the production function, in a particular way for analytic purposes. But what about the industries we study? If one is producing a drug (or a computer program), the fixed costs of development are extraordinarily high. The marginal costs of producing another batch of pills or another shrink-wrapped box of disks are pretty trivial, and do not rise with output level, at least over a very large range. Average cost per unit will then fall with output, while exceeding marginal cost, over any conceivable output range -- except for marketing costs. So how do you price at marginal cost?

You don't. A large proportion, probably most, of the product price is quasi-rent, covering development and marketing cost. Hence the extraordinary efforts

---

[33] It also raises a question as to why, if Americans are getting what they want while people in all other countries are having their desires suppressed by "rationing," it is the *Americans* who are so unhappy about their situation (Blendon *et at.,* 1990)?

[34] There may be other arguments, good or bad, for markets and for private enterprise (Nelson, 1981). But the stories that we tell on the basis of *economic theory* require that prices correspond to the opportunity cost of resources.

Things get a little fuzzier in the hypothetical "long run." Sometimes we use the traditional argument that co-ordination costs (or something) lead to a U-shaped average cost curve; other times we fall back on constant returns to scale and let the equilibrium firm size dangle. It does not matter, of course, because so long as firms can enter freely *at any scale, no matter how small*, the threat of entry will hold prices at marginal cost in the long run, even if the industry is monopolized. Public policy to promote competition -- anti-trust, anti-combines, whatever -- is thus superfluous if not actually harmful.... So the "technological assumption" of constant returns to scale becomes politically significant. Maybe one should try to find out?

pharmaceutical firms put into marketing their products, and suppressing competition through political investments in anti-competitive regulation.[35] They have a very high "demand for regulation" (Stigler, 1971), with exceptional willingness, and ability, to pay. A world of perfect competition, with free entry and prices driven down to marginal costs, would be catastrophic.

Competition among firms is Schumpeterian, taking the form of new product development, which in his famous description bears about as much relation to price competition as an artillery bombardment does to forcing a door. Ranitidine did not simply "compete" with cimetidine -- Glaxo convinced physicians that it was a better drug and cimetidine's market collapsed. (SmithKline has reacted by getting regulatory permission, in the United States, to sell it over the counter.)

So what is the "supply curve" for such an industry?

Even if the technology were cooperative, the supply curve and its underlying cost curves and production function all depend for their relevance on the assumption that "firms," or whatever the producing units are, operate *on* their cost functions. Why should they? Well, cost-minimization is a necessary condition for profit-maximization, which is enforced by competition in either or both of product and capital markets.... But most "firms" in the health care sectors of most countries are not-for-profit, operating in highly regulated markets, and nothing like price competition occurs. Even where services are provided by independent, fee-for-service practitioners, these typically work under some collectively negotiated fee schedule. When practitioners do have some discretionary power over their own fees, there is typically a good deal of collusion -- as one would expect of rational self-interested transactors with highly developed communication skills.

The United States has for a number of years been offered as a counter-example, a system that is, or rather is about to become or has just become, highly price-competitive. But even if that were true, presumably health economics has to be something more than a theory of the American health care system.

Furthermore, if it is the case, as it seems to be, that prices for health care (relative to other commodities) are much higher in the United States than elsewhere, does this mean that the opportunity costs are correspondingly higher? How is it that other countries appear to be able to elicit the necessary resources at lower -- sometimes much lower -- (regulated) prices? So what *do* the American prices indicate? *A priori* assumptions about markets are not too helpful; again one

---

[35] Members of the industry prefer to speak of "protection of intellectual property." But the label does not matter; the process is the same.

has to go and find out where the money is going, to whom and for what.

Are higher prices primarily a distributional phenomenon -- yielding higher levels of economic rent? To what extent do they ration access to health services, and with what implications for the use patterns, and the health outcomes, of people in different income classes? Do higher prices reflect higher levels of resource input to perform functions that are carried out in a less costly way in other countries -- technical inefficiency? Or are there differences in "quality," as perceived and valued by patients, behind the higher prices? All these effects may be at work; the interesting question is the mix.

All of this discussion, however, has to do with the technology of health *care* production. If we consider instead the production of health, or at least some contribution to health, then any notion of a monotonic positive relationship between inputs and outputs flies out the window. A diagnostic or therapeutic manoeuvre may as easily damage health as improve it -- or simply have no effect at all. Health care *can* make you sick -- powerful interventions have powerful side-effects. That's why even we economists, in our private lives, rely on clinicians.

And that's why the whole area of clinical epidemiology, technology assessment in health care, and various forms of program evaluation, and behind them the study of why practitioners choose or reject particular techniques, have become critical aspects of health policy. If health status were simply a monotonic positive function of health care input, as some of its marketers would have us believe,[36] no one would be celebrating the work of Archie Cochrane or participating in the extraordinary new international initiative of the Cochrane Collaboration. But it isn't, and they are.

This is also an area to which health economists have made important contributions, both methodologically and in applied studies. But the work is multi-disciplinary to its core; the economist alone, relying only on the tools of economics, would be fortunate simply to have no impact.

The way around Ken Bassett's Problem, short of going off to do a Ph.D. in something else, thus appears trivially simple. All one needs to do, is to fill in the [and...] terms in our "If...then" propositions with sound information derived from other clinical and social disciplines -- or from direct observation. In other words, build this information into the heart of our own models. And the best way of doing this, in that it provides both access to the necessary information and incentive to

---

[36] Or, more shameless yet, a monotonic function of health *spending*!

force one to use it, is truly joint research (not partitioned projects) with people from other disciplines.

So if that is so obvious, why do we keep on repeating old errors?

Well, making things up permits us to control the structure of our models, preserving analytic tractability and simplicity, and facilitating translation into the language of mathematics. Many economists seem to view mathematics much the way medieval scholars viewed Latin, as a language that confers special authority on statements that have been written in it. (Users of these languages were/are able to get away with a good deal of nonsense by avoiding the vernacular.)

Schooling, force of habit, and herd instincts are also powerful conditioners. We make the assumptions that we were taught, that we have always made, and that everyone else makes. Moreover, there is considerable economy in communication when everyone can use the same code. You do not have to explain in detail, let alone justify, what you are doing. An outsider, especially one with substantive knowledge in related fields, might make very trenchant criticisms. But "peer" review and disciplinary self-reference permit one to avoid exposure to such criticism, or to ignore it without penalty. So long as we all make the same assumptions, we cannot be criticized by reviewers.

Quite the contrary, skilful manipulation of an intellectual framework shared by peer reviewers and editors leads to prestigious publication, reputation, research grants, academic promotion, etc. etc. The whole apparatus of a learned discipline comes into play, to preserve the intellectual *status quo*. In the sciences, experiment and empirical observation periodically force more or less radical revision of the dominant frameworks. But economics is not a science. Or rather, we approximate a science most closely when we "go and find out," and are most vulnerable when we make things up.

There is also another dimension, one that we rarely discuss openly. Whether we wish it or not, the choices we make to fill in the [and...] terms in our analyses have powerful ideological and political content. Other people with important interests at stake inevitably give considerable attention to how we "make up" the content of these terms, and the analytic results. We have already noted above the way that "technology," in the abstract, has been and is being used as an argument both to explain and to justify ever-growing health care spending.

Such claims emanate from sectors of the health care industry and from their spokesmen.[37] Health expenditures, from whatever source, are their sales revenues and incomes, so they have every reason to resist and subvert public and private efforts at cost control. So long as discussion can be focused on "technology" in the abstract -- rather expensive but overall a GOOD THING, and certainly something on which a progressive society should be spending more -- such claims cannot be tested in detail. They reduce to "Day by day, in every way, we're getting better and better. Send more money."

But the same interests are involved in the detailed structure of our formal models, again whether we like it or not. Different assumptions about the arguments of individual utility functions, for example, map directly into alternative political programs with powerful (and very different) redistributional effects. If we formulate economic models that embody the observations that users of care really want health, not health care *per se*, and that they are concerned about each other's health, and that they cannot deal comfortably or very successfully with decision-making under uncertainty, we will be led to a certain "world-view."

Evaluating and improving the effectiveness of health care will be an important public concern, and questions about the distribution of burdens and benefits among the different members of a society will be central to the organization and financing of health care systems. Individual "consumer" choices in private markets will appear not only as unsuitable guides for resource allocation, but in a fundamental sense as undefined.

On the other hand once one has adopted a standard individualistic, commodity-based utility function, with uncertainty captured in the expectations operator, one is led naturally into a concern with the "efficiency" of "markets" for this commodity. "Optimality" of resource allocation will be achieved by some appropriate structuring of private markets, including private insurance markets. One may add some surrounding textual comment about imperfect information or redistributional concerns, but that is mere window-dressing. The central analytic construct holds the centre of the stage.[38]

---

[37] Recall that NERA's proposals to re-ignite the international escalation in health care costs, that has been largely damped since the late 1970s, were commissioned by the international pharmaceutical industry (Note 31 above).

[38] It is only from the second perspective that it becomes possible to raise questions like: "We do not make groceries free: why should the government provide "free" health care?" or: "Not everyone can afford a Cadillac; why should everyone get Cadillac-style care?" or even: "We don't need a special economic theory for car repair, and what really makes medicine different?" and be taken even half-seriously. From the perspective of the first world-view such questions are so crashingly stupid that

In the realm of actual public policy, it is clear that the first view is dominant in the industrialized world outside the United States (Abel-Smith and Mossialos, 1994; White, 1995). Within the United States both policy and the public appear to be quite schizophrenic. But the second view is nowhere completely absent, because the policies that follow from different world-views *do* have such important differences in their implications for the distribution of income and wealth.

As we all know even if we do not always talk about it -- and rarely admit it in formal models -- the wealthy and healthy are relatively much better off under private forms of finance, while the unhealthy and unwealthy are better off with public tax-based financing (Evans *et al.*, 1994, 1995). (There is more, but this much is obvious, fundamental, and beyond contention.) Well-defined and self-aware interest groups in every society thus have a strong economic interest, in addition to their ideological orientation, in the content of the "world-views" that govern health policy (Evans, 1996a, 1997a).

It follows that these same groups have an interest in the structure and content of the economic frameworks that contribute towards -- though they are far from dominating -- the formulation of those world-views. And, as economists, we have a particular professional interest in the way in which economic interests are expressed in action.

Or to put it more bluntly, if economists can choose their assumptions in ways that are crucial to the results of their analysis, and if other people have a strong economic interest in those results, cold-blooded economic analysis itself would seem to predict that economic inducements will be offered to steer those choices. And if so, cold-blooded economic analysis also predicts that some of us, at least, will accept.

Is this happening? That's an empirical question, and is left for the reader.

But to the extent that it *could* happen -- and I would welcome any demonstration that it is *not* an obvious economic prediction -- this possibility underscores the importance of placing the contents of the [and...] terms of our analyses on a firmer empirical foundation, and of exposing our work to a wider range of professional criticism. We are going to *need* the input of others, to protect us from external subversion, and from ourselves. And health economists, though I believe we are at the forefront in cross-disciplinary, truly *applied* economics, are also going to come, are already coming, under the heaviest external pressure.

---

their being asked at all suggests a deliberate act of intellectual sabotage.

Indeed this may be a back-handed form of compliment -- our work has actually been quite useful, so we are worth subverting. We're going to need more allies.

What role might be played by an organization like iHEA? By linking health economists from many countries and institutional environments more closely together, it could encourage and promote intellectual and methodological variety -- providing a larger garden in which a hundred flowers might bloom. This will be the more likely if we encourage membership and participation from non-economists who have interests parallel to ours. On the other hand, iHEA could become a vehicle for the enforcement of ideological and methodological hegemony -- defining what is and is not "real" health economics on the basis of who does it and/or what methodologies and conventional assumptions (including normative ones) are employed. Such an organization would then become more closely aligned with and supportive of a particular set of ideological and economic interests, interests that are increasingly operating internationally.[39]

It may be worth reflecting upon the fact that iHEA gives an annual prize in the name of Kenneth Arrow, one of the most distinguished theorists of his generation -- and indeed his classic 1963 paper is widely and justly cited. But there is another classic paper in this field, "Price Discrimination in Medicine" by Reuben Kessel (1958), that for many years was more widely cited, and that was and is much more important for anyone trying to understand the economics of health care.

Unlike Arrow the theoretician, Kessel went out and studied the actual behaviour of U.S. physicians in considerable detail, and then described and interpreted that behaviour from an economic perspective. Many of his insights are still valid, and not surprisingly they did not and do not all fit comfortably within conventional price theory. His contribution to *our* field, in substance and particularly in method, was far greater than Arrow's single paper, however theoretically elegant. But we do not give a Kessel Prize. Maybe we should.

REFERENCES

Abel-Smith, B. (1985) Who is the odd man out: the experience of western Europe in containing the costs of health care. *Milbank Memorial Fund Quarterly* 63: 1-17.

---

[39] The list of contributors to the founding of iHEA makes interesting reading, though Willie Sutton would have understood.

Abel-Smith, B. and Mossialos, E. (1994) Cost containment and health care reform: A study of the European Union. *Health Policy* 28:89-132.

Arrow, K.J. (1963) Uncertainty and the welfare economics of medical care. *American Economic Review* 53(5):941-973.

Arrow, K.J. (1973) Welfare Analysis of Changes in Health Coinsurance Rates, R-1281-OEO Santa Monica, CA: The Rand Corp.; republished in Rosett, R., editor, *The Role of Health Insurance in the Health Services Sector*. New York: National Bureau of Economic Research, 1976, pp. 3-23.

Bassett, K. (1996) Anthropology, clinical pathology and the electronic fetal monitor: lessons from the heart. *Social Science and Medicine* 42(2):281-292.

Bator, F.M. (1957) The simple analytics of welfare maximization. *American Economic Review* 47(1):22-59.

Blendon, R.J., Leitman, R., Morrison, I., and Donelan, K. (1990) Satisfaction with health systems in ten nations. *Health Affairs* 9(2):185-192.

Culyer, A.J. (1991) The normative economics of health care finance and provision. In McGuire, A., Fenn, P., and Mayhew, K., editors, *Providing Health Care: The Economics of Alternative Systems of Finance and Provision* Oxford: Oxford U. Press, pp. 65-98.

Culyer, A.J., and R.G. Evans (1996) Normative Rabbits from Positive Hats: Mark Pauly on Welfare Economics. *Journal of Health Economics* 15(2):243-251.

Davey Smith, G. (1996) Income inequality and mortality: why are they related? *British Medical Journal* 312(7037):987-988.

Editor's choice (1996) The Big Idea. *British Medical Journal* 312(7037):985-986.

Evans, R.G., Barer, M.L. and Stoddart, G.L. (1994) *Charging Peter to Pay Paul: Accounting for the Financial Effects of User Charges*. Toronto:The Premier's Council on Health, Well-being and Social Justice, June.

Evans, R.G., Hodge, M., and Pless, I.B. (1994) If not genetics, then what? Biological pathways and population health. In Evans, R.G., Barer, M.L., and Marmor, T.R., editors, *Why Are Some People Healthy and Others Not?* New York: Aldine de Gruyter, pp. 161-188.

Evans, R.G., Barer, M.L., and Stoddart, G.L. (1995) User fees for health care: why a bad idea keeps coming back (or, what's health got to do with it?). *Canadian Journal on Aging* 14(2):360-90.

Evans, R.G. (1996a) Marketing the market, regulating regulators: Who gains? Who loses? What hopes? What scope? In *Health Care Reform: The Will to Change* OECD Health Policy Studies No. 8, Paris: OECD, pp. 95-114.

Evans, R.G. (1996b) Health, hierarchy, and hominids. In Culyer, A.J. and

Wagstaff, A., editors, *Reforming health care systems: experiments with the NHS* Aldershot: Edward Elgar, pp. 35-64.

Evans, R.G. (1997a) Going for the gold: the redistributive agenda behind market-based health care reform. *Journal of Health Politics, Policy and Law* 22(2):423-466.

Evans, R.G. (1997b) Coarse correction -- and way off target. *Journal of Health Politics, Policy and Law* 22(2):503-508.

Feldstein, M.S. (1973) The welfare loss of excess health insurance. *Journal of Political Economy* 81(2, Part 1):251-280.

Frank, R.H. (1985) *Choosing the Right Pond: Human Behaviour and the Quest for Status.* New York: Oxford.

Frank, R.H. and Cook, P.J. (1995) *The Winner-Take-All Society.* New York: Free Press.

Friedman, M. (1953) The methodology of positive economics. In Friedman, M., editor, *Essays in Positive Economics.* Chicago: University of Chicago Press, pp. 3-43.

Fuchs, V.R. (1996) Economics, Values, and Health Care Reform. *American Economic Review* 86(1):1-24.

Fuchs, V.R. and Hahn, J.S. (1990) How does Canada do it? A comparison of expenditures for physicians' services in the United States and Canada. *New England Journal of Medicine* 323(13):884-90.

Gaynor, M. and Vogt, W.B. (1997) What does economics have to say about health policy anyway? -- A comment and correction on Evans and Rice. *Journal of Health Politics, Policy and Law* 22(2):475-496.

Gerdtham, U-G., and Jönsson, B. (1991) Price and quantity in international comparisons of health care expenditure. *Applied Economics* 23:1519-28.

Giacomini, M. *et al.* (1996) *Financial Incentives in the Canadian Health Care System -- Executive Summary* Hamilton, Ont.: McMaster University Centre for Health Economics and Policy Analysis, 42 p.

Hammond, P.J. (1982) Utilitarianism, uncertainty and information. In Sen, A. and Williams, B., editors *Utilitarianism And Beyond* Cambridge: Cambridge University Press, pp. 85-102.

Hammond, P.J. (1983) Ex-post optimality as a dynamically consistent objective for collective choice under uncertainty. In Pattanaik, P. K. and Salles, M. editors, *Social Choice and Welfare* Amsterdam: North-Holland, pp. 175-205.

Harberger, A.C. (1971) Three basic postulates for applied welfare economics: An interpretive essay. *Journal of Economic Literature* 9:785-797.

Hoffmeyer, U.K., and McCarthy, T.R. (1994) *Financing Health Care* (two vols.) Dordrecht: Kluwer Academic Publishing.

Judge, K. (1995) Income distribution and life expectancy: a critical appraisal. *British Medical Journal* 311:1282-1285.

Kaplan, G.A., Pamuk,, E.R., Lynch, J.W. *et al.* (1996) Inequality in income and mortality in the United States: analysis of mortality and potential pathways. *British Medical Journal* 312(7037):999-1003.

Kennedy, B.P., Kawachi, I., and Prothrow-Stith, D. (1996) Income distribution and mortality: cross section ecological study of the Robin Hood index in the United States. *British Medical Journal* 312(7037):1004-1007.

Kessel, R.A. (1958) Price discrimination in medicine. *Journal of Law and Economics* 1(2):20-53.

Krugman, P.R. (1992) The right, the rich, and the facts: deconstructing the income distribution debate. *The American Prospect* 11(Fall):10-31.

Manning, W.G. Newhouse, J.P., Duan, N., *et al.* (1987) Health Insurance and the demand for medical care: evidence from a randomized trial. *American Economic Review* 77(3):251-77.

Molloy, W. and Guyatt, G. (1991) A comprehensive health care directive in a home for the aged. *Canadian Medical Association Journal* 145 (4):307-11.

Morone, J. (1986) Seven laws of policy analysis. *Journal of Policy Analysis and Management* 5(4):817-819.

Nair, C., Karim, R., and Nyers, C. (1992) Health care and health status: a Canada-United States statistical comparison. *Health Reports* 4:2 (October) Ottawa: Statistics Canada (Cat. no. 82-003), pp. 175-83.

Nelson, R.R., (1981) Assessing private enterprise: an exegesis of tangled doctrine. *Bell Journal of Economics* 12(1):93-111.

OECD (1996) *OECD Health Data 96* Paris: Organization for Economic Cooperation and Development.

Pauly, M.V. (1994a) Editorial: A re-examination of the meaning and importance of supplier-induced demand. *Journal of Health Economics* 13(3):369-72.

Pauly, M.V. (1994b) Reply to Roberta Labelle, Greg Stoddart, and Thomas Rice. *Journal of Health Economics* 13(4):495-496.

Pauly, M.V. (1996) Reply to Anthony J. Culyer and Robert G. Evans. *Journal of Health Economics* 15(2):253-254.

Pauly, M.V. (1997) Who was that straw man anyway? A comment on Evans and Rice. *Journal of Health Politics, Policy and Law* 22(2):467-474.

Redelmeier, D.A. and Fuchs, V.R. (1993) Hospital expenditures in the United

States and Canada. *New England Journal of Medicine* 328(11):772-778.

Reinhardt, U.E. (1992) Reflections on the meaning of *efficiency*: can efficiency be separated from equity? *Yale Law & Policy Review* 10(2):302-315.

Reinhardt U.E. (1998) Abstracting from distributional effects, this policy is efficient. In: Barer, M.L., Getzen, T.E., and Stoddart, G.L., editors, *Health, Health Care and Health Economics: Perspectives on Distribution* London: John Wiley & Sons, Ltd.

Rice, T.H. (1997a) Can markets give us the health system we want? *Journal of Health Politics, Policy and Law* 22(2):383-422.

Rice, T.H. (1997b) A reply to Gaynor and Vogt, and Pauly. *Journal of Health Politics, Policy and Law* 22(2):497-502.

Rice, T.H. (1998) The desirability of market-based health reforms: a reconsideration of economic theory. In: Barer, M.L., Getzen, T.E., and Stoddart, G.L., editors, *Health, Health Care and Health Economics: Perspectives on Distribution* London: John Wiley & Sons, Ltd.

Smeeding, T.M. and Gottschalk, P. (1995) *The International Evidence on Income Distribution in Modern Economies: Where Do We Stand?* Working Paper #13, Maxwell School of Citizenship and Public Affairs, Syracuse University, Syracuse, New York.

Stigler G.J. (1971) The theory of economic regulation. *The Bell Journal of Economics and Management Science* 2(1):3-21.

Support Principal Investigators, The. (1995) A controlled trial to improve care for seriously ill hospitalized patients. The study to understand prognoses and preferences for outcomes and risks of treatment (SUPPORT). *Journal of the American Medical Association* 274(20):1591-1598.

Towse A., editor (1995) *Financing Health Care in the U.K.: A Discussion of NERA's Prototype Model to Replace the NHS.* London: Office of Health Economics. p. 47.

van Doorslaer, E. and Wagstaff, A. (1998) Equity in the finance and delivery of health care: an introduction to the ECuity project. In: Barer, M.L., Getzen, T.E., and Stoddart, G.L., editors, *Health, Health Care and Health Economics: Perspectives on Distribution* London: John Wiley & Sons, Ltd.

Wennberg, J.E. (1992) Innovation and the policies of limits in a changing health care economy. In Gelijns, A.C., editor, *Technology and Health Care in an Era of Limits*. Vol. III of "Medical Innovation at the Crossroads, Institute of Medicine Committee on Technological Innovation in Medicine. Washington, DC: National Academy Press, 9-33.

White, J. (1995) *Competing Solutions: American Health Care Proposals and International Experience.* Washington, DC: Brookings.

Wilkinson, R.G. (1994) *Unfair Shares.* Ilford: Barnardo's.

Williams, A. (1998) If we are going to get a fair innings, someone will need to keep the score! In: Barer, M.L., Getzen, T.E., and Stoddart, G.L., editors, *Health, Health Care and Health Economics: Perspectives on Distribution* London: John Wiley & Sons, Ltd.

Woolhandler, S. and Himmelstein, D.U. (1991) The deteriorating administrative efficiency of the U.S. health care system. *New England Journal of Medicine* 324(18):1253-1258.

APPENDIX

INTERNATIONAL HEALTH ECONOMICS ASSOCIATION

INAUGURAL CONFERENCE
May 19-23, 1996

Hyatt Regency Hotel
Vancouver, British Columbia, Canada

PROGRAMME

SCIENTIFIC PROGRAMME

SUNDAY, MAY 19

09:30-16:30

Critical Appraisal of Clinical Intervention Literature
Faculty: Sam Sheps, Robin Hanvelt

13:30-16:30

Advances in Health Econometrics
Faculty: Willard Manning, Mark McClellan, John Mullahy

The Health Utilities Index and Its Applications
Faculty: George Torrance, William Furlong, David Feeny, Lauren Cuddy

Determinants of Health Populations
Faculty: Clyde Hertzman, Michael Wolfson

Risk-Adjustment: The Achilles Heel of Market Oriented Health Care Reform
Faculty: Wyand van de Ven

Determinants of Health of Populations
Faculty: Clyde Hertzman, Michael Wolfson

MONDAY, MAY 20

08:30-09:00

Opening Remarks
Morris Barer

Welcome on Behalf of the Province of British Columbia
Chris Lovelace

Welcome on Behalf of *i*HEA
Joseph Newhouse

09:00-10:00

Plenary

The New Social Contract for Health Care:
Should Economists Write It or Merely Describe It?
Speaker: Uwe Reinhardt
Chair: Thomas Getzen

10:30-12:00

Concurrent Sessions

Addiction and Youths
Chair: Willard Manning

Christine Godfrey, Matthew Sutton
Young People and Heavy Drinking: Economic and Social Influences
Michael Grossman, Frank Chaloupka, Charles Brown
An Empirical Analysis of Cocaine Addiction
Jody Sindelar, John Mullahy
Employment, Alcohol and Single Mothers

Theoretical Foundations of CEA and CUA in Health Care
Chair: J.-M. Graf von der Schulenburg
Discussant: Amiram Gafni

Joan Rovira
Theoretical Foundations of CEA and CUA in Health Care:
Conclusions of a EU Project
Milton Weinstein, Alan M. Garber, George Torrance
Welfare Economics as a Theoretical Foundation of
Cost-Effectiveness Analysis

Economic Evaluation Methods
Chair: Jeff Richardson

Clive Pritchard
QALYs versus HYEs: Another Look at the Standard Gamble
Walter Ried
QALYs versus HYEs—What's Right and What's Wrong

Janelle Seymour, Alan Shiell, Sue Cameron
Can You Count on HYEs?

Economic Burden of Illness
Chair: Peter Zweifel

Raymond Hutubessey, Maurits van Tulder, Hinrik Vondeling
Indirect Costs of Back Pain in the Netherlands:
Human Capital or Friction Cost Method?
Christian Krauth, Reinhard Busse, Friedrich Schwartz
Indirect Costs of Illness in the Last Year of Life
Elizabeth Savoca
Measuring the Effect of Mental Illness on Earnings

Hospital Costing Applications
Chair: James Butler

Mlika Linna
A Comparative Application of Translog and DEA Methods: The Productive
Efficiency of Finnish Hospitals
Dale McMurchy
Efficiency Studies in South African Public Sector Hospitals
Petia Sevil, Terri Jackson
Medical Costs in DRG-Based Funding Policy: An Evaluation Using Clinical
Costing Data—Australian Perspective

Physician Requirements

Jean M. Mitchell, Jack Hadley
The Effect of Managed Care on Physician Labor Market Behavior
Jack Reamy
Physician Resource Management: The New Brunswick Experience
Ronald Wall, Noralou Roos, David Patton
Needs Based Planning for Manitoba Physicians

Health Care Reform
Chair: Dov Chernichovsky

Tamás Angelus
Health Care Reforms in Hungary

Maureen Lewis
Health Reform in Brazil: Lessons of Reform

Pharmaceutical Sector
Chair: Patricia Danzon

F. Antoñanzas, Joan Rovira, Laura Cabiedes
The Pharmaceutical Reforms in the Context of the Single European Market
Jørgen Clausen
Pharmaceutical Expenditures in OECD Countries—Theoretical Foundations
and Empirical Analysis
Paul Grootendorst, Bernie O'Brien, Geoffrey Anderson
On Becoming 65 in Ontario: Effects of Drug Plan Eligibility on Utilization of
Prescription Medicines

Health Care System Reforms
Chair: Alan Maynard

Colleen Flood
Performance and Prospects of New Zealand's Reformed Health Care System
Peter Hatcher
A Comparative Analysis of New Managed Care Models
Resulting from Reform of British National Health Service
Jenny Hughes, Colm Harmon, Joseph Durkan
Health Service Utilisation Pre and Post Reforms

Health Care Financing—International Approaches
Chair: Jacques van der Gaag

Kieke Okma
Financial Dilemmas in Health Care Policies in The Netherlands
Allan Maslove
Financing Canadian Health Care: New Roads and Dead Ends

13:30-15:00

Concurrent Sessions

Beyond Health Outcomes (Part 1)
Chair: Gavin Mooney

Jan Abel Olsen
Beyond Health Outcomes: For Which Types of Care Might
Which Actors be Willing to Pay?
Mandy Ryan
Using Conjoint Analysis to Go Beyond Health Outcomes:
An Application to In Vitro Fertilization
Alan Shiell
The Value of Community

Economic Evaluation Applications (WTP)
Chair: Robert Woodward

Glenn Blomquist, Rich O'Connor
Eliciting Preferences for Asthma Treatments from Asthmatics
and Non-Asthmatics
Julie Ratcliffe, Mandy Ryan
Using the Closed Ended Willingness to Pay Technique to
Value Alternative Models of Antenatal Care
Marcia Weaver, Michael Chapko, Robert Ndamobiss
Willingness to Pay: A Comparison of Contingent
Valuation and Two-Stage Model Estimates of Health Care Demand

Quality of Life Measurement: Issues and Applications
Chair: George Torrance

Jane Hall
Genetic Screening: Problems in Economic Evaluation
Susanne Wähling, J.-M. Graf von der Schulenburg, Matthias Stoll
Cost and Quality of Life Evaluation of Oral Ganciclovir in
Treating CMV Retinitis

Costing Issues and Applications
Chair: Charles Normand

Susan Bronskill, Marsha Cohen
Diagnostic D&C: Cost Implications of Patterns of Practice
Franco Sassi
The Opportunity Cost of Shared Resources in Joint Production Processes

Myra Siminovitch, Alan Hochstein
Outpatient Physiotherapy Services: An Economic Interpretation
Marjon van der Pol, John Cairns
Economic Analysis of Blood Donor Services in the North of Scotland

Physician Behaviour
Chair: Norman Thurston

Marina Pascali, Morris L. Barer, Robert G. Evans
Cost Control and Physician Behaviour in British Columbia, 1979-90
Randolph Quaye
Doctoring as Business in Sweden
Ronald Wall, Noralou Roos, John Horne
Payment-Modality and Physician Behaviour in Rural Manitoba

Effects of Managed Care
Chair: Michael Morrisey

Laurence Baker
Competition in Health Care Markets: Empirical Evidence from
the US Medicare Program
Patricia Born, Carol Simon, Phillip Kletke
The Impact of Managed Care on Physician Supply
Deborah Freund, Thomas Kniesner, Anthony LoSasso
A Comparison of Count Data Methods Applied to Medicaid Managed Care with
Implications for Health Reform

Technology and Health Care
Chair: Bengt Jönsson

Pedro Barros
Technology Levels and Efficiency in Health Care
Wija Oortwijn, Hindrik Vondeling
Setting Priorities for Health Technology Assessment: The Dutch Discussion
Peter Poulsen
Economic Models of Innovation in the Field of Medical Technology
Development
Hindrik Vondeling, David H. Banta
Cosmetic or Medically Necessary? Reimbursement of Dye-Laser Treatment of
Port Wine Stains and Excimer Laser Treatment of Nearsightedness in the
United States and in the Netherlands

User Fees in Health Care Financing
Chair: Dov Chernichovsky

Stefan Felder
Cost of Dying: Alternatives to Rationing
Marty Makinen, Abdo Yazbeck
User Fees: Findings from Ukraine and Kazakstan
Gerald Rosenthal
How Free is "Free" Care?

Health Insurance and Malpractice Insurance, U.S.

Randall Ellis
Health Premium Payment Systems for State Employees
Timothy Hylan, Maureen Lage, Michael Treglia
Physician Liability Premiums and Statutory Limits to Recovery:
An Empirical Assessment
Richard Miller
Estimating Compensating Differentials for Employer-Provided
Health Insurance Benefits

New Research on Health Policy in the Developing World:
Reports from Three Countries
Chair: Alex Herrin
Discussants: Jacques Van der Gaag, Paul Gertler

Michael Alba
Some Aspects of the Structure of Costs and Production of
Philippine Hospitals:
Inferences from Translog Variable Cost Function Estimates
John Anyanwu
Markets for Health Care in Nigeria: A Demand Analysis
Gaspard Munishi
Response to Privatization of Health Care in Tanzania

15:30-17:00

Concurrent Sessions

Economic Evaluation Methods
Chair: Alan Williams

Christa Claes, J.-M. Graf von der Schulenburg, Wolfgang Greiner
The German Version of the EuroQol Questionnaire—
A Tool for Quality of Life Research in Cost-Utility-Analyses
Julia Fox-Rushby, Melissa Parker
Cross-Cultural Measures of Health-Related Quality of Life: The Ultimate
Outcome Measure for Health Economists?
Harri Sintonen
Why To Use the 15D in Economic Evaluation of Health Programs?

Economics Evaluation Applications
Chair: Alan Maynard

Philippe Beutels, Pierre van Damme, Eddy van Doorslaer
Cost-Effectiveness Analysis of Hepatitis B in Belgium
Douglas Bradham, Andrea Ebbers, Margaret Dailey
Cost Analysis of Teen Sexual Activity and Pregnancy for a Rural Country
Stirling Bryan, Jacqueline Brown, Ruth Warren
Efficiency in the Delivery of Mammography Screening Programmes: An
Empirical Investigation

Comparative Health System Reforms
Chair: Alexander Preker

Kenneth Cahill, Kathryn Langwell
Health Sector Reform in Emerging Market Countries:
Similar Problems, Different Paths
Amparo Gordillo, Ruben Suarez
Efficiency and Equity of National Health Systems in Latin America: A
Comparative Study
Holly Wong
The Policy Process: Achieving Health Sector Reforms

Beyond Health Outcomes (Part 2)
Chair: Robert G. Evans, Gavin Mooney

Jan Abel Olsen, Mandy Ryan, Alan Shiell
Panel Discussion

Economic Stress and Health
Chair: Cameron Mustard

Timothy McBride
Uninsured Spells for the Poor: Impact of Spells
on Health and Health Utilization
Roger Roberge, J.M. Berthelot, M.C. Wolfson
Calculating Population Health Status: A Population Health Index

Health Care Reforms in China and Taiwan
Chair: William Hsiao

Gerald Bloom, Xing-yuan Gu
The Need for Strategic Analysis of Reform Options: Lessons from China
Chunhuei Chi, Jwo-Leun Lee
An Evaluation of Taiwan's National Health Insurance's
Impact on Health Care Utilization
Xiao-wan Wang
Overview of Chinese Workers' Medical Insurance Reform

International Comparison of Health Care System Performance
Chair: Jean-Pierre Poullier

Pedro Barros
The Black Box of Health Care Expenditure Growth Determinants
David Parkin, Mark Deverill, Dennis O'Mullane
Designing a Health System: A Model of the Production of
Dental Care and Dental Health
Joan Rovira, Ian Blasco, Karin de Wildt
Defining a Standard Framework for Describing Health Care
Systems from an Economic Perspective

Modelling
Chair: Michael Morrisey

Derek DeLia
Positive Aspects of Health Insurance Purchase and Maintenance
Neil Rickman, Alistair McGuire
The Optimal Regulation of Physician Effort
in a Mixed Market for Health Care
Ed Westerhout, Frank Van Tulder, Kees Folmer
A Model for the Dutch Health Care Sector

Issues in Costing in Economic Appraisal
Chair: Frans Rutten
Discussant: Evi Hatziandreu

Michael Drummond
Issues in the International Transferability of Cost Data
Marc Koopmanschap, L. van Roijen
Indirect Costs: From Aggregate to Study Specific Estimates
Ben van Hout, J. Al Maiwenn, Eddy van Doorslaer
Taking Account of Prior Knowledge in the Assessment of Costs
Alongside a Clinical Trial

Recent Advances in Econometrics
Chair: Andrew Jones

John Mullahy
Instrumental Variable Estimation of Count Data Models—
Applications to Models of Cigarette Smoking Behaviour
Volker Ulrich
An Econometric Model of the Two-Part Decision Making Process
in the Demand for Health Care

TUESDAY, MAY 21

8:30-10:00

Plenary

Equity in the Finance and Delivery of Health Care in Europe and the U.S.: Preliminary Results from an International Comparison
Speaker: Adam Wagstaff, Eddy van Doorslaer
Chair: Andrew Jones

Conceptual Issues Concerning the Equity/Efficiency Trade-Off
Speaker: Alan Williams
Chair: Andrew Jones

10:30-12:00

Concurrent Sessions

Hospital Productivity and Quality of Care
Chair: Pierre-Jean Lancry

B. Dervaux, G. Escano, H. Leleu, et al.
Measuring and Explaining Efficiency in French Hospitals with Quality
Assessments (Part 1)
Stephane Jacobzone, Y. Merliere
Measuring and Explaining Efficiency in French Hospitals with Quality
Assessments (Part 2)
J.F. Burgess, P.W. Wilson
Impact of Measuring Quality of Care on Malmquist
Decompositions of Hospital Productivity Changes
P. Roos
Index Approaches for the Measurement of Hospital Productivity,
Efficiency and Quality

Reconsidering the Theoretical Foundations of Health Economics
Chair: Anthony Culyer
Discussant: Uwe Reinhardt

Jeremiah Hurley
Welfarist and Extra-Welfarist Approaches to Evaluative Economic
Analysis in the Health Sector
Gavin Mooney
A Communitarian Critique of Health Economics
Thomas Rice
The Desirability of Market-Based Health Reforms:
A Reconsideration of Economic Theory

**The Economic Impacts of Government Policies on
Women's Reproductive Choices**
Chair: Deborah Haas-Wilson
Discussant: Robert Ohsfeldt

Deborah Haas-Wilson
Women's Reproductive Choices: The Impact of Federal
and State Reproductive Policies
Catherine Jackson, Jacob Klerman
Welfare and American Fertility
David Ribar, Stephen Matthews
The Effects of Economic Conditions and Access
to Reproductive Health Services on State Abortion and Birth Rates

Economic Evaluation Applications
Chair: Bill Furlong

Herman Ader, Hindrik Vondeling
Confidence Intervals for Cost-Effectiveness Ratios: The Case of a RCT
Comparing Epidural and Intramuscular Pain Treatment
Mária do Rosário Giraldes, Maria de Fátima Geada
Economic Evaluation of Prevention of Diabetic Nephropathy in Portugal
Sandra Vick, John Cairns
An Economic Evaluation of Antenatal Anti-D Prophylaxis in Scotland

Economic Evaluation Methods
Chair: Glenn Blomquist

Han Bleichrodt, Magnus Johanneson
Experimental Results on the Ranking Properties of QALYs

James Butler
Measuring Preferences Over Health State: QALYs and Willingness-to-Pay
Pekka Rissanen, Seppo Aro
Production of HRQOL in Hip and Knee Replacements

Comparative Economic Strategy in Reforming Health Care for Low Income Populations
Chair: Dean Jamison
Discussant: Jacques Van der Gaag

Max Price
Should National Health Insurance Fund Primary or Hospital Care? Health
Financing Reform Strategies in Post Apartheid South Africa
Yuanli Liu
Is Community Financing Necessary and Feasible for Rural China?
Gaspard Munishi
Title Unavailable

HMOs: Performance and Effects
Chair: Willard Manning

Patricia Born
Profit Status and the Operating Performance of
Health Maintenance Organizations
Jean Mitchell, Jack Hadley
The Effect of Economic and Other Nonclinical Factors on
Treatment Choice for Breast Cancer

Health Insurance—International Experience
Chair: Randall Ellis

Frederik Schut, René van Vliet
Premium Elasticities of Health Insurer Choice
Carlos Antonio Tan, Orville Solon, Paul Gertler
Estimating the Welfare Effects of Insurance Coverage
Norman Thurston
A Normative Approach to Evaluating the Decline in
Employment-Based Health Insurance

Work and Health
Chair: Clyde Hertzman

Stan Finkelstein, Ernst Berndt
Occupation-Illness Mapping
Paul Greenberg, Ernst Berndt, Stan Finkelstein
Objective Evidence of the Effects of Health Status on Worker Productivity
Winfried Pohlmeier, Sikandar Siddiqui
The Impact of Health on Retirement Behaviour:
Empirical Evidence from West Germany

12:00-13:30

Arrow Award Presentation
Chair: Richard J. Arnould
Presentation of Award: Mark Pauly
Award Recipients: Martin Gaynor, Paul Gertler
"Moral Hazard and Risk Spreading in Partnerships"
RAND Journal of Economics, Vol. 26

13:30-15:00

Concurrent Sessions

Risk Adjustment: Part 1: The State of the Art
Chair: Wynand van de Ven
Discussants: Mark Hornbrook, Peter Zweifel

Joseph Newhouse
Reimbursing Health Plans and Health Providers:
Selection versus Efficiency in Production

Access to Care
Chair: J.-Matthias Graf von der Schulenburg

Nancy Breen
Race, Class and Access to Breast Cancer Care
Anupama Ramabhadran
Problem of Urban-Rural Inequity in Access to Health Care in the US

Economic Evaluation Applications
Chair: Douglas Bradham

Urpo Kiiskinen
Economic Evaluation of Health Promotion Activities:
Incorporating Epidemiologic and Economic Perspectives
Bupendra Makan, Max Bachmann, Dale McMurchy
An Economic Evaluation of Community Health Worker (CHW)
Programmes in the Western Cape Provinces in South Africa
Jacqueline Roberts, Gina Browne, Carolyn Byrne
Lessons From Studies Examining Community Approaches to Care: More
Effective and Less Expensive
Marion Haas, Jane Hall, Rosalie Viney
Applying Economic Evaluation to Health Care Reform

Distributional Considerations in Health Care Financing—
International Experience
Chair: Pedro Barros

David Mayston
Disadvantaged Populations and the Distribution of Health Care Financing
Diane McIntyre, Gerald Bloom
Inequities in Health Care Financing and Expenditure in South Africa
Abdo Yazbeck, John Langenbruner
Who is Paying for Health Care in Kazakstan?
Results from a Household Survey in South Kazakstan

Guidelines for Cost-Effectiveness in Health and Medicine:
The Washington Panel
Chair: George Torrance

Joseph Lipscomb
Time Preference and Discounting
Bryan Luce
Measurement of Costs
Willard Manning
Uncertainty, Sensitivity Analysis and Statistical Analysis
George Torrance
Measurement of Outcomes

Milton Weinstein
Components Belonging in the Numerator and the Denominator of a Cost-
Effectiveness Ratio

Hospital Efficiency and Financing
Chair: Gerald Rosenthal

Eulalia Dalmau-Matarrodona, Jaume Puig-Junoy
Market Structure and Hospital Efficiency: An Evaluation of
the Potential Effects of De-Regulation in a National Health Service
Philip Jacobs, Judith Lave, Kyung Bay
The Economic Impact of Case Mix Funding in Canada
Elena Sanchez-Ruano, David Vivas
Efficiency and Quality Measurement in Hospital Acute Units:
A Multi-Criteria Model

Technology, Research and the Policy Process
Chair: Steve Fox

Stephen Lewis, Catherine Fooks
Great Product, Few Sales: Strategies for Marketing Research
Hannu Valtonen, Pirjo Koivukangas
Welfare Cluster—A New Conceptualization of Relations in the Health Field

Pricing in Health Care Markets
Chair: Jean-Pierre Poullier

Luke Connelly, Darrel Doessel
The Effect of Producer Concentration on the Prices of General Practitioner
Services: Theory and Australian Evidence
Patricia Danzon
Pharmaceutical Price Inflation: A Cross-National Comparison
John Brooks, Avi Dor, Herbert Wong
The Hospital-Insurer Interaction as a Bargaining Process: An Empirical
Investigation of Appendectomy Pricing

Quality of Life and Utility
Chair: Ariel Beresniak
Discussant: Marie-Odile Carrere

G. Duru, M.O. Carrere, A. Beresniak, et al.
Multi-Attribute Utility Theory: Validation Methods and Studies
L. Eeckhoudt
Multidimensional Utility, Multiple Risks and the Health Risk Premiums
S. Haddad, D. Reinharz, A. Beresniak, et al.
The Development and Evaluation of an Analytical Grill for
Measuring Quality of Life and Social Preferences
Y. Yfantopoulos, N. Nicoloyannis, A. Beresniak, et al.
The Construction of a Cardinal Utility Based on Profiles Obtained
in a Quality of Life Questionnaire—Applied to SF36

Economic Appraisal in Developing Countries
Chair: Julia Fox-Rushby
Discussant: John Hutton

Moses Aikins, J. Fox-Rushby, A. Mills
Cost-Effectiveness Analysis of the Gambian National
Impregnated Mosquito Net Programme
David B. Evans
Research and Development Priorities and Cost-Effectiveness Analysis: An
Application to Vaccine Development
Joses Kirigia
A Cost-Utility Decision Analysis Model:
Applied to Schistosomiasis Problem in Kenya

Physician Behaviour
Chair: Martin Gaynor

David Dranove, Carol Simon, William White
Physician Earning Under Managed Care
Christopher Ferrall, Allan Gregory, William Tholl
Endogenous Work Hours and Practice Patterns of Canadian Physicians
Tami Mark, Martin Gaynor
Contracting with Health Plans and Physician Practice Patterns
Sherwin Rosen, Thomas Tenerelli
The Market for Physicians

15:30-17:00

Concurrent Sessions

Risk Adjustment: Part 2: New Empirical and Theoretical Studies
Chair: Wynand Van de Ven

Susan L. Ettner, Richard Frank, Thomas McGuire, et al.
Risk Adjustment of Mental Health and Substance Abuse Payments
Leida M. Lamers
The Predictive Accuracy of Risk-Adjusted Capitation Payments Based on
Diagnostic Information: An Empirical Evaluation Using Both Claims and
Health Survey Data
Thomas McGuire, Jacob Glazer
Optimal Risk Adjustment of Health Insurance Premiums for Managed Care

Economic Burden of Illness
Chair: Charles Normand

Nicholas Graves, Rosalind Plowman, Jennifer Roberts
How Can Information on the Extent and Distribution of the
Economic Burdens of Nosocomial Infections
Assist Purchasers and Providers of Health Care to
Realise Their Objectives?
Rosanna Tarricone, Giovanni Fattore
The Economic Burden of Major Depression

Health Care Reform—Eastern Europe and Former Soviet Union
Chair: Alexander Preker

Dov Chernichovsky
Incquality of Health Finance, Resources and Mortality in Russia: Potential
Implications for Health and Medical Care
Marty Makinen, Alexander Telyukov
The Fund Flow Analysis for Mandatory Health Insurance:
The Case of Issyk-Kul Oblast, Kyrgyzstan

Regionalization and Redistribution: International Experiences
Chair: Anne Mills

Peter Bundred, Peter Todd
The Economics and Equitable Distribution of Cardiac Interventions
in the British Health Service:
How One Health District Approached These Problems
Joseph Capuno
Decentralization, Efficiency and the Public Choice Aspect of Local Health
Expenditures in the Philippines
Jane Doherty, Alex van den Heever
Territorial Justice in South Africa: The Role of a Formula

Physician Decision-Making
Chair: David Feeny

William Johnson, Marjorie Baldwin, Antonio Campos
Physician Career Decisions: The Pathways to Practice
Raymond Pong, Karatholuvu Nagarajan
Equal Access?: A Comparative Study of Rural Physician
Recruitment Strategies Among Canadian Provinces
Douglas Bunn
The Referral Decision: Is Quality of Care Being Compromised?

Evaluations of U.S. Health Care Policies
Chair: Anthony T. LoSasso

Patricia Born, Sara Thran
The Impact of CLIA-88 on Physician Office Laboratories
Gestur Davidson, Shawn Welch, George Hoffman
The Impact of Subsidized Health Insurance on Welfare
Sally Stearns, Thomas Mroz
Patterns of Care and Effects of Case Management for
Persons with Chronic Diseases

Determining Values for Economic Evaluation:
The Use of the Person Trade-Off
Chair: Alan Williams

Erik Nord
Why Measure with the Person Trade-Off?

Jan Abel Olsen
Applying the PTO to Derive Equity Weights:
The Case of Remaining Life Years
Jose-Luis Pinto
The Validity of the Person Trade-Off Technique
as a Measure of Social Value
Jeff Richardson, Erik Nord
Personal Versus Impersonal Perspective: A Comparison of Four Instruments

Internal Markets
Chair: Stuart Altman

Toni Ashton
Contracting for Health Services in New Zealand: Early Experiences
Bengt Jönsson, Clas Rehnberg
Internal Markets in the Swedish Health Care System
Alan Maynard, Karen Bloor
Health Care Reform in the UK National Health Service

Equity Implications of Health Care Reforms
Chair: Eddy van Doorslaer

Michael Gerfin, Robert E. Leu
Changing Inequity in the Finance and Delivery of Health Care in Switzerland
During the 1980s
Jan Klavus, Unto Häkkinen
Micro-Level Analysis of Distributional Changes in Health Care Financing
Hattem van der Burg, Eddy van Doorslaer, René van Vliet
Distributional Consequences of Proportional Copayments:
An Analysis of Their Proposed Introduction
in the Dutch Public Health Insurance
Adam Wagstaff, Eddy van Doorslaer
Equity and Health Care Reform: Reforms to Date and Their
Likely Equity Consequence

Guidelines Standards for Economic Evaluation
Chair: Michael Drummond

Tom Jefferson, Michael Drummond
Guidelines for Peer Review of Economic Submissions to Medical Journals

Jean-Francois Baladi, Nick Otten, Devidas Menon
Guidelines and Pharmacoeconomic Studies:
The First Year's Experience in Canada
Bryan Luce
Existing Guidelines and Standards: Areas of Consensus and Debate
Joan Rovira
Harmonization of Guidelines: The European Approach

National Health Accounts
Chair: Thomas Getzen
Discussant: Charlotte Leighton

Peter Berman
National Health Accounts in Developing Countries:
Appropriate Methods and Recent Applications
Alejandro Herrin, Orville Solon, Rachel Racelis
The Philippine National Health Accounts: Lessons Learned
William McGreevey
The Development of National Health Accounts
in the People's Republic of China
Jean-Pierre Poullier
The Development of Methods and Standards
for International Comparative Health Expenditure Statistics
Daniel Waldo
Title Unavailable

WEDNESDAY, MAY 22

8:30-10:30

Concurrent Sessions

Issues in Resource Allocation
Chair: Eddy van Doorslaer

Joanna Coast, Richard Smith
Implicit Rationing: Utility of Ignorance

Brian Ferguson, Russell Mannion, Kirsteen Smith
The Nature of the Commodity "Social Care" and its Efficient Allocation
Sujha Subramanian
How Homogeneous is the Distribution of New AIDS Cases in Tanzania?

Economic Evaluation Applications
Chair: Karatholuvu Nagarajan

Tami Axcell, Wendy Young
Cost Savings Resulting from a Shift from Inpatient to Outpatient Service
for Same Day Surgery
Qing Chen, Robert Kane
The Cost Effectiveness of Institutional Post-Hospital Care for Medicare
Beneficiaries with Stroke and Hip Fractures
Joyce Huber, Margo Rosenbach, Mary Lawrence Cawthon
Prenatal Substance Abuse Treatment and Infant Medical Costs
in a Medicaid Population
Mingliang Zhang, Kathryn Rost, John Fortney
The Economic Utilization Analysis of Government Health Expenditure
in 114 Poor Rural Counties of China

Economic Evaluation Methods
Chair: Robert Woodward

Andrew Briggs, Bernie O'Brien
A Portfolio Approach to Cost-Effectiveness League Tables
Douglas Coyle, Michael Drummond
Analysing Differences in the Costs of Treatment Across Centres Within
Economic Evaluations
Dorte Gyrd-Hansen, Jes Søgaard
Discounting Life-Years: Whither Time Preference

Physician Service Use and Expenditures
Chair: David Kindig

Sajal Chattopadhyay
Utilization of Physicians' Services in the United States: 1960-1993
Vivian Hamilton, Barton Hamilton, Harry J. Paarsch
Access, Utilization and Equity in Canada and the US:
An Empirical Model of Physician Visits

Jeffrey Stoddard, Bradley Gray, David Kindig
Specialists and US Health Expenditures

Demand/Choice of Provider
Chair: David Bunting

John Fortney, Kathryn Rost, Mingliang Zhang
Modelling the Decision to Seek Treatment for Depression
and Choice of Provider Sector
David Hotchkiss
The Tradeoff Between Price and Quality: An Empirical Analysis
of the Demand for Obstetric Care in Cebu, Philippines
Winnie Yip, Peter Berman
Quality as a Determinant in Patients' Choice of Provider in Egypt

Incentives and Organizational Behaviour
Chair: Timothy Hylan

V.K. Chetty
Value of Life in a General Equilibrium Model with Strategic Behaviour
Ravinder Dhawan
Encouraging HMO Use—A Multi Sector Analysis
Rajiv Sharma
Cost Incentives in Health Care

Health System Reforms in Former Socialist Economies
Chair: Dov Chernichovsky
Discussant: James Rice

Antonio Campos, Richard Saltman
Health Reform in Western Former Soviet Union:
Foreseeing the Outcome and Neglecting the Process
Dov Chernichovsky, Tatiana Kirsanova, Elena Potapchik
Basic Financial and Administrative Mechanisms Necessary
to Achieve Health System Reform
Under the Russian Health Insurance Legislation
William McGreevey
Chinese Puzzles

Alexander Preker
The Transition and the Health Sector:
Trends in Health Services and Health Care Financing
in Central and Eastern Europe During the 1990s

Social Exclusion and Access to Health Care
Chair: Pierre-Jean Lancry
Discussant: Lise Rochaix

Marie-Christine Closon
How to Avoid a Risk of Social Exclusion
in a Hospital Prospective Payment System
Jacob Feldman, Diane M. Makuc
Socioeconomic Differentials in Heart Disease Services and Survival
Lise Rochaix, Andree Mizrahi, Ari Mizrahi
Effects of Health Insurance Coverage on Access to Care

13:30-15:00

Concurrent Sessions

The Economic Impacts of Proposed Medicare Reforms
Chair: James Rodgers
Discussant: Robert Helms

Allen Dobson
The Financial Future of the American Hospital Industry
Kurt Gillis
The Impacts of Medicare Payment Reforms on Physicians
Jack Rodgers
Distributional Analysis of Medicare Reforms
Physician Decision-Making: Motivations and Incentives
Chair: Albert Okunade

Ivar Sonbo Kristiansen
Understanding the Motivation of Doctors:
A Review of Economic Modelling of Doctors' Behaviour
Anthony Scott
Agency, Incentives and Doctor Behaviour:
What Do We Want Doctors to Do and How Do We Get Them to Do It?

Norman Thurston
Physician Behavioral Responses to Variations
in Marginal Income Tax Rates: Longitudinal Evidence

Determinants of Risk
Chair: Konstantin Beck

Mark Hornbrook
Ambulatory Dispensed Drugs as Predictors of Medical Risk
Murielle Lona, Paul Kestens, Jean-Mar Laasman
Belgium: A Long Way to the Reforms

Income and Health
Chair: Cameron Mustard

Terkel Christiansen
Socio-Economic Inequalities in Health: Results from Two Danish Surveys
Gun Sundberg, Ulf-G. Gerdtham
Measuring Income-Related Health Inequalities in Sweden
Thomas Wan, Charles Shasky, George Wan
Racial and Socioeconomic Disparities
in Health Status and Health Services Use

Health Human Resources
Chair: Ronald Wall

Bupendra Makan, Max Bachmann, Dale McMurchy
Health Care Human Resources:
The Issue of Differential Salaries and Options for Parity
Dennis Shea, Bruce Stuart
Rural Physician Use and Measures of Physician Availability

Approaches to Distributing Treatment Capacity
Chair: Michael Farnworth

Paul Boumbulian, Scott Rowand
Pushing the Boundaries of Health Care: The Journey Upstream
Peter Todd, Peter Bundred, Helen Forbes
Modelling the Consequences of Service Development
Within the UK "Internal" Health Market

Jerry Vila
Hospital Referral System: A Tool for Equitable Distribution of
Health Care Resources

Hospital Costs, Quality and Reimbursement
Chair: Jack Boan

Reiner Hellbrück
Quality Assurance in Germany and Resource Allocation
Katrien Kesteloot, Natalie Voet
Incentives for Cooperation in Quality Improvement Among Hospitals—
Impact of the Reimbursement System
Neil Soderlund, Alastair Gray, James Raftery
The Impact of the British NHS Reforms on Hospital Costs—
An Analysis of the First 3 Years

Economic Evaluation: Applications
Chair: Anne Mills

Dyna Carol Arhin
Health Insurance Demand in Ghana: A Contingent Valuation
Frank Sloan, Kip Viscusi, Harrell Chesson, et al.
Alternative Approaches to Valuing Intangible Loss From Multiple Sclerosis

Economic Analysis of China's Health Care
Chair: Teh-Wei Hu
Discussant: Shan Cretin

Xingzhu Liu, Ningshan Chen, Shushan Dong
Estimation of Unit Cost of Medical Services
Yuanli Liu, Winnie Yip, Wei Ying
Investigating Efficiency in Health Care for China's Rural Poor: A Stochastic
Frontier Approach
Hong Wang, Winnie Yip
Analysis of Demand in Poor Rural China: Implications for Financing and
Organizing Health Care
Winnie Yip, William Hsiao
Urban Health Finance Reform in China

Economic Evaluation Applications
Chair: Frans Rutten

Phil Shackley, John Cairns
Using Decision Analysis to Value the Benefits of Antenatal Screening
Saradha Suresh
Cost Effectiveness of Two Regimens of Treatment
for Pulmonary Tuberculosis in the Community

15:30-17:00

Concurrent Sessions

Economic Evaluation Methods
Chair: Pierre-Jean Lancry

Han Bleichrodt
Health Utility Indices and Equity Considerations
Han Bleichrodt, Magnus Johannesson, Peter Wakker
Characterizing QALYs By Means of Risk Neutrality
Paul Dolan, Angela Robinson
The Allocation of Benefits in Health Care: Does Equity Matter?

Approaches to Risk Adjustment
Chair: Peter Zweifel

Konstantin Beck, Peter Zweifel
Cream-Skimming in Deregulated Social Health Insurance: Evidence from
Switzerland
Emmett Keeler, Grace Carter, Joseph Newhouse
A Model of the Impact of Reimbursement Schemes on Health Plan Choices
Erik Van Barneveld, Leida Lamers, René Van Vliet
Mandatory Pooling Arrangements as a Supplement
to Capitation Payments for Competing Health Insurers
Wynand Van de Ven, Erik Van Barneveld, Frederik Schut
Risk-Adjustment: A Necessary Complement to Open Enrollment and
Rate-Banding in a Competitive Health Insurance Market

Competitive Health Care Reforms
Chair: Peter Hatcher

Robert Leu, Jürg Sommer
Competitive Reforms in Health Care: The Case of Switzerland
Claude Schneider-Bunner
Equity in Managed Competition

Patient Decision-Making
Chair: Winnie Yip

Raisa Deber, Nancy Kraetschmer
Patient or Consumer? What Role do Sick People Wish to Play in Making
Treatment Decisions?
Ulrika Enemark
The Role of Regret in Medical Decision-Making

Economics of Pharmaceuticals
Chair: Aslam Anis

Joanna Coast, Richard Smith, Michael Millar
Resistance: The Opportunity Cost of Antibiotic Treatment
Marisa Domino
The Role of Prices in the Demand for Pharmaceuticals
Christine Huttin, Jerry Avorn
Drug Expenditures for Hypertension:
An Empirical Test of a Disease-Economic Model in a French Population
Naoki Ikegami, Hiroki Kawai, Seiritsu Ogura
The Paradox of Decreasing Prices and Increasing Costs for Drugs in Japan

Age and the Use of Health Care
Chair: Sikandar Siddiqui

Dorota Girard
Time Profiles of Medical Consumption of Elderly
Volker Ulrich, Manfred Erbsland, Walter Ried
The Impact of Double Aging on Health Care Expenditure and
the Contribution Rate: Simulation Results for the
German Statutory Health Insurance

Issues in U.S. Hospital Financing
Chair: Norman Thurston

Billie Ann Brotman, Morris Roberts
Charity Care Funded by Georgia Hospitals
Cyril Chang
Uncompensated Hospital Care Before and After TennCare

Nursing Home Economics
Chair: Jack Boan

Craig Copeland, Richard Arnould, Lawrence DeBrock
Excess Capacity and Equilibrium Quality Choice in Nursing Homes
Laura Miller, Sabrina Su, Ronald Ozminkowski
Fair Rental Systems and the Asset Value of Nursing Homes

Approaches to Health Care Reform in Transition Economies
Chair: Alexander Preker

Dov Chernichovsky, William Hsiao, Alexander Preker
Panel Discussion

THURSDAY, MAY 23

08:30-10:00

Concurrent Sessions

Economic Evaluation Applications
Chair: Frans Rutten

Eddy Adang, Cor Baeten, Gerard Engel
Cost-Effectiveness of Dynamic Graciloplasty in The Netherlands
Marjorie Baldwin, William Johnson
The Relative Cost Effectiveness of Chiropractic and Physician Care in the
Treatment of Back Pain
Nobuo Koinuma
Cost-Benefit Analysis of Stomach-Cancer Treatment

Economic Evaluation Methods
Chair: Frank Sloan

Han Bleichrodt
Explaining the Disparity Between Extreme and Assorted Gambles
Philip Clarke
Cost Benefit Analysis of Mammographic Screening:
A Travel Cost Approach
Robert Woodward, Larry Kvols, Mark Schnitzler
Reduced Uncertainty as a Benefit in the Cost-Effectiveness of Diagnostic
Procedures: Detecting Carcinoid Tumors

Hospital Costing Applications
Chair: Franco Sassi

Peter Coyte, Wendy Young
Estimated Hospital Costs for Patients Receiving Home Care
Following Joint Replacements
Keith Tolley, Marlene Gyldmark, Max Good
Cost Standardisation, Diagnosis Related Groups and the Financing
of HIV/AIDS Hospital Care Within the European Nation
Wendy Young, Marsha Cohen
Costs for Hospitals for Hysterectomies Vary by Surgical Approach

Changing Drug Prescribing Behaviour
Chair: Aslam Anis

Patricia Danzon
Reference Pricing and Physician Drug Budgets: Lessons from Germany
James Wright, Carl Whiteside, Malcolm Maclure
Impact of Educational Interventions on Drug Prescribing

Effects of Fee Schedule Reform
Chair: David Kindig

Niccie McKay, Fred Dorner
Volume Effects of a Change in the Texas Medicaid Fee Schedule
Albert Okunade, Ann Patterson
Medicare Physician-Payment Reform and
the Utilization of Cardiovascular Procedures

J.M. Porter, Peter Coyte, Jan Barnsley
The Effects of Fee Item Restructuring on Dental Utilization

Economic Issues in Breast Screening
Chair: Jane Hall

Martin Brown
Direct and Induced Costs of Mammography: An International
Perspective
Karen Gerard, Kathy Johnston, Alison Morton
From Trial to Policy: Evaluation of Options for the UK Breast Screening
Programme
Tamara Stoner, Bryan Dowd
Do Vouchers Reduce Financial Barriers to Mammography?

Changes in Patterns of Health Care Use in Finland
Chair: Harri Sintonen

Unto Häkkinen, Gunnar Rosenqvist, Seppo Aro
Economic Recession and the Use of Physician Services
Kalevi Luoma, Maijo-Liisa Järviö, Ilpo Suoniemi
Financial Incentives and Productivity Change in
Finnish Health Centres, 1989-1993

Diverse Economic Strategies in Reforming the Health Sector

Tung-Liang Chiang
Recent Health Care Reform in Taiwan:
Searching for an Efficient and Socially Affordable
Universal Health Insurance Program
William Hsiao
Can Medical Savings Accounts Contain Cost Inflation—The Singaporean
Experience
Juan Luis Londoño
Managed Competition in the Tropics?

The Organization of Medical Practice
in the Brave New World of Managed Care
Chair: Richard Hirth

Jose Escarce
Economies of Scale in Physician Practice
Martin Gaynor, James Rebitzer
Rational Incentives for a Not Quite Rational World:
Group Norms and Optimal Pay Systems in Physician Groups
Frank Mathewson, Carol Simon
An Empirical Analysis of Buying Groups in Medicine

10:30-12:00

Concurrent Sessions

Economic Evaluation Methods
Chair: Han Bleichrodt

Lieven Annemans
Combining Willingness to Pay of Individuals and Private/Public Payers to
Estimate Optimal Price and Reimbursement Ranges for New Drug Therapies
Stefan Felder, Markus Meier
Demand for Health Care Services in the Last Years of Life
Walter Ried
Willingness to Pay, Cost of Illness, and the Human Capital Approach
in Health Care—A Comparative Study for Pure Morbidity Effects

Income and Health Care Use—International Experience
Chair: Thomas Getzen

Xing-Yuan Gu, Sheng-Lan Tang
Equity of Utilization of Health Services in China
Cameron Mustard, Marian Shanahan
Consumption of Insured Health Care Services in Relation to Household Income
in a Canadian Province
Kailas Sarap
Factors Affecting Access to Health Care: An Analysis Based on Primary Data
from Two Villages in Orissa, India

Smoking Behaviour
Chair: Naoki Ikegami

Dave Buck, Matt Sutton
An Economic Model of Variations in Smoking Behaviour
Sandra Decker, Amy Schwartz
Cigarettes, Alcohol and Taxation: Complementarities in Consumption
Heini Salo, Markku Pekurinen
Rational Addiction and the Demand for Cigarettes in Finland:
An Empirical Analysis

Waiting Lists
Chair: Andrew Jones

Michael Farnworth
An Equilibrium Model of Waiting Lists
Barton Hamilton, Vivian Hamilton, Dana Goldman
Queuing for Surgery: Is the US or Canada Worse Off?
Ronald Ozminkowski, Andrea Hassol, Alan White
Access to Multiple Waiting Lists for Kidney Transplants

Economic Evaluation Applications
Chair: David Feeny

Krista Huybrechts, Eric Souêtre
Economic Evaluation of Risperidone in the Context of an International
Schizophrenia Clinical Trial
Xiao-wan Wang, Kan Yang
A Comparing Research of Two Antihypertensive Drugs on
the Patient's Quality of Life and Cost-Effectiveness

Child Health Production
Chair: Gavin Mooney

David Bishai
Quality Time: How Parental Schooling Affects Child Health Through its
Interaction with Childcare Time in Bangladesh
David Salkever, Alison Jones, Deborah Miller
Parental Alcohol Use and Child Health Production

International Studies of Demand
Chair: Charles Normand

David Bunting
Distribution and the Income Elasticity of Demand for Health Care
Chee-Ruey Hsieh, Shin-Jong Lin
Health Information and Preventive Care for the Elderly in Taiwan
Stephane Jacobzone, Pascale Genier
Risk Bearing, Demand for Preventive Care and Human Capital

Issues in Long Term Care Financing

August Österle
Equity in the Finance of Long-Term Care and
the Role of Informal Care-Giving
James Reschovsky
The Use of Paid Home Care by the Disabled Elderly:
A Simultaneous Equations Approach
Shelley White-Means, Gong-Soog Hong
Health and Well-Being of Adult Child Caregivers

The Behaviour and Potential of the Private Health Sector in Developing Countries
Chair: Anne Mills
Discussant: Peter Berman

Sara Bennett, Viroj Tangcharoensathien
The Nature of Competition Amongst Private Hospitals in Bangkok
M.R. Bhatia
Contracting Out of Dietary Services by Public Hospitals in Bombay, India
Jonathan Broomberg
To Purchase or to Provide? The Relative Efficiency of Contracting Out versus
Direct Public Provision of Hospital Services in South Africa

13:15-15:00

Plenary

Toward a Healthier Economics
Speaker: Robert G. Evans

Index

Page numbers followed by *n* refer to footnotes.

income (*cont.*)
    health inequalities related to 192–8, 469
        cross-national comparisons 195–8, 203–4
        measurement 193–5
        principles 192–3
        in rural China 238–9
        in Sweden 119–36
        in US 196–8, 486
        inequality, in Finland 149, 150, 152
        and insured health care use, in Canada 23–
            4, 157–75
        in Manitoba, Canada 165–6
        Medicare health plan choice and 225,
            227
        redistribution 426–9
        relative 422–3, 469
Income Distribution Statistics (IDS) 146
incremental analysis 347
individuals 365, 399
    preferences, *see* preferences, individual
    tastes, *see* tastes
inequity, *see* equity
infant health, Australian Aborigines 65–6
infant mortality
    Australian Aborigines 55–6
    in China 235, 237
infectious diseases, in Australian Aborigines
    57–8, 61–2
information
    consumer choice and 441–4, 482
    use by higher income groups 135–6
Infrafamily Food Distribution and Feeding
        Practices Survey (Bangladesh) 90–1
inpatient care, *see* hospital inpatient care
insurance, *see* health insurance; social
        insurance
"interests functions" 408
international comparisons, *see* cross-national
        comparisons
International Health Economics Association
        (iHEA) 495
Ireland 185*n*

jargon, professional 7–8, 20–1, 470
Jensen, N.E. 340
justice
    distributive 385–7
    evaluative economics and 384–8
    procedural 387
    see also equity

Kakwani's progressivity index 148, 183
Kakwani, Wagstaff and van Doorslaer (KWV)
        formula 194–5
Kaldorian (Kaldor-Hicks) criterion 30–3, 419,
        471
    see also potential Pareto improvement
Ken Bassett's problem 465–95
Kessel, R. 495
Keynes, J.M. 364
Kirsanova, T. 253–68
Klavus, J. 139–52

labour, augmentation 466
lagged instrument fixed effect (LIFE)
        technique 98, 99
Lagrange Multiplier (LM) tests 113
land, Australian Aborigines 59–61
Landsburg, S. 31, 50–1
language, of economists 7–8, 20–1, 470
Leamer, E. 391
Le Grand, J. 122, 304, 305–6
leprosy 58
Level of Living Survey (LNU) (Sweden) 123
liberal equity 297, 301–3
liberalism 297
    in quasi-markets 310
    "redistributive" 301–2, 303, 315
libertarianism 301, 302–3, 440–1
life expectancy
    Australian Aborigines 54–5
    in China 235
    quality adjusted, *see* quality-adjusted life
        expectancy at birth
    in Russia 261*n*, 268
    social class effects 323–4, 325
    in US 437*n*
lifestyle, Australian Aborigines 59, 60–4
life-years 321
likelihood ratio tests 113
Liu, Y. 231–49
local entities, in Russia 255
local taxes
    changes in Finland 149, 150
    financing health care 185–6
    in rural China 234, 236
    in Russia 257
Lorenz curves 122, 258
lotteries 346, 388
low-income groups
    diseases, in Sweden 130, 133–5

Index compiled by Liza Weinkove